Virology Research Progress Series

HERPESVIRIDAE: VIRAL STRUCTURE, LIFE CYCLE AND INFECTIONS

Virology Research Progress Series

Insect Viruses: Detection, Characterization and Roles
Christopher I. Connell and Dominick P. Ralston (Editors)
2009. ISBN: 978-1-60692-965-0

Herpesviridae: Viral Structure, Life Cycle and Infections
Toma R. Gluckman (Editor)
2009. ISBN: 978-1-60692-947-6

Virology Research Progress Series

HERPESVIRIDAE: VIRAL STRUCTURE, LIFE CYCLE AND INFECTIONS

TOMA R. GLUCKMAN
EDITOR

Nova Biomedical Books
New York

For permission to use material from this book please contact us:
Telephone 631-231-7269; Fax 631-231-8175
Web Site: http://www.novapublishers.com

Library of Congress Cataloging-in-Publication Data

Herpesviridae viral structure, life cycle, and infections / [edited by] Toma R. Gluckman.
p. ; cm.
Includes bibliographical references and index.
ISBN 978-1-60692-947-6 (hardcover)
1. Herpesviruses. 2. Herpesvirus diseases. I. Gluckman, Toma R.
[DNLM: 1. Herpesviridae--pathogenicity. 2. Herpesviridae Infections--microbiology. QW 165.5.H3 H5632 2009]
QR400.H37 2009 614.5'812--dc22
2009017706

Published by Nova Science Publishers, Inc. ✦ New York

Contents

Preface

The Herpesviridae are a large family of DNA viruses that cause diseases in animals, including humans. The members of this family are also known as herpesviruses. Members of the herpesviridae family include oral and genital herpes, chickenpox, Kaposi's sarcoma herpesvirus (most often seen in people with HIV), and the Epstein-Barr virus (which causes infectious mononucleosis). There are eight known herpesviruses out of 100 known herpesviruses that infect humans. Herpesviruses are currently being researched for use in medical treatment, especially in the areas of gene therapy and oncology. Research is also being done into interactions between viral and host proteins, the mechanisms involved in gene regulation, and to find out how herpesviruses establish, maintain, and reactivate latency. The herpesviruses vary greatly in genomic sequence and proteins synthesized, but they all share similar genome and virion structures. This new book presents the latest research from around the world in this field.

Chapter 1 - Bioluminescence imaging (BLI), like fluorescence imaging, enables the visualization of genetic expression and physiological processes at the molecular level in living tissues and animals. It can be used to detect much lower levels of light due to the clean background. BLI has become a powerful technique in the study of herpesvirus pathogenesis, both *in vitro* and *in vivo*. Its major advantage over traditional techniques is that BLI can be used to monitor viral growth *in vivo* and enables real-time detection of the spatial and temporal progression of viral growth in living cultures or animals. Two human herpes viruses, HSV-1 and VZV, have been successfully engineered to express luciferase enzymes from insects and sea pansies. This mini-review highlights some approaches that have been developed and some results that have been achieved by using this versatile technology in herpesvirus studies. The authors expect that the application of BLI to the study of the pathogenesis of herpesviruses will provide new insights into disease processes.

Chapter 2 - Herpesviruses infect members of all groups of vertebrates and 9 equid herpesviruses (EHV) have been identified so far. Equine herpes virus-1 (EHV-1) to EHV-5 infect horses, EHV-6 to EHV-8 infect donkeys and are also called asinine herpesvirus-1 (AHV-1) to AHV-3 and EHV-9 or gazelle herpesvirus (GHV) infects Thomson's gazelles. Of the list of presently known equid herpes viruses, EHV-1 and EHV-4 are clinically and epidemiologically the most important and most studied viruses. EHV-1 infection induces clinical signs of disease ranging in severity, from mild respiratory distress to abortion in pregnant mares, neonatal foal death and in more extreme cases neuropathogenic disorders. EHV-4 infection, by contrast, induces mainly a mild respiratory disease. It is estimated that 80-90% of horses have been exposed to either EHV-1 or EHV-4 by two years of age and these equid herpesviruses, in common with other herpesviruses, have unique life cycles adapted to infect and persist latently the host. EHV-1 presents a particular problem in this regard as recrudescence of latent viral infection can result in active and/or silent transmission from brood mares to foals and subsequently between foals. Recrudescence of latent EHV-1 can also result in neurological disease and this viral state appears to be on the increase. Together, these viruses have a major economic and welfare impact on all sectors of the horse industry worldwide. This chapter will overview all equid herpesviruses with a specific focus on EHV-1/4 and EHV-2/5. Our current understanding of the life cycle, pathogenicity and protective humoral and cellular immune responses stimulated by natural EHV-1 infection will be discussed along with several different strategies of vaccination that have been investigated and developed over the past decades to fight and contain these pathogens.

Chapter 3 - The purpose of this article is to review the results and conclusions of our group in previous studies of herpesvirus infections in three different musculoskeletal diseases: rheumatoid arthritis, giant cell arteritis and osteoarthritis. The presence of Epstein-Barr virus (EBV) and human herpesvirus 6 (HHV-6) genomes in blood, synovial fluid, and serum samples of patients with rheumatoid arthritis in a higher proportion than in healthy donors; the presence of HHV-6 and Varicella-zoster virus (VZV) in temporal artery biopsies of patients with giant cell arteritis; and the higher viral DNA prevalence of VZV in mesenchymal stem cells of osteoarthritis patients than in healthy controls, all these results take together suggested a possible involvement of the herpesviruses in the pathogeny of these diseases. Furthermore, recent insights have added new value information that should be analyzed to better understand those previous results; in the last years, a huge number of articles have been published on this topic, and different possible mechanisms have been suggested to explain the role of the herpesviruses in the musculoskeletal diseases; a review of these new hypothesis will also be performed.

Chapter 4 - MicroRNAs (miRNAs) are a class of small non-coding functional RNAs that mediate post-transcriptional regulation of target mRNAs in a sequence-specific manner. They affect a wide variety of cellular processes, ranging from cellular differentiation, proliferation, apoptosis, metabolism, and infection to cancer. Over the past few years, miRNAs have been shown to be encoded in a number of herpesvirus genomes. These DNA viruses utilize the highly conserved host machinery to produce their own virally encoded miRNAs. These viral-encoded miRNAs are important regulators in both viral life cycle and virus-host interaction, specifically viral oncogenesis.

Chapter 5 - Human alphaherpesviruses include types 1 and 2 herpes simplex virus (HSV) and varicella zoster virus (VZV). All human alphaherpesviruses are neurotropic. After primary infection, these viruses become latent in cranial nerve ganglia (HSV-1 and VZV), in dorsal root ganglia (VZV), in sacral ganglia (HSV-2 and VZV) and in autonomic ganglia (VZV). During latency, virus gene expression is restricted and no infectious virus is produced.

Primary HSV-1 infection usually occurs in childhood and results in few lesions in the head and neck, but primary infection can also be asymptomatic. The classical diseases of

HSV-1 reactivations are fever blisters and ocular herpes. Recent reports demonstrating frequent shedding of shedding of HSV-1 DNA in the absence of disease, suggests that a small percentage of neurons reactivate to yield virus that is detected on ocular and oral surfaces.

Primary HSV-2 infection typically develops in sexually active individuals. Primary infections range from asymptomatic seroconversion to typical primary disease (i.e., genital herpes). HSV-2 shedding, both symptomatic and asymptomatic, are more frequent in the first couple of years after seroconversion. Asymptomatic virus shedding can be divided into two groups: unrecognized shedding, in which symptoms or lesions are present but go un-noticed or are misdiagnosed; and strict asymptomatic shedding, in which the subject has no symptoms and even a skilled clinician is unable to note any abnormality on physical exam. Therapies that reduce symptomatic recurrences may be less effective against strict asymptomatic shedding and transmission (Corey and Wald, 2008). Herein, data concerning the contribution of asymptomatic shedding to HSV transmission as well as the biology of HSV-2 shedding are reviewed.

Primary VZV infection typically results in childhood varicella (chickenpox). VZV reactivation, predominately in the elderly, most often results in zoster (shingles), but virus may spread to the spinal cord to cause myelitis or to blood vessels of the brain to cause vasculopathy. VZV reactivation often produces prolonged pain after zoster (post herpetic neuralgia). While the clinical features of VZV reactivation are well recognized, subclinical VZV reactivation and shedding has recently been reported in astronauts. Physical and physiological stressors associated with spaceflight (Taylor et al., 1992; White and Averner, 2001; Williams, 2003) appear to induce virus reactivation and subsequent shedding of VZV in saliva (Mehta et al., 2004; Cohrs et al., 2008). Herein, asymptomatic VZV reactivation during space flight, in ground-based space flight analogs, and in the general population will be reviewed as well as a mathematical model estimating the contribution of asymptomatic VZV reactivation to virus epidemiology presented.

Chapter 6 - Periodontitis has traditionally been ascribed to bacterial activity. However, herpesviruses, particularly Epstein-Barr virus (EBV) and cytomegalovirus (CMV), are found in clinical samples from both apical and marginal periodontitis. Reported prevalence are typically in the range 30-70 % while the viruses are found more sporadically in material taken from healthy sites in the mouth. These observations have led some scientists to suggest that the viruses play a role in the etiology of periodontitis. Several lines of investigation have been pursued in an attempt to clarify the issue: Quantification of viruses in clinical samples, methods suggesting local viral activity, associations between virus and bacteria to indicate possible synergism, and the treatment of patients with antiviral medication to see whether a subsequent decrease in viral titer may impact on the periodontitis. The conclusion based on the present review of the literature is that these viruses can in some cases impact on the pathogenesis, but that in the majority of patients their detection probably does not reflect any clinical role. Yet, particularly in cases with advanced or chronic periodontitis, viral analysis is called for. If there are signs of local viral activity, for example a high viral load, antiviral therapy may be tried as an adjunct to conventional periodontal treatment.

Chapter 7 - Human herpesvirus-6 (HHV-6) is a β-herpesvirus first recognized in 1986. Recent studies have shown a pathogenic role for HHV-6 in immunosuppressed patients, including transplant recipients. HHV-6 latently infects the body after the primary infection and reactivates after introduction of immunosuppressive therapy or another form of stimulation. The clinical sequelae of HHV-6 may range from asymptomatic infection, febrile illness to tissue-invasive, life-threatening disseminated disease. Several severe complications of viral infection in transplant recipients have been reported including encephalitis, interstitial pneumonitis, bone marrow suppression and hepatitis. Prospective studies suggest, however, disease associations are rare. HHV-6 infection has been documented in 31-66% of kidney transplant recipients. The clinical impact of HHV-6 is being investigated. The role of HHV-6 as an immunomodulatory virus that may facilitate acute rejection episodes and chronic nephropathy is discussed. According to DNA sequence homology and similar clinical features between cytomegalovirus and human herpesvirus-6, the association and correlation in both CMV and HHV-6 activity is also discussed.

Chapter 8 - Gammaherpesviruses comprise a subfamily (*Gammaherpesvirinae*) of the *Herpesviridae* genus; they fall into two genera: Rhadinovirus and Lymphocryptovirus. Human gammaherpesviruses encompass the Epstein-Barr virus (EBV, HHV-4) and the Kaposi´s sarcoma herpesvirus (KSHV, HHV-8). Their genomes as well as the genomes of several mammalian gammaherpesviruses were fully sequenced. The gammaherpesvirus genes may be grouped according to several criteria. As a rule, non-structural and structural genes can be distinguished. Another commonly used classification is related to transcription kinetics, distinguishing immediate-early, early, early-late and late genes. Genes which expression is inevitable for productive virus replication *in vitro* are usually referred to as essential ones. The non-structural early gammaherpesvirus genes encode enzymes for viral DNA synthesis and specify polypeptides involved in immune evasion and in complement regulation. These also modulate or hamper the effects of cytokines and/or disregulate interferon action. During latency, which can be defined as non-productive maintenance of the circularized episomal dsDNA genome, a few (or at least one) latency-associated gene(s) are (is) expressed. Comparative sequence analysis of herpesvirus genomes throughout all subfamilies revealed the group of herpesvirus common genes (showing relatively wide sequence homologies), which encode structural as well as non-structural proteins with related functions. An important group of genes was found gammaherpesvirus specific (γ-specific). Finally, about 10 – 15 genes may be unic for each gammaherpesvirus. Such genes, present in the given gammaherpesviruses only, may encode proteins, which act in analogical manner though being different in their sequence. The products of gammaherpesvirus specific genes are often virus-coded counterparts of cellular genes; such proteins usually promote cell division and/or cause false intracellular signaling. The latter are believed to represent pirated cellular genes, which have been modified by evolution when becoming virus genome components. Viral oncogenes and virus-coded immune regulation proteins act in accord with infected lymphocytes. Since gammaherpesviruses remain latent in lymphatic tissues and may be associated with lymphoproliferation, comparison of their DNA sequences and functional analysis of corresponding proteins are of special interest.

Chapter 9 - The human papilloma virus (HPV) is a DNA virus that can be the cause of many carcinomas. This DNA virus has been proven as a DNA tumor virus. Cervical carcinoma is the main carcinoma that relates to HPV infection. Screening for HPV DNA is a new laboratory analysis in gynecology, and a vaccine for HPV is presently available. In this work, current knowledge on HPV laboratory diagnosis, therapy and prevention are reviewed and discussed. In addition, the author also performs a meta-analysis of the previous reports on cervical carcinoma, the most common female carcinoma in Thailand, and HPV virus infection in Thailand.

Short Commentary - Human herpesvirus-6 (HHV-6) is a lymphotropic virus, which was first isolated from immunocompromised patients. Two variants of HHV-6 have been categorized: HHV-6A and HHV-6B, of which the variant B is the most common. HHV-6B causes *exanthema subitum,* febrile seizures and other infectious syndromes of early childhood. The clinical symptoms are usually mild and self-limitted, but complications such as encephalitis and hepatitis have been described. Infection with HHV-6A appears to be much less frequent, but is suggested to be more neurotropic than HHV-6B. In the adult population, there is a high HHV-6 seroprevalence of 90-95%. Like other herpesviruses, after primary infection, HHV-6 persists in latency for life time and may reactivate later.

Acute liver failure (ALF) is a significant cause of liver transplantation. Common causes of ALF are hepatitis B, drug toxicity and vascular disorders. The etiology of ALF remains often unknown, but viral infections are thought to be involved. HHV-6 has been demonstrated to cause acute hepatitis as a complication of primary infection. HHV-6 DNA is also frequently detected in hepatocytes of liver of children with various liver diseases. Also cases of HHV-6-related acute liver failure in immunocompetent adults have been reported. In our study, HHV-6 was found in most explanted livers of adult patients with ALF of unknown origin ending-up with liver transplantation. HHV-6 antigens were demonstrated in the explants with numerous positive inflammatory cells and even in a few hepatocytes. No other viruses but HHV-6 were found in these explanted livers. This indicates, that ALF and hepatocyte necrosis may be caused by HHV-6. On the other hand, it is also possible, that the hepatocyte necrosis seen in this and other studies, is not caused by HHV-6 directly, but the immunoresponse triggered by the virus leads to destruction of hepatocytes. On the other hand, the impact of HHV-6 infection on the immunological events of the liver and triggering inflammation could be one of the mechanisms of HHV-6 to enhance acute liver failure. Despite the lack of definitive evidence of the direct causality of HHV-6 in liver failure, these observations strongly support its involvement in some cases, and probably a systematic research in cases of unexplained ALF could be recommended.

Short Commentary – The authors investigated the role of herpesviruses in human chronic pathologies such as cancedrf and autoimmune diseases. Our first focus was on HHV6 and HHV1 role in the susceptibility to sporadic skin cancers. HHV6 (31.7%) and HHV1 (23.8%) fragments were detected more frequently in 120 skin cancer patients cancer than in 41 normal control individuals (14.6% and 5%, respectively). The risk of presenting a Basal Cell Carcinomas (BCC) was more than 3 times higher for HHV6 infected patients (OR= 3.182; 95% CI: 1.125-8.997). The risk for HHV1 infected individuals of presenting BCC and SCC was increased 8 and 6 times, respectively (OR= 8.125; 95% CI: 1.735-38.043 and OR= 6.290; 95% CI: 1.283-30.856, respectively). Because a subset of immunocompromised patients appeared to be more susceptible to HHV-associated skin cancer, the authors further investigated the influence of the variants of codon 72 and codon 47 of exon 4 on the susceptibility to HHV6 and 1 HHV1 infection in immunosuppressed patients. They examined 78 renal transplant recipients and 151 controls. HHV6 infection was more frequent among the renal transplant patients (35.89%) than in the control population (11.25%). HHV1 infection rate was similar in renal transplant patients (7.28%) and controls (2.56%). HHV6 positive cases were more frequent among patients with codon 72 of *p53* variants (60.71%) than among wild-type *p53* patients (28.20%) despite the higher frequency of codon 72 of *p53* wild-type variant in renal transplant patients compared to controls (64.1% *versus* 36.4%; $p< 0.001$). The presence of a codon 72 of *p53* germ line variant genotype increased the risk for HHV6 infection more than 5 times (OR= 5.479; 95% CI= 1.992-15.069). More recently, the authors have aimed to study the relationship between HHV6 and HHV7 infection, p53 apoptotic ability as represented by 72p53 polymorphisms, and Graves Disease (GD) susceptibility. Sixty GD patients were paired to 60 controls. Both viruses infection demonstrated to increase the risk for GD, especially HHV7 that was more frequent among GD (64.64%) than in controls (38.73%). Patients presenting 72TP53 Pro/Pro variants had more chance to develop GD and to be infected by HHV7.

Short Commentary - Human herpesvirus-6 (HHV-6) is a causative virus of exanthema subitum which is characterized by high fever followed by rash in young children. HHV-6 infection is associated with variety of acute and chronic neurologic diseases, including febrile seizure, encephalitis, meningitis, facial palsy, Guillain-Barré syndrome and multiple sclerosis, possibly through immune-mediated reactions [1, 2]. Although cerebral infarctions have been also reported following HHV-6 infection on rare occasions, the underlying mechanism has not yet been elucidated [4, 5].

Antiphospholipid syndrome (APS) is an autoimmune disease characterized by thrombosis, repeated abortions, or thrombocytopenia associated with elevated antiphospholipid antibodies (aPL) [6]. APS often appears in association with autoimmune diseases or infections, while the cause of aPL induction is obscure in many patients with APS. Anticardiolipin antibodies (aCL) are the most common aPL and are one of the risk factors for cerebral vascular disease or myocardial infarctions in both adults and children [7-13]. Recent epidemiologic studies suggested that the infectious environment in infancy influence the likelihood producing aCL [14].

In: Herpesviridae Viral Structure, Life Cycle and Infections ISBN 978-1-60692-947-6
Editor: Toma R. Gluckman

Chapter 1

Bioluminescence Imaging for Herpesvirus Studies *in vivo*

***Qiyi Tang*[1], *Zhen Zhang*[2] *and Hua Zhu*[2,*]**
[1]Department of Microbiology/AIDS program, Ponce School of Medicine, 395 Zona Industrial, Reparada 2, Ponce, PR 00716-2348
[2]Department of Microbiology and Molecular Genetics, UMDNJ-New Jersey Medical School, 225 Warren Street, Newark, NJ 07101, USA

Abstract

Bioluminescence imaging (BLI), like fluorescence imaging, enables the visualization of genetic expression and physiological processes at the molecular level in living tissues and animals. It can be used to detect much lower levels of light due to the clean background. BLI has become a powerful technique in the study of herpesvirus pathogenesis, both *in vitro* and *in vivo*. Its major advantage over traditional techniques is that BLI can be used to monitor viral growth *in vivo* and enables real-time detection of the spatial and temporal progression of viral growth in living cultures or animals. Two human herpes viruses, HSV-1 and VZV, have been successfully engineered to express luciferase enzymes from insects and sea pansies. This mini-review highlights some approaches that have been developed and some results that have been achieved by using this versatile technology in herpesvirus studies. We expect that the application of BLI to the study of the pathogenesis of herpesviruses will provide new insights into disease processes.

Keywords: Herpesvirus; pathogenesis; bioluminescence imaging.

* Correspondent author: Phone: 973 972-4483, ext. 2-6488; Fax: 973 972-8981 E-mail: zhuhu@umdnj.edu

Introduction

Herpes viruses consist of 8 human pathogens: human herpes virus (HHV) 1-8. They are classified into 3 different categories. Herpes Simplex Virus-1 (HSV-1), herpes Simplex Virus-2 (HSV-2) and Varicella-zoster virus (VZV) are in alpha subfamily of herpesvirinae; human cytomegalovirus (HCMV), HHV-6 and HHV-7 belong to beta subfamily; the gamma subfamily includes Epstein Bar virus (EBV) and Kaposi's sarcoma-associated herpesvirus (KSHV). The viruses cause a plethora of diseases: oral and/or genital herpes; chickenpox and shingles; infectious mononucleosis, Burkitt's lymphoma, CNS lymphoma in AIDS patients, post-transplant lymphoproliferative syndrome (PTLD), nasopharyngeal carcinoma, and HIV-associated hairy leukoplakia; infectious mononucleosis-like syndrome and retinitis; roseola infantum (or *exanthem subitum*); and Kaposi's sarcoma, primary effusion lymphoma, and some types of multicentric Castleman's disease [1-6].

These herpes viruses are able to infect large populations, sometimes remaining latent (or intermittently latent) for the entire lifetime of the host, only becoming active should the host's immune system be or become compromised. During the active infection phase, the viruses can infect and replicate in different types of cells and tissues, altering their functions and causing disease. A number of biological techniques have contributed greatly to the current knowledge regarding HHV pathogenesis; bio-imaging methods based on fluorescence and luciferase have been among the most successful. With them, it has become possible to study the sites of infected viral particles and the interaction of viral and cellular proteins, detect gene function, and do real-time studies of viral life cycles. There are two kinds of fluorescence-based imaging (FRI) that allow researchers to study the interaction of a given virus with its host: immunofluorescence (which uses dye-conjugated antibodies to show target proteins) and direct fluorescence (which uses a fusion of fluorescent proteins (FP) in order to visualize target proteins). The former can only detect respective proteins in fixed cells; the latter can visualize the protein in live cells but with a high background. Both methods need a UV excitation light source, an expensive microscope, and a system for creating images from the results.

Developed in the last decade, bioluminescence imaging (BLI) is an important technique that promises to supersede other methods. Using luciferin as a substrate, BLI detects luciferase activity. With the luciferase gene integrated into the viral genome, one can detect viral gene expression directly and viral replication indirectly. BLI has been demonstrated to be a powerful tool in DNA viral studies, both *in vitro* and *in vivo*, and appears to have even greater potential in the development of animal models. A BLI system equipped with a CCD (cooled charge-coupled device) camera [7, 8] is faster and less expensive than many other imaging systems. The relative amounts of bioluminescence produced *in vivo* can be quantified by computer-based analysis.

BLI clearly has some advantages. First of all, the substrate for firefly luciferase, D-luciferin, can cross both the cell membrane and the blood-brain barrier [7, 9, 10] so that it can permeate all of the tissues in the living animal. More importantly, D-luciferin has very low toxicity, which allows for multiple applications in the same animal [7, 9]. Furthermore, BLI is very sensitive, detecting luciferase activity with a much lower background than fluorescence imaging. BLI can detect as little as 10^{-15}-10^{-17} M of luciferase *in vivo* [11].

Finally, BLI has been increasingly applied to gene therapy [12], pathogen detection [13], cancer research [10, 14-17], viral gene regulation [18-20], and protein-protein interaction [21] studies.

This review summarizes the achievements of BLI techniques in virology studies, especially in herpesviruses, and its application in small animal models for the study of herpesvirus pathogenesis. A few disadvantages along with many potential advantages will be discussed.

Bioluminescence Imaging System

Bioluminescence is the production and emission of light by a living organism. It results from a chemical reaction in which chemical energy is converted to light energy [22, 23]. Ninety percent of deep-sea marine life is estimated to produce bioluminescence in one form or another. Because blue and green wavelengths travel most easily through water, it perhaps comes as no surprise that most marine light-emission belongs to that spectrum. Non-marine bioluminescence is less widely distributed, but a larger variety in colors is seen. Though fewer in number, land-based bioluminescent species have a greater variety of colors; fireflies and glow worms are the best-known forms, but bioluminescent abilities can be found in other insects and some insect larvae, annelids, arachnids, and several species of fungi [24, 25]. Many areas of research target these bioluminescent organisms, and in fact, luciferases are used as reporter genes in genetic engineering and are widely applied in biomedical research.

Luciferase is an enzyme that is frequently used in bioluminescence imaging systems; in addition, it is a versatile and common reporter gene. One such, the luciferase of the North American firefly (*Photinus pyralis*), is the most widely employed, and when exposed to the appropriate luciferin substrate, it catalyzes the substrate's bioluminescent oxidation, producing light. Because the bioluminescence wavelength generated by firefly luciferase can penetrate tissues efficiently, it is an excellent indicator to be utilized for *in vivo* studies.

Firefly luciferase is one of several luciferase genes that have been cloned from different organisms; it can be expressed in mammalian cells by inserting it under the control of a promoter (e.g., a CMV promoter). Luciferase that is produced by mammalian cells (either in cell culture or in animals) can—as previously described—catalyze a reaction that emits visible light when luciferin, oxygen, and ATP are added into the reaction system. The light's intensity varies depending on the amount of luciferase that the cells or tissues generate, and this intensity makes it possible to monitor the activities of the promoter that mediates gene regulation. Finally, because the emitted light is visible to the human eye, it can be used to posit gene expression, which would be very useful for showing the sites of viral infection.

Luciferase can be produced in the lab through genetic engineering and can serve a number of purposes. Luciferase genes can be synthesized and inserted into organisms or transfected into cells. Mice, silkworms, and potatoes are just a few organisms that have already been engineered to produce the protein [26, 27]. For the detection of luciferase activity, several Imaging devices and detection systems have been produced. The equipment for luciferase detection is much less expensive than that which is required for fluorescence detection.

Ex-vivo imaging is a very powerful technique for studying cell populations outside of the organism. Different types of cells (e.g., bone marrow stem cells, T-cells) can be engineered to express a luciferase allowing for non-invasive visualization inside a live animal using a sensitive CCD camera. Light is emitted when luciferase is exposed to the appropriate luciferin substrate. Photon emission can be detected by a light sensitive apparatus, such as a luminometer or a modified optical microscope. This allows the observation of, for example, biological processes and stages of infection. Luciferase can be used in blood banks to determine whether red blood cells are starting to break down.

BLI can be used to study (in animal models, i.e., *in vivo*) both viral infection and therapy in small animal models. BLI can capture the light emitted from luciferase enzymes to detect sites of viral infection and quantify viral replication in the context of a living animal. Small animals are the preferred *in vivo* models. The more tissue between the bioluminescence-emitting and -detecting site, the more signal is lost to absorption and from the scattering of optical photons. If larger animals, such as rats and rabbits, are needed, luciferase expression is restricted to subcutaneous tissue sites in order to achieve a high sensitivity of signal detection. Other factors, including dark fur and heavy pigmentation of the skin, may block or attenuate the optical signal. Therefore, nude or severe combined immunodeficiency (SCID) mice are ideal for *in vivo* bioluminescence detection due to their small size and lack of pigment.

The application of BLI for *in vivo* and *in vitro* studies requires a substrate, luciferin. There are different kinds of luciferins produced by different organisms: 1) Firefly luciferin is the luciferin found in fireflies; it is the substrate of firefly luciferase [28]; 2) Bacterial luciferin is a type of luciferin found in bacteria, some squid, and fish. It consists of a long-chain aldehyde and a reduced riboflavin phosphate [29]. 3) Dinoflagellate luciferin is a chlorophyll derivative and is found in dinoflagellates, which are often responsible for the phenomenon of nighttime ocean phosphorescence [30]. A very similar type of luciferin is found in some types of euphausiid shrimp. Firefly luciferin has been the most commonly used for biological studies.

Firefly luciferin is ideal for the *in vivo* application of BLI since it has a minimal level of toxicity and is able to distribute throughout the body (including brain tissue) [7, 9, 10]. After i.p. injection of luciferin, bioluminescence reaches a peak level in as little as 10 min and begins to fade after 30 min [16].

Although the bioluminescent photons (emitted from the luciferase-expressing site) that pass through the host tissue are extremely dim, advances in the development of ultra-sensitive photon detecting devices (such as those based on CCD cameras) have made the observation and quantitative detection of bioluminescence in living animals possible [31]. There are several bioluminescence-detecting devices commercially available for *in vivo* BLI in small animals. The key components of these systems consist of a sensitive CCD camera and a low background imaging chamber where the imaging of bioluminescence takes place (Figure 1). In our laboratory, we have used the IVIS™ imaging system from Xenogen/ Caliper Life Science, Waltham, MA (Figures 1C and D). Mice need to be anesthetized (injectable or gaseous anesthetics) and injected with luciferin (Figures 1A and B). In the IVIS™ imaging system, a sensitive CCD camera is mounted on top of a light-tight, low background imaging chamber (Figure 1C). Within the chamber, a manifold maintains delivery of anesthetic gas to the mice while bioluminescence is measured. The stage inside the chamber is heated and movable, which makes the system preferable for *in vivo* BLI. A grey-scale reference image of the animal is taken first, and the bioluminescence signal is measured within, from seconds up to several minutes depending on the signal strength. The software for IVIS™ imaging system has been designed specifically for *in vivo* BLI. The bioluminescence signal intensity is presented as a pseudo-color image and imposed on the grey-scale reference image (Figure 1D). The cumulative bioluminescence from a designated "region of interest" (ROI) can then be quantified by using the system software.

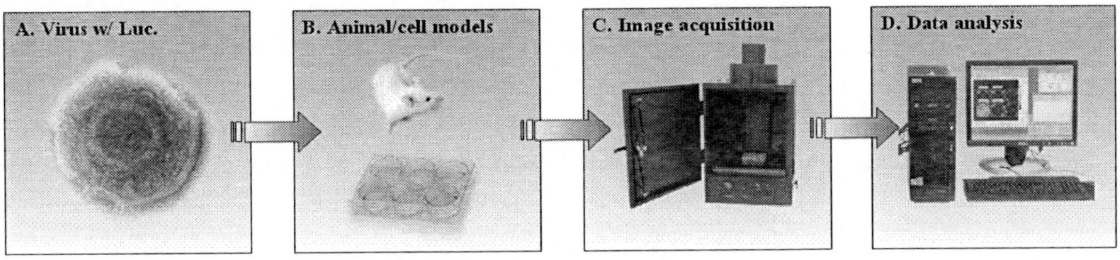

Figure 1. Schematic of application of bioluminescence imaging modality in a study of herpesvirus pathogenesis. (A) Virus can be tagged with a bioluminescence reporter gene (Fluc). (B) Small modeling animals/tissue cultures can be infected with Fluc gene-labeled viruses. (C) After administration of enzyme substrate, luciferin, bioluminescence emitting from living animals/cultured cells can be detected and monitored by using a bioluminescence imaging system (a CCD camera mounted on top of a light-tight low background imaging chamber). (D) Data can be stored in a connected PC and quantified by using region-of-interest analysis.

Bioluminescence Imaging in Herpesvirilogical Studies

Eight herpes viruses are defined as being human pathogens. They contain genomes measuring between 125 and 250 kilobase pairs (kb) and which putatively encode 70 to 200 proteins [32-35]. Even though anti-herpes drugs (including viral DNA replication inhibitors) are effective on acute infection, the diseases caused by them have not yet been controlled, largely due to the fact that the mechanisms that herpes viruses use for setting up latency and for being activated are unknown. A herpes virus infection has a typical life cycle in host cells: contacting and entering cells with the stimulation of multiple signal transduction pathways; viral genomic DNA's entrance into the nucleus; immediate gene expression/early gene expression/DNA replication/late gene expression; viral particle packaging and releasing to the Golgi body for enveloping [36, 37].

Different herpes virus infections occur in different sites of body: HSV-1/2 infect oral and genital epithelial cells (HSV-1 is also a neurophilic virus); HCMV causes infection in multiple organs, including the lungs, blood, bone marrow, the salivary gland, and probably the heart; VZV infection is related to neuron cells and causes shingles and chicken pox. The BLI technique can detect not only gene expression regulation (reflected by luciferase activity), but also this method is able to clarify the gene expression sites that can be used to stand for viral infection sites because they are where viral genomic DNA docks. Therefore, BLI is now accepted as the method of choice for small-animal model studies of viral replication, gene regulation, and pathogenesis. When using BLI to study herpesvirus pathogenesis, either the virus or its host can be engineered to express luciferase as a reporter. Thus, viral infection can be followed and analyzed both *in vitro* and *in vivo* (Figure 1).

Bioluminescence Imaging in HSV-1 Studies

HSV-1 causes herpes simplex. Infection with the herpes virus is categorized into one of several distinct disorders based on the site of infection. Although some disorders have significantly different rates of infection by type, HSV-1 generally infects 80% of the adult population. Herpes simplex is not typically life-threatening for immunocompetent people. Following primary infection, the virus enters the nerves (at the site of the primary infection), migrates to the cell body of the neuron, and becomes latent in the ganglion that may later be (occasionally) reactivated.

Although fluorescence techniques have played a vital role in the investigation of HSV DNA replication, the interactions of viral genomes with subnuclear compartments, and the molecular interactions of viral proteins and cellular proteins [38-40], there are several drawbacks to their use. First, immunofluorescence can be used only to detect biological activities in fixed cells, and the antibodies required for the experiments are extremely expensive, so this technique cannot be used for *in vivo* studies. Immunofluorescence has been used in live-cell studies for HSV-1 [41], but is not suitable for animal models. Second, the fluorescent proteins—such as green fluorescent protein (GFP)—used for fusion with the proteins of interest can cause a high background. Last, fluorescence detection requires expensive equipment such as a confocal fluorescent microscope.

Normally, experimental animals must be sacrificed in order to detect viral load in viral, toxic, or pathogenic experiments. This is an expensive prospect since it requires a large number of animals. Another problem is that using such a large number of—different—animals can cause statistical errors in the generated data. In addition, kinetic studies and investigations into disease progression in the same animal are unlikely. A non-invasive bio-imaging technique that would allow a time course transgenic analysis, viral pathogenic studies, and viral titer detection would be considered revolutionary in the field of virology.

Utilizing the BLI technique in mice (using a CCD camera to visualize luciferase reporter protein expression) made it possible for researchers to generate an *in vivo* image. Since luciferin is nontoxic to small animals and can be distributed throughout their systems, BLI can be used as a non-invasive bio-imaging technique in small animal models. Luker et al. [42], propelled by their previous work in which BLI was used for *in vivo* imaging studies [7, 8, 43], developed a non-invasive methodology for detecting HSV-1 infection *in vivo* [42]. First, a recombinant HSV-1 (KOS strain), KOS/Dlux/oriL (which expresses both luciferase reporter genes from UL 29 and UL30 promoters) was constructed; the luciferase gene-expressing cassette was inserted between the UL49 and UL50 regions. This recombinant virus has the same growth phenotype as the wild-type strain. Then, this recombinant HSV-1 was inoculated into mice, and wild-type HSV-1 was used as control. BLI of luciferase activity in the living mice was performed at 3 days postinfection. Bioluminescence could be detected in mice infected with KOS/Dlux/oriL, while the mice infected with wild-type HSV-1 showed insignificant amount of background bioluminescence.

In the experiments, KOS/Dlux/oriL was injected into the mice through different sites: via the footpad, i.p., i.c., and corneal routes. Although the luciferase activity was detectable in all inoculation sites, the BLI luciferase assay was able to define the spread of the HSV-1 from the inoculation sites because the foci of increased bioluminescence were seen in different places around them.

Importantly, BLI-detected luciferase activity correlated with viral titer. *In vitro* luciferase assays using homogenized tissues were proportional to titers of KOS/Dlux/oriL. This investigation demonstrates the viability of utilizing a BLI time-course study as a real-time, noninvasive method of monitoring viral replication and spread during infection.

Since luciferase activity detected by BLI correlates with viral titer and kinetic luciferase activities obtained in BLI during infection in mice were proportional to viral replication, BLI appears to be a valuable tool for monitoring the effects of anti-viral therapy, which was also demonstrated by Luker et al. [42]. In their experiments, they used the BLI technique to monitor the effects of valacyclovir on the replication of KOS/Dlux/oriL and showed that changes in photon flux from BLI can be used to quantify relative differences in therapeutic efficacy.

Another BLI study from the same group combined the recombinant HSV with IFN receptors-knockout (ko) mice in order to investigate the effects of type I and type II interferon on replication and tropism of HSV-1 in mice [44]. The results showed that type I interferon receptors were essential to limit systemic dissemination of HSV-1. By contrast, in wild-type mice and mice lacking receptors for type II interferons, viral infection remained localized at the epithelial site of infection and in the sensory neurons. This information suggested that type I and II IFNs are involved in limiting systemic dissemination of HSV-1 and proved again that BLI is a great tool in detecting virus infection in unanticipated sites.

Recently, more studies using BLI uncovered valuable information regarding HSV-1 pathogenesis in living mice. One of them explored the use of *in vivo* bioluminescence imaging to monitor the replication and tropism of KOS strain HSV-1 viruses expressing the luciferase reporter gene in hematogenously infected mice [45]. Following intraperitoneal inoculation, HSV-1 DNA concentrations by real-time PCR (after sacrificing the experimental animals) and *in vivo* bioluminescence emissions in living mice were compared. It was noted that HSV-1 spread preferentially to the ovaries and adrenal glands after infection. PCR and bioluminescence methods consistently showed low viral loads in the nervous system. The results demonstrated that BLI can be used for non-invasive, real-time monitoring of HSV-1 hematogenous infection in living mice.

A transgenic mouse model has been engineered to express Fluc (firefly luciferase) under the control of the HSV-1 thymidine kinase promoter as an alternative approach to monitor viral infection using BLI [46]. These mice produced light at the site of the HSV-1 infection due to the activation of the luciferase gene. The authors concluded that by using a reporter mouse instead of a reporter virus, multiple strains or mutants of HSV-1 can be studied without producing new Fluc-expressing recombinant viruses for each experiment, thus avoiding the possibility that the virus may be attenuated by the insertion of a reporter. However, this study also showed certain limitations to the reporter-mouse strategy. The lower limits of viral detection were an input titer of $1X10^3$ PFU, which is approximately 10-fold less sensitive compared with the reporter-virus method [42]. Additionally, the HSV-1 reporter mouse had much higher background luminescence in the body extremities due to the instability of the luciferase protein at cooler temperatures (near the surface of the body).

A different study demonstrated that the introduction of Fluc under the control of a strict-late promoter provided successful non-invasive imaging and real-time monitoring of HSV-1 replication *in vitro* and *in vivo*. By taking advantage of two distinct promoters (immediate-early and strict-late promoters), the results from this study suggested HSV-1 infection and replication can be separately monitored non-invasively and *in vivo*, thereby allowing the study of various factors and conditions that determine both infection and replication of oncolytic HSV-1 vectors in animal models [17].

Bioluminescence Imaging in VZV Studies

VZV is one of eight herpes viruses known to infect humans (and other vertebrates). It commonly causes chickenpox in children and both shingles and postherpetic neuralgia in adults. Primary infection of VZV leads to varicella (chicken pox). VZV establishes lifelong latency in the host, specifically in the trigeminal and dorsal root ganglia. The sequelae of VZV reactivation is herpes zoster (shingles), which can lead to chronic postherpetic neuralgia [47, 48]. VZV infection is highly cell associated in cell culture. Various *in vitro* and *in vivo* systems have been developed to analyze VZV replication and pathogenesis [49].

Previously, we have reported that we developed a BLI technique to study VZV pathogenesis by generating a recombinant virus expressing luciferase, VZV_{Luc}. The recombinant virus contains a firefly luciferase gene in the intergenic region between ORF65 and ORF66 of the VZV_{BAC} (recombinant VZV generated from a bacterial artificial system) genome [50], and the insertion of the reporter gene had minimal effects on the natural pathogenesis of the virus. Growth curve analysis was first performed and showed that VZV-expressing luciferase grew like its parental VZV_{BAC}. The luciferase activity from infected cells was then measured (Figure 2A). Bioluminescence from VZV_{Luc}-infected cells was visualized and quantified using the IVIS™ imaging system [51]. MeWo cells were grown in six-well culture dishes and infected with either VZV_{BAC} (Figure 2B, upper panel, two left wells) or VZV_{Luc} (Figure 2B, upper panel, two right wells). Three days post-infection, many green fluorescent plaques were observed in all wells under fluorescence microscopy (Figure 2B, lower panel), indicating that the cells were efficiently infected by both viruses, since VZV_{Luc} was also tagged with a GFP marker. When the substrate of luciferase, D-luciferin, was added to the culture medium, strong bioluminescence was detected only from the VZV_{Luc}-infected cells (Figure 2B, upper panel, two right wells), and not from the VZV_{BAC}-infected cells (Figure 2B, upper panel, two left wells).

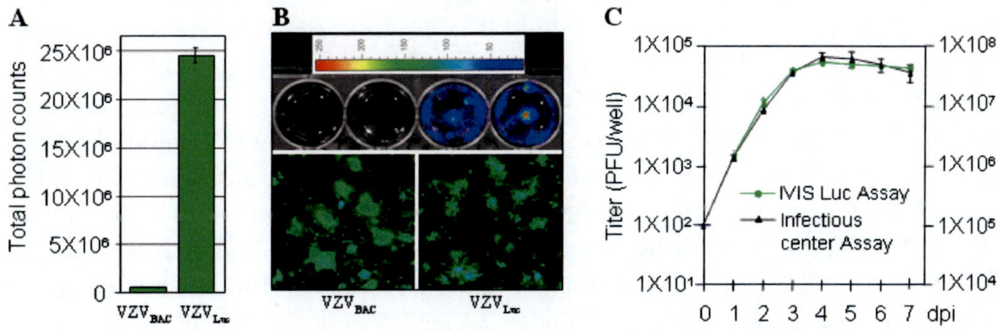

Figure 2. Generation and analysis of the VZVLuc strain. (A) Luciferase assay. MeWo cells were infected with VZVLuc or VZVBAC for 2 days and luciferase activity was measured. The cells infected with VZVLuc showed a high level of luciferase activity, while the parental VZVBAC strain had no activity. (B) Bioluminescence measurement. Two wells of a six-well dish of MeWo cells were infected with VZVBAC (upper left) and two were infected with VZVLuc (upper right). Two days post-infection, D-luciferin substrate was added to the cultured wells, and bioluminescence was measured using IVIS imaging. Bioluminescence could be detected only in VZVLuc-infected cells. The intensities were indicated as pseudo- colors, as shown by an intensity scale bar at the top; higher intensity is represented by a warmer color, and lower intensity is represented with a cooler color. The infection of these wells was verified by showing GFP-positive plaques (bottom panel). (C) Correlation of luminescence and plaque numbers. Growth curves generated by an infectious center assay (black curve and left scale) and a bioluminescence assay (green curve and right scale) were compared.

We investigated whether bioluminescence intensity correlated with viral titers. As shown in Figure 2C (green curve), the growth kinetic analysis based on conventional infectious center and luciferase activity assays demonstrated that the intensities of bioluminescent signals correlated with viral titers. This enables subtle detection of viral replication as well as location over the course of infection in a real-time and non-invasive manner *in vivo*. Moreover, the presence of luciferase activity indicates viral replication in cells and not free viral particles, which makes it suitable for studies of this cell-associated virus under tissue culture condition.

The development of the severe combined immunodeficient mouse with human tissue xenograft (SCID-hu) model greatly facilitates the investigation of VZV pathogenesis *in vivo*. Results from histopathological studies have shown that this tissue-graft strategy is an accurate representation of VZV pathogenesis in human tissues [52-54]. However, acquiring data has been hampered by having to euthanize mice in order to measure viral growth. Sampling VZV-infected thymus/liver implants in the SCID-hu model has usually been done weekly or at most every 4 days. Moreover, the implants are different in size, so viral titers vary widely from animal to animal. Titration of VZV from the implants does not accurately reflect viral spread. The skin tissue is too hard to be dispersed to a single-cell suspension. Thymus/liver implants contain many dead T cells that are killed by VZV infection and are no longer infectious. In previous studies, the titer of VZV from infected implants (skin and thymus/liver) was not considered quantitative, and the kinetics of VZV replication was unclear. These factors have impeded efforts to study large numbers of VZV variants and made it difficult to discern minor phenotypic differences leading to pathogenesis.

To increase the sampling frequency and accuracy, and more importantly, to directly monitor VZV growth in live animals, we applied BLI to measure VZV spread *in vivo*, each day for one week in the same mouse. Three SCID-hu mice with thymus/liver implants were inoculated by direct injection of a VZV-infected cell suspension. At different days post-inoculation, VZV spread was observed using the IVIS system at 10 minutes after i.p. injection of the SCID-hu mice with luciferin substrate. Bioluminescence was easily detected over the left flank of each of three infected SCID-hu mice (where the thymus/liver implants were located, under the kidney capsule), demonstrating that the replication of VZVLuc virus can be monitored in living animals. Photon emissions from the infected implants were converted into a pseudo-colored image (Figure 3A). VZV was detected in the thymus/liver implants and did not transfer into the peritoneum or other organs, which was expected of this human-restricted virus. Notably, the average background emissions were similarly low for uninfected areas of the inoculated mice and over the kidney of a mock-inoculated control mouse. The boundaries of a region of interest were manually set to closely border the luminescent area in each mouse. Measurements of total photon flux were used as an indicator of VZV infection.

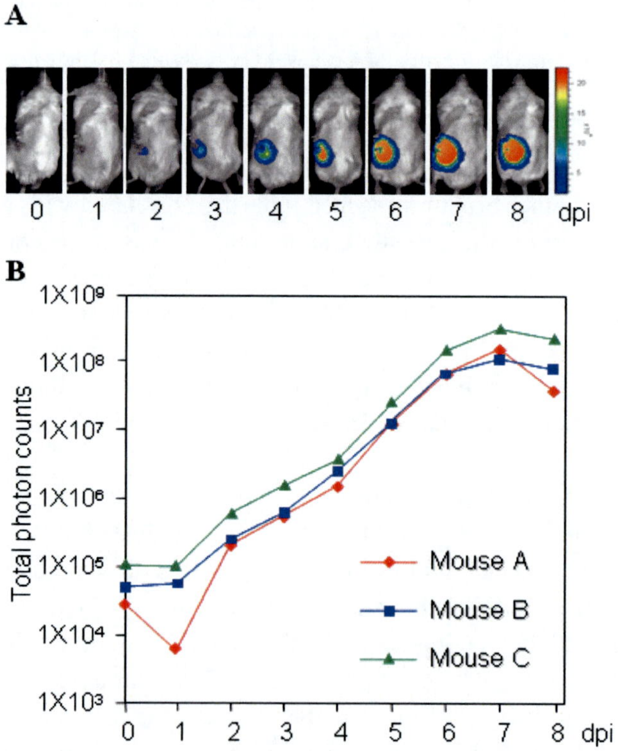

Figure 3. Measuring VZVLuc virus replication in SCID-hu mice. (A) Replication and progression of VZVLuc in human thymus/liver implants in SCID mice. Three SCID-hu mice implanted with thymus/liver implants were inoculated with VZVLuc. Using the IVIS Imaging System, each mouse was scanned daily (from day 0 to day 8). Measurements were taken 10 minutes after i.p. injection with D-luciferin substrate. Only images from mouse C are shown. Warmer colors indicate higher viral load; colder colors indicate lower viral load. (B). VZV growth curves in vivo. Bioluminescence from three SCID-hu mice in the above experiment was measured, and VZV growth curves in human thymus/liver implants were generated.

This result demonstrates that VZV_{Luc} virus spread can be monitored and quantified *in vivo* using the IVIS system. The kinetics of VZV_{Luc} spread in three mice were similar, and showed a general trend of exponential growth from day 1 to day 6 or 7, then growth slowed or reached a steady state due to the fact that the viral infection within the limited implants had reached saturation (Figure 3B). Based on these growth curves, it can be seen that VZV grew rapidly in human T cells *in vivo*, doubling approximately every 12 hrs, with maximal replication at 7 days post-infection. VZV_{Luc} viruses were also tested for their spread and detection in human fetal skin xenografts *in vivo* (our unpublished data).

Furthermore, ORFs 0 to 4 were individually deleted from the VZV_{Luc} genomes, and the phenotype of each viruses been studied by BLI, both *in vivo* and *in vitro*. Results have indicated that ORF 1, 2, and 3 were dispensable for VZV replication, both *in vitro* and *in vivo,* while ORF 0 could be a potential virulence factor. This work has validated and justified the use of the novel luciferase VZV BAC system to efficiently generate recombinant VZV variants and facilitate subsequent viral growth kinetic analysis, both *in vitro* and *in vivo* [50]. A detailed protocol has been established exploiting the new luciferase VZV BAC system to rapidly isolate and characterize VZV ORF deletion mutants by growth curve analysis [55].

Bioluminescence Imaging in Other Herpesviruses Studies

Pseudorabies virus (PrV) is a member of the herpesvirus family and is a close relative of human VZV and HSV. It is a natural pathogen of pigs in which it causes Aujeszky's disease. A recombinant pseudorabies virus (PrV) was constructed by inserting luciferase gene into the nonessential glycoprotein G gene region under the control of the gG promoter [56]. The results showed that the detection of luciferase expression in organ extracts of mice infected with luciferase recombinant PrV is a sensitive way to examine viral spread [56]. Luminescence in cells infected by a recombinant luciferase-expressing pseudorabies virus can be visualized macroscopically and microscopically with photon-counting devices coupled to image processors with a resolution at the single-cell level [57]. These early studies revealed the great potentials of using bioluminescence detection to observe herpesvirus pathogenesis, even though the more advanced CCD camera devices were not available at that time.

Herpes-based viral vectors have also been developed for use in a variety of immunization strategies. Replication-defective viruses have been used for immunization against herpes infections [58, 59]. BLI has been applied to examine the kinetics and spatial expression of HSV amplicon gene products with the goal of further developing these as immunization vectors [60].

Conclusion

The BLI technique has been experimentally demonstrated as being a promising tool for biological studies *in vivo*. This mini-review summed up recent applications of BLI in studies of pathogenesis and virus-host interactions of HSV-1 and VZV in living animal models.

Many small animal models of human disease caused by different pathogens have been investigated successfully using BLI. As demonstrated by us and other groups, BLI has apparent advantages over conventional methods that require sacrifice of animals and harvesting of tissues at multiple time points. Traditionally, large groups of animals need to be infected with the viral pathogen. During the course of viral infection, subsets of animals need to be sacrificed at defined time points in order to collect tissues for a determination of viral load and localization of infection. Non-invasive BLI requires much smaller groups of animals and the same set of animals can be kept alive and examined extensively, which dramatically reduces the number of animals required in experiments in order to achieve statistically meaningful results. Since signals from the same animals can be measured repeatedly, the animals serve as their own controls during the entire infection course, making it possible to overcome inter-animal variation and increase overall data reliability and reproducibility. Moreover, BLI enables the entire animal to be monitored for viral replication, thereby minimizing the possibility of overlooking unexpected sites of viral replication because tissues were not sampled.

Although BLI has increasingly been used for studying viral pathogenesis, there are also certain limitations to this modality. The sensitivity for detecting bioluminescence with BLI is determined by the combination of signal strength and anatomical location. Hair and overlying tissues can scatter and absorb light, while darkly pigmented organs and tissues can attenuate photon transmission [61]. Therefore, bioluminescence signals measured by computer analysis of emitted photons only allow relative quantification, given that expression levels of the luciferase enzyme by relative numbers of viruses or cells correlate linearly with the bioluminescence signal intensities. In addition, BLI is typically a two-dimensional imaging technique, with a spatial resolution of 2–3 mm. Even with advanced instrumentation (e.g., three-dimensional imaging systems using signal reconstruction techniques), it remains difficult to separate photons produced by two immediately adjacent photon-emitting sites.

Although BLI has been used in different studies and has successfully obtained semi-quantitative results regarding the biological process in animal models, it cannot completely replace conventional assays. The luciferase reaction is a complex one, and it needs ATP, oxygen, and luciferin, so the photon produced from the reaction also depends on the maintenance of those substances; if any are missed or decay, the false negative results would interfere with the whole experiment. Another drawback is that photons emitted as a result of BLI have a greater level of intensity in the shallower parts of the animal body, which can make it difficult when comparing infection in different sites *in vivo*. Therefore, the important results should be verified by complementary methods, such as traditional plaque assays. BLI rather serves as an easy to use alternative approach to traditional assays and can be superimposed on the existing animal model to allow more information to be obtained. *Ex vivo* examination of tissues can confirm the exact origin of the luciferase-expressing cells.

Acknowledgments

This study was supported by the Research Center for Minority Institutes (RCMI) program (grant #G12RR003050) of the Ponce School of Medicine and a start-up fund from the Ponce School of Medicine to Q.T., NIH grant AI050709 to HZ. We acknowledge Bob Ritchie for English editing.

References

[1] Sauerbrei, A.; Wutzler, P., Herpes simplex and varicella-zoster virus infections during pregnancy: current concepts of prevention, diagnosis and therapy. Part 2: Varicella-zoster virus infections. *Med Microbiol Immunol*, 2007. 196(2): p. 95-102.

[2] Streblow, D.N.; Dumortier, J., Mechanisms of cytomegalovirus-accelerated vascular disease: induction of paracrine factors that promote angiogenesis and wound healing. *Curr Top Microbiol Immunol*, 2008. 325: p. 397-415.

[3] Szajerka, T. and Jablecki, J. Kaposi's sarcoma revisited. AIDS Rev, 2007. 9(4): p. 230-6.

[4] Posnett, D.N., Herpesviruses and autoimmunity. *Curr Opin Investig Drugs*, 2008. 9(5): p. 505-14.

[5] Brady, G., MacArthur, G. J., Epstein-Barr virus and Burkitt lymphoma. *J Clin Pathol*, 2007. 60(12): p. 1397-402.

[6] Caselli, E. and Di Luca, D. Molecular biology and clinical associations of Roseoloviruses human herpesvirus 6 and human herpesvirus 7. *New Microbiol*, 2007. 30(3): p. 173-87.

[7] Contag, C.H.; Spilman, S. D., Visualizing gene expression in living mammals using a bioluminescent reporter. *Photochem Photobiol*, 1997. 66(4): p. 523-31.

[8] Wu, J.C., Sundaresan, G., Noninvasive optical imaging of firefly luciferase reporter gene expression in skeletal muscles of living mice. *Mol Ther*, 2001. 4(4): p. 297-306.

[9] Rehemtulla, A., Stegman, L. D., Rapid and quantitative assessment of cancer treatment response using in vivo bioluminescence imaging. *Neoplasia*, 2000. 2(6): p. 491-5.

[10] Rehemtulla, A., Hall, D. E., Molecular imaging of gene expression and efficacy following adenoviral-mediated brain tumor gene therapy. *Mol Imaging*, 2002. 1(1): p. 43-55.

[11] Massoud, T.F. and Gambhir, S.S. Molecular imaging in living subjects: seeing fundamental biological processes in a new light. *Genes Dev*, 2003. 17(5): p. 545-80.

[12] Soling, A., Theiss, C., A dual function fusion protein of Herpes simplex virus type 1 thymidine kinase and firefly luciferase for noninvasive in vivo imaging of gene therapy in malignant glioma. *Genet Vaccines Ther*, 2004. 2(1): p. 7.

[13] Wiles, S., Pickard, K. M., In vivo bioluminescence imaging of the murine pathogen Citrobacter rodentium. *Infect Immun*, 2006. 74(9): p. 5391-6.

[14] Huang, Q., Shan, S., Noninvasive visualization of tumors in rodent dorsal skin window chambers. *Nat Biotechnol*, 1999. 17(10): p. 1033-5.

[15] Wetterwald, A., van der Pluijm, G., Optical imaging of cancer metastasis to bone marrow: a mouse model of minimal residual disease. *Am J Pathol*, 2002. 160(3): p. 1143-53.

[16] Paroo, Z., Bollinger, R. A., Validating bioluminescence imaging as a high-throughput, quantitative modality for assessing tumor burden. *Mol Imaging*, 2004. 3(2): p. 117-24.

[17] Yamamoto, S., Deckter, L. A., Imaging immediate-early and strict-late promoter activity during oncolytic herpes simplex virus type 1 infection and replication in tumors. *Gene Ther*, 2006. 13(24): p. 1731-6.
[18] White, M.R., Masuko, M., Real-time analysis of the transcriptional regulation of HIV and hCMV promoters in single mammalian cells. *J Cell Sci*, 1995. 108 (Pt 2): p. 441-55.
[19] Collaco, A.M., Rahman, S., Circadian regulation of a viral gene promoter in live transgenic mice expressing firefly luciferase. *Mol Imaging Biol*, 2005. 7(5): p. 342-50.
[20] Fan, S., Maguire, C. A., Valproic acid enhances gene expression from viral gene transfer vectors. *J Virol Methods*, 2005. 125(1): p. 23-33.
[21] Contag, C.H. and Bachmann M.H. Advances in in vivo bioluminescence imaging of gene expression. *Annu Rev Biomed Eng*, 2002. 4: p. 235-60.
[22] Hastings, J.W., Biological diversity, chemical mechanisms, and the evolutionary origins of bioluminescent systems. *J Mol Evol*, 1983. 19(5): p. 309-21.
[23] Kurfurst, M., S. Ghisla, and Hastings, J.W. Bioluminescence emission from the reaction of luciferase-flavin mononucleotide radical with O2. *Biochemistry*, 1983. 22(7): p. 1521-5.
[24] Alipour, B.S., Hosseinkhani, S., Molecular cloning, sequence analysis, and expression of a cDNA encoding the luciferase from the glow-worm, Lampyris turkestanicus. *Biochem Biophys Res Commun*, 2004. 325(1): p. 215-22.
[25] Fraga, H., Firefly luminescence: a historical perspective and recent developments. *Photochem Photobiol Sci*, 2008. 7(2): p. 146-58.
[26] Luker, G.D. and Luker, K.E. Optical imaging: current applications and future directions. *J Nucl Med*, 2008. 49(1): p. 1-4.
[27] Luker, K.E. and Luker, G.D. Applications of bioluminescence imaging to antiviral research and therapy: multiple luciferase enzymes and quantitation. *Antiviral Res*, 2008. 78(3): p. 179-87.
[28] Denburg, J.L., Lee, R.T., McElroy, Substrate-binding properties of firefly luciferase. I. Luciferin-binding site. *Arch Biochem Biophys*, 1969. 134(2): p. 381-94.
[29] Davison, J.A. and Fynn, G.H. The assay of ATP by the luciferin-luciferase method. Interference by a bacterial phosphatase enzyme stable to perchlorate treatment. *Anal Biochem*, 1974. 58(2): p. 632-7.
[30] Suzuki, C., Nakajima, Y., A new additional reporter enzyme, dinoflagellate luciferase, for monitoring of gene expression in mammalian cells. Gene, 2005. 344: p. 61-6.
[31] Oshiro, M., Cooled CCD versus intensified cameras for low-light video--applications and relative advantages. *Methods Cell Biol*, 1998. 56: p. 45-62.
[32] Chee, M.S., Bankier, A. T., Analysis of the protein-coding content of the sequence of human cytomegalovirus strain AD169. Curr Top Microbiol Immunol, 1990. 154: p. 125-69.
[33] Dolan, A., Jamieson, F. E., The genome sequence of herpes simplex virus type 2. *J Virol*, 1998. 72(3): p. 2010-21.
[34] McGeoch, Dalrymple, M. A., The complete DNA sequence of the long unique region in the genome of herpes simplex virus type 1. *J Gen Virol*, 1988. 69 (Pt 7): p. 1531-74.

[35] Russo, J.J., Bohenzky, R. A., Nucleotide sequence of the Kaposi sarcoma-associated herpesvirus (HHV8). *Proc Natl Acad Sci U S A*, 1996. 93(25): p. 14862-7.
[36] Mocarski, E.S., Jr., Biology and replication of cytomegalovirus. *Transfus Med Rev*, 1988. 2(4): p. 229-34.
[37] Fortunato, E.A., McElroy, A. K., Exploitation of cellular signaling and regulatory pathways by human cytomegalovirus. *Trends Microbiol*, 2000. 8(3): p. 111-9.
[38] Tang, Q., Li, L., Determination of minimum herpes simplex virus type 1 components necessary to localize transcriptionally active DNA to ND10. *J Virol*, 2003. 77(10): p. 5821-8.
[39] Everett, R.D. and Murray, J. ND10 components relocate to sites associated with herpes simplex virus type 1 nucleoprotein complexes during virus infection. *J Virol*, 2005. 79(8): p. 5078-89.
[40] Weller, S.G., Sakai, A. K., Predicting the pathway to wind pollination: heritabilities and genetic correlations of inflorescence traits associated with wind pollination in Schiedea salicaria (Caryophyllaceae). *J Evol Biol*, 2006. 19(2): p. 331-42.
[41] Liu, W.W., Goodhouse, J., A microfluidic chamber for analysis of neuron-to-cell spread and axonal transport of an alpha-herpesvirus. *PLoS ONE*, 2008. 3(6): p. e2382.
[42] Luker, G.D., Bardill, J. P., Noninvasive bioluminescence imaging of herpes simplex virus type 1 infection and therapy in living mice. *J Virol*, 2002. 76(23): p. 12149-61.
[43] Luker, G.D., Sharma, V., Noninvasive imaging of protein-protein interactions in living animals. *Proc Natl Acad Sci U S A*, 2002. 99(10): p. 6961-6.
[44] Luker, G.D., Prior, J. L., Bioluminescence imaging reveals systemic dissemination of herpes simplex virus type 1 in the absence of interferon receptors. *J Virol*, 2003. 77(20): p. 11082-93.
[45] Burgos, J.S., Guzman-Sanchez, F., Non-invasive bioluminescence imaging for monitoring herpes simplex virus type 1 hematogenous infection. *Microbes Infect*, 2006. 8(5): p. 1330-8.
[46] Luker, K.E., Schultz, T., Transgenic reporter mouse for bioluminescence imaging of herpes simplex virus 1 infection in living mice. Virology, 2006. 347(2): p. 286-95.
[47] Arvin, A.M., Varicella-zoster virus: molecular virology and virus-host interactions. *Curr Opin Microbiol*, 2001. 4(4): p. 442-9.
[48] Gilden, D.H., Kleinschmidt-DeMasters, B. K., Neurologic complications of the reactivation of varicella-zoster virus. *N Engl J Med*, 2000. 342(9): p. 635-45.
[49] Shiraki, K., Yoshida, Y., Pathogenetic tropism of varicella-zoster virus to primary human hepatocytes and attenuating tropism of Oka varicella vaccine strain to neonatal dermal fibroblasts. *J Infect Dis*, 2003. 188(12): p. 1875-7.
[50] Zhang, Z., Rowe, J., Genetic analysis of varicella-zoster virus ORF0 to ORF4 by use of a novel luciferase bacterial artificial chromosome system. *J Virol*, 2007. 81(17): p. 9024-33.
[51] Rice, B.W., Cable, M.D., Nelson, In vivo imaging of light-emitting probes. J Biomed Opt, 2001. 6(4): p. 432-40.
[52] Besser, J., Sommer, M. H., Differentiation of varicella-zoster virus ORF47 protein kinase and IE62 protein binding domains and their contributions to replication in human skin xenografts in the SCID-hu mouse. J Virol, 2003. 77(10): p. 5964-74.

[53] Ku, C.C., Besser, J., Varicella-Zoster virus pathogenesis and immunobiology: new concepts emerging from investigations with the SCIDhu mouse model. *J Virol*, 2005. 79(5): p. 2651-8.

[54] Zerboni, L., Ku, C. C., Varicella-zoster virus infection of human dorsal root ganglia in vivo. *Proc Natl Acad Sci U S A*, 2005. 102(18): p. 6490-5.

[55] Zhang, Z., Huang, Y., A highly efficient protocol of generating and analyzing VZV ORF deletion mutants based on a newly developed luciferase VZV BAC system. *J Virol Methods*, 2008. 148(1-2): p. 197-204.

[56] Kovacs, F. and Mettenleiter, T.C. Firefly luciferase as a marker for herpesvirus (pseudorabies virus) replication in vitro and in vivo. *J Gen Virol*, 1991. 72 (Pt 12): p. 2999-3008.

[57] Mettenleiter, T.C. and Grawe, W. Video imaging of firefly luciferase activity to identify and monitor herpesvirus infection in cell culture. *J Virol Methods*, 1996. 59(1-2): p. 155-60.

[58] Da Costa, X.J., Jones, C.A., Immunization against genital herpes with a vaccine virus that has defects in productive and latent infection. *Proc Natl Acad Sci U S A*, 1999. 96(12): p. 6994-8.

[59] Jones, C.A. and Knipe, D. Herpes simplex virus vaccines. *Pediatr Infect Dis J*, 2003. 22(11): p. 1003-5.

[60] Santos, K., Simon, D. A., Spatial and temporal expression of herpes simplex virus type 1 amplicon-encoded genes: implications for their use as immunization vectors. *Hum Gene Ther*, 2007. 18(2): p. 93-105.

[61] Contag, C.H. and Ross, B.D. It's not just about anatomy: in vivo bioluminescence imaging as an eyepiece into biology. *J Magn Reson Imaging*, 2002. 16(4): p. 378-87.

In: Herpesviridae Viral Structure, Life Cycle and Infections ISBN 978-1-60692-947-6
Editor: Toma R. Gluckman

Chapter 2

Herpes Virus Infection in Equid Species

R. Paillot, E. Sharp, R. Case and J. Nugent
Animal Health Trust, Centre for Preventive Medicine, Lanwades Park,
Newmarket, CB8 7UU, UK

Abstract

Herpesviruses infect members of all groups of vertebrates and 9 equid herpesviruses (EHV) have been identified so far. Equine herpes virus-1 (EHV-1) to EHV-5 infect horses, EHV-6 to EHV-8 infect donkeys and are also called asinine herpesvirus-1 (AHV-1) to AHV-3 and EHV-9 or gazelle herpesvirus (GHV) infects Thomson's gazelles. Of the list of presently known equid herpes viruses, EHV-1 and EHV-4 are clinically and epidemiologically the most important and most studied viruses. EHV-1 infection induces clinical signs of disease ranging in severity, from mild respiratory distress to abortion in pregnant mares, neonatal foal death and in more extreme cases neuropathogenic disorders. EHV-4 infection, by contrast, induces mainly a mild respiratory disease. It is estimated that 80-90% of horses have been exposed to either EHV-1 or EHV-4 by two years of age and these equid herpesviruses, in common with other herpesviruses, have unique life cycles adapted to infect and persist latently the host. EHV-1 presents a particular problem in this regard as recrudescence of latent viral infection can result in active and/or silent transmission from brood mares to foals and subsequently between foals. Recrudescence of latent EHV-1 can also result in neurological disease and this viral state appears to be on the increase. Together, these viruses have a major economic and welfare impact on all sectors of the horse industry worldwide. This chapter will overview all equid herpesviruses with a specific focus on EHV-1/4 and EHV-2/5. Our current understanding of the life cycle, pathogenicity and protective humoral and cellular immune responses stimulated by natural EHV-1 infection will be discussed along with several different strategies of vaccination that have been investigated and developed over the past decades to fight and contain these pathogens.

Abbreviations

ADCC:	antibody dependent cell-mediated cytotoxicity
AHV:	asinine herpesvirus
APC:	antigen presenting cell
BVDV:	Bovine viral diarrhea virus
BHV:	bovine herpes virus
CCL3:	chemokine (C-C motif) ligand 3
CF:	complement fixing
CG:	chorionic gonadotrophine
CMI:	cell mediated immunity
CMV:	cytomegalovirus
CSF:	cerebro spinal fluid
CTL:	cytotoxique T lymphocyte
CTLp:	cytotoxique T lymphocyte precursor
CXCL:	chemokine (C-X-C motif) ligand
DC:	dendritic cells
EIV:	equine influenza virus
EHM:	equine herpesvirus myeloencephalitis
EHV:	equine herpesvirus
ER:	endoplasmic reticulum
gB, gC…:	glycoprotein B, glycoprotein C …
GHV:	gazelle herpesvirus
GM-CSF:	granulocyte-macrophage colony stimulating factor
GPCR:	G protein-coupled receptors
HSV:	herpes simplex virus
ICP:	infected cell polypeptide
IE:	immediate-early
Ig:	immunoglobulin
IFN:	interferon
IL:	interleukin
ISCOM:	immuno-stimulating complex
LAT:	latent-associated transcript
L-particles:	light particles
Mϕ:	Macrophage
MALT:	mucosal associated lymphoid tissue
MHC:	major histocompatibility complex
Mo:	Monocyte
mRNA:	messenger RNA
MVA:	modified vaccinia Ankara
NALT:	nasal associated lymphoid tissue
NK:	natural killer cell
NPC:	nucleopore complex
ORF:	open reading frame
PBMC:	peripheral blood mononuclear cells

PBL:	peripheral blood lymphocyte
PCR:	polymerase chain reaction
PREP:	pre-viral DNA replication particles
PRV:	pseudorabies
RPLN:	retropharyngeal lymph node
SMLN:	submandibulary lymph node
TAP :	transporter associated with antigen processing
Tc: T	cytotoxique
TCR:	T cell receptor
TGFβ:	transforming growth factor
Th:	T helper
TK:	thymidine kinase
TNF:	tumor necrosing factor
T_{reg}:	lymphocyte T regulator
Ts:	temperature sensitive
vCKBP:	viral chemokine binding protein
VN:	virus neutralising
VP:	virus protein
WNV:	West Nile virus
XCL:	chemokine (C motif) ligand

Introduction

Herpes is a Latin word coming from the Greek word *herpein*, which means to creep. Herpesviruses induce a chronic, latent and recurrent infection. In humans, herpesvirus is the leading cause of disease, in front of influenza and cold viruses. Herpesviruses infect members of all groups of vertebrates and some invertebrates. Around 120 herpesviruses have been identified and isolated. The *Herpesviridae* family is divided into three lineages. Historically, assignment of members to the family *Herpesviridae* was based on virion morphology. Biological criteria, such as their tissue tropism, pathogenicity and behaviour in tissue culture (Table 1) were then used to make assignments to three subfamilies, the *Alpha-, Beta-* and *Gammaherpesvirinae* (α, β and γ) [1, 2]. However, sequence comparisons are now the primary approach for evaluating phylogenetic and taxonomic relationships among herpesviruses, and for identifying newly characterised viruses as members of the *Herpesviridae*. Tables 2 to 4 illustrate the current taxonomic assignment of a number of herpesviruses. Notably Equine herpesvirus-2 and Equine herpesvirus-5 are currently assigned to the *Rhadinovirus* genus of the subfamily *Gammaherpesvirinae* on the basis of sequence similarity with other members of this genus.

It has become apparent that in contrast to mammalian/avian/reptilian herpesviruses which can all be assigned to the three current herpesvirus subfamilies, piscine, amphibian and the single known invertebrate herpesvirus (of bivalve molluscs) belong to unrelated groups. Thus proposals of The *Herpesviridae* Study Group of the International Committee on Taxonomy of Viruses to revise higher-level taxonomic arrangements for herpesviruses, have recently been reported [3].

Table 1. Sub-divisions of the family Herpesviridae and their associated biological properties

Sub-family	Biological Properties
Alphaherpesvirinae	Variable host range; relatively short reproductive cycle; rapid spread of virus in culture; efficient destruction of infected cells; ability to establish latency primarily but not exclusively within sensory ganglia.
Betaherpesvirinae	Restricted host range; long reproductive cycle; slow spread of infection in culture.
Gammaherpesvirinae	Host range generally restricted to the family or order to which the natural host belongs; specificity for T- or B-lymphocytes.

Table 2. Current genera of the *Alphaherpesvirinae* showing a selection of assigned herpesviruses [adapted from the Index of viruses-Herpesviridae (2006) at www.ncbi.nlm.nih.gov/ICTVdp]. Asterisk mark tentative species in the genera

Sub-family	Genus	Species name	Common name
Alpha-herpesvirinae	Simple-xvirus	*Human herpesvirus 1* (HHV-1)	Herpes simplex virus type 1
		Human herpesvirus 2 (HHV-2)	Herpes simplex virus type 2
		Cerocopithecine herpesvirus 1	Herpesvirus simiae (B virus)
		Cerocopithecine herpesvirus 2	Simian agent 8 (SA8)
		Cerocopithecine herpesvirus 16	Baboon herpesvirus 2
		Saimiriine herpesvirus 1	Marmoset herpesvirus
		Bovine herpesvirus 2 (BHV-2)	Bovine mammillitis virus
		Ateline herpesvirus 1	Spider monkey herpesvirus
	Varicell-ovirus	*Human herpesvirus 3* (HHV-3)	Varicella-zoster virus (VZV)
		Cercopithecine herpesvirus 9	Simian varicella virus (SVV)
		Equid herpesvirus 1 (EHV-1)	Equine abortion virus
		Equid herpesvirus 3 (EHV-3)	Equine coitalexanthema virus
		Equid herpesvirus 4 (EHV-4)	Equine rhinotracheitis virus
		Equid herpesvirus 6 (EHV-6)*	Asinine herpesvirus 1 (AsHV-1)
		Equid herpesvirus 8 (EHV-8)	Asinine herpesvirus 3 (AsHV-3)
		Equid herpesvirus 9 (EHV-9)	Gazelle herpesvirus (GHV-1)
		Bovine herpesvirus 1 (BHV-1)	Infectious bovine rhinotracheitis virus
		Bovine herpesvirus 5 (BHV-5)	Bovine encephalitis virus
		Bubaline herpesvirus 1	Waterbuffalo herpesvirus
		Canid herpesvirus 1 (CHV-1)	Canine herpesvirus
		Cervid herpesvirus 1	Red deer herpesvirus
		Cervid herpesvirus 2	Reindeer herpesvirus
		Felid herpesvirus 1 (FHV-1)	Feline viral rhinotracheitis virus
		Phocid herpesvirus 1	Harbour seal herpesvirus
		Suid herpesvirus 1	Pseudorabies virus (PRV)
	Mar-s diviru	*Gallid herpesvirus 2* (GaHV-2)	Marek's disease herpesvirus 1
		Gallid herpesvirus 3 (GaHV-3)	Marek's disease herpesvirus 2
		Meleagrid herpesvirus-1	Turkey herpesvirus
	Iltovirus	*Gallid herpesvirus I*	Infectious laryngotracheitis virus (ILTV)

Table 3. Current genera of the *Betaherpesvirinae,* showing a selection of assigned herpesviruses [adapted from the Index of viruses-Herpesviridae (2006) at www.ncbi.nlm.nih.gov/ICTVdp]. * mark tentative species in the genera

Sub-family	Genus	Designation	Common name
Beta-herpesvirinae	Cyto-megalovirus	*Human herpesvirus 5* (HHV-5)	Human cytomegalovirus (HCMV)
		Cercopithecine herpesvirus 5	African green monkey simian cytomegalovirus (SCMV)
		Cercopithecine herpesvirus 8	Rhesus Monkey cytomegalovirus (RhCMV)
		Pongine herpesvirus 4	Chimpanzee cytomegalovirus (CCMV)
		*Aotine herpesvirus 1**	Herpesvirus aotus 1
		*Aotine herpesvirus 3**	Herpesvirus aotus 3
	Muro-megalovirus	*Murid herpesvirus 1*	Mouse cytomegalovirus (MCMV)
		Murid herpesvirus 2	Rat cytomegalovirus (RCMV)
	Roseolovirus	*Human herpesvirus 6* (HHV-6)	
		Human herpesvirus 7 (HHV-7)	

Table 4. Current genera of the *Gammaherpesvirinae* showing a selection of assigned herpesviruses [adapted from the Index of viruses-Herpesviridae (2006) at www.ncbi.nlm.nih.gov/ICTVdp]

Sub-family	Genus	Designation	Common name
Gamma-herpesvirinae	Lymphoc-ryptovirus	*Human herpesvirus 4* (HHV-4)	Epstein-Barr Virus (EBV)
		Cercopithecine herpesvirus 12	Baboon herpesvirus
		Cercopithecine herpesvirus 14	African green monkey EBV-like virus
		Cercopithecine herpesvirus 15	Rhesus EBV-like virus
		Callitrichine herpesvirus 3 (CHV-3)	Marmoset lymphocryptovirus (MarLCV)
		Pongine herpesvirus 1	Herpesvirus pan
		Pongine herpesvirus 2	Orangutan herpesvirus
		Pongine herpesvirus 3	Gorilla herpesvirus
	Rhadinovirus	*Human herpesvirus 8* (HHV-8)	Kaposi's Sarcoma Associated herpesvirus (KSHV)
		Saimiriine herpesvirus 2	Herpesvirus Saimiri (HVS)
		Cercopithecine herpesvirus 17	Rhesus rhadinovirus (RRV)
		Equid herpesvirus 2 (EHV-2)	Equine herpesvirus-2
		Equid herpesvirus 5 (EHV-5)	Equine herpesvirus-5
		Equid herpesvirus 7	Asinine herpesvirus 7 (AHV-2)
		Mustelid herpesvirus 1	Badger herpesvirus

Table 4. (Continued)

Sub-family	Genus	Designation	Common name
		Murid herpesvirus 4	Mouse herpesvirus strain 68 (MHV-68)
		Bovine herpesvirus 4 (BHV-4)	Movar virus
		Alcelaphine herpesvirus 1 (AlHV-1)	Wildebeest malignant catarrhal fever virus
		Alcelaphine herpesvirus 2 (AlHV-2)	Hartebeest malignant catarrhal fever virus
		Ateline herpesvirus 2	Herpesvirus ateles (HVA)
		Hippotragineherpesvirus 1	Roan antelope herpesvirus
		Ovine herpesvirus 2	Sheep-associated malignant catarrhal fever of cattle virus
		Leporid herpesvirus 1	Cottontail rabbit herpesvirus (CRHV)
		Porcine lymphotropic herpesvirus-1 (PLHV-1)	
		Porcine lymphotropic herpesvirus-2 (PLHV-2)	
		Porcine lymphotropic herpesvirus-3 (PLHV-3)	

Membership of the family *Herpesviridae* will be restricted to viruses that belong to the *Alpha-, Beta-* and *Gammaherpesvirinae* subfamilies on the basis of their gene contents and sequences. The group of piscine and amphibian herpesviruses will be assigned to a new family, the *Alloherpesviridae*, and the single known invertebrate herpesvirus to another new family, the *Malacoherpesviridae*. All three families will be grouped in a new higher-level taxon, the order *Herpesvirales*.

Additionally, three new genera of the *Herpesviridae* are proposed. *Proboscivirus* in the *Betaherpesvirinae* will contain elephant endothelial herpesvirus (EEHV). In the *Gammaherpesvirinae*, the genus *Rhadinovirus* will become more tightly demarcated so that the lineage containing *alcelaphine herpesvirus-1* (AlHV-1) among other artiodactyle herpesviruses will form the genus *Macavirus*, and notably, the lineage containing *Equid herpesvirus-2* (EHV-2), *Equid herpesvirus-5* (EHV-5) and certain other perissodactyl and carnivore herpesviruses will form the genus *Percavirus*. As these changes have yet to be formally accepted, the current assignment of EHV-2 and EHV-5 to the genus *Rhadinovirus* will be employed throughout this chapter.

To summarise, 9 equid herpesviruses have been identified (Table 5). Equine herpes virus-1 (EHV-1) to EHV-5 infect horses, EHV-6 to EHV-8 infect donkeys and are also called asinine herpesvirus (AsHV, AsHV-1 to 3), 3 others asinine herpesvirus (AsHV-4 to 6) have been recently described [4, 5]. EHV-9 or gazelle herpesvirus (GHV) infects Thomson's gazelles [6-8]. A majority of horses have been exposed to either EHV-1 or EHV-4 by two years of age. These two equine herpesviruses have a major economic and welfare impact on all sectors of the horse industry worldwide and have been the subject of most researches. Therefore this chapter will concentrate mainly on EHV-1 and EHV-4.

Table 5. Summary of Equid herpesviruses and associated disease

Host species	Name	Other name/relationship	Subfamily	Disease
Equus caballus	EHV-1	Eq. abortion virus	α2	Respiratory, abortion, neurological
	EHV-2	Eq. cytomegalovirus	γ	NA
	EHV-3	Eq. coital exanthema virus	α	Coital exanthema
	EHV-4	Eq. rhinopneumonitis virus	α2	Respiratory
	EHV-5	Eq. cytomegalovirus	γ	NA
Equus asinus	AsHV-1/EHV-6	Related to EHV-3	α	Coital exanthema
	AsHV-2/EHV-7	Related to EHV-2	γ	NA
	AsHV-3/EHV-8	Related to EHV-1	α	Rhinitis
Gazella thomsoni	GHV-1/EHV-9	Similar to EHV-1/EHV-8	α	Ga.andEq. neurological

Eq. = equine; Ga. = gazelle; NA= not associated.

Equine Herpes Virus Type 1 and Type 4 (EHV-1; EHV-4)

EHV-1 and EHV-4 are ubiquitous in domestic and wild equid populations throughout the world. EHV-1 also infects zebras (*Equus grevyi* and *Equus burchelli*) and onager (*Equus hemionus onager*) [9-11]. It is estimated that 80 to 90% of horses have been exposed to EHV-1, or the closely related EHV-4, by two years of age [12]. EHV-1 can cause a respiratory disease that is most commonly seen in young animals, abortion (sporadic abortion and abortion storms) and neurological disease in horses.

Structure of EHV-1 and EHV-4

EHV-1 is composed of an icosahedral nucleocapsid containing the viral genome, surrounded by an amorphous envelope, which contains several glycoproteins (Figure 1). The majority of EHV-1 proteins share extensive homology with human simplex virus (HSV), which is the prototype virus of the *Alphaherpesvirinae* subfamily.

The entire linear double strand DNA genome of a plaque purified clone of EHV-1 strain Ab4 has been sequenced [14]. It is divided into a unique long (U_L) and a unique short (U_S) region. U_S is flanked by an inverted internal and terminal repeat sequence (I_R and T_R). The genome (150 223 bp) contains 80 open reading frames (ORFs), which encode 76 unique genes and four ORFs duplicated in the I_R and T_R (Table 6) [6, 14, 15]. U_L contains genes 1 to 63, U_S contains genes 68 to 76, I_R and T_R contain genes 64 to 67 and 67 to 64, respectively. The list of genes is presented in Table 6. EHV-4 is closely related to EHV-1 [1, 2], its genome is 145 kb in size, encodes 76 genes and possesses the same organisation than EHV-1.

The tegument corresponds to the space between the nucleocapsid and the envelope. This is composed of 12 viral proteins and enzymes involved in the initiation of viral replication. Nucleocapsids and tegument are surrounded by an envelope presenting 12 viral glycoproteins on its surface (Table 7). The eleven glycoproteins of EHV-1 (i.e. gB-gp14, gC-gp13, gD-gp18, gE, gG, gH, gI, gK, gL, gM and gN) are conserved in other alpha herpesvirus and therefore named according to the nomenclature established for HSV-1. Glycoproteins are essential in infection processes including virus adsorption, penetration, and cell-to-cell spread. Compared to HSV-1 and the majority of other alpha herpesviruses, EHV-1 encodes an additional glycoprotein, gp2, with homologues present only in EHV-4 and AsHV-3.

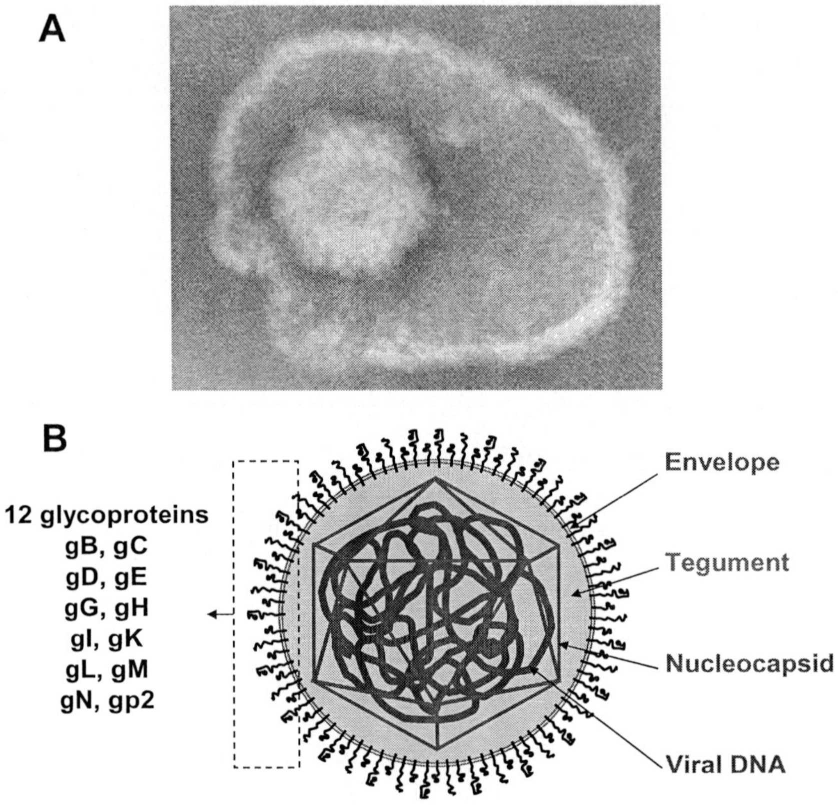

Figure 1. Equine herpesvirus-1 [13]. (A) Transmission electron microscopy of whole EHV-1 (Animal Health Trust), (B) schematic of EHV-1 structure.

Table 6. Open Reading Frames (ORFs) of EHV-1, name and function of their genes products

ORF	Location	Amino acids	Name/Function
1	U_L	202	Unknown
2	U_L	205	Unknown
3	U_L	257	Unknown
4	U_L	200	Unknown
5	U_L	470	EIVP 27, transactivator
6	U_L	343	Envelope glycoprotein (gK)
7	U_L	1081	DNA helicase-primase
8	U_L	245	Unknown

ORF	Location	Amino acids	Name/Function
9	U_L	326	Deoxyuridine triphosphatase
10	U_L	100	UL49.5 (glycoprotein gN)
11	U_L	304	Tegument protein
12	U_L	449	ETIF, transactivator of IE, α-TIF homolog
13	U_L	871	Tegument protein
14	U_L	747	Tegument protein
15	U_L	227	Tegument protein
16	U_L	468	Envelope glycoprotein (gC)
17	U_L	401	unknown
18	U_L	405	DNA polymerase
19	U_L	497	Host shut-off factor
20	U_L	321	Ribonucleotide reductase
21	U_L	790	Ribonucleotide reductase
22	U_L	465	Capsid protein
23	U_L	1020	Tegument protein
24	U_L	3421	Tegument protein
25	U_L	119	Capsid protein
26	U_L	275	unknown
27	U_L	140	DNA packaging protein
28	U_L	620	DNA packaging protein
29	U_L	326	unknown
30	U_L	1220	DNA polymerase
31	U_L	1209	DNA-binding protein
32	U_L	775	DNA packaging protein
33	U_L	980	Envelope glycoprotein (gB)
34	U_L	160	Virus egress
35	U_L	646	Capsid protein
35.5	U_L	329	Capsid protein
36	U_L	587	DNA packaging protein
37	U_L	272	unknown
38	U_L	352	Thymidine kinase (TK)
39	U_L	848	Envelope glycoprotein (gH)
40	U_L	530	Tegument protein
41	U_L	239	unknown
42	U_L	1376	Capsid protein
43	U_L	314	Capsid protein
44	U_L	734	DNA packaging protein
45	U_L	706	unknown
46	U_L	370	Tegument protein
47	U_L	358	unknown
48	U_L	317	unknown
49	U_L	594	Tegument protein
50	U_L	565	Deoxyribonuclease

Table 6. (Continued)

ORF	Location	Amino acids	Name/Function
51	U_L	74	Tegument protein
52	U_L	450	Envelope glycoprotein (gM)
53	U_L	887	Oringin-binding protein
54	U_L	751	DNA helicase-primase
55	U_L	303	unknown
56	U_L	753	Capsid protein
57	U_L	881	DNA helicase-primase
58	U_L	225	unknown
59	U_L	179	unknown
60	U_L	212	unknown
61	U_L	312	DNA glycosylate
62	U_L	218	Envelope glycoprotein (gL)
63	U_L	532	ICP0, early gene, transactivator
64	I_R and T_R	1487	IE (immediate early gene), transactivator
65	I_R and T_R	293	Possible late regulatory gene
66	I_R and T_R	236	Late gene, homolog of H_SV US10
67	I_R and T_R	272	EICP22, unique early gene, transactivator
68	U_S	418	Late gene
69	U_S	382	Serine-threonie protein kinase
70	U_S	411	Envelope glycoprotein (gG)
71	U_S	797	Envelope glycoprotein (gp2)
72	U_S	402	Envelope glycoprotein (gD)
73	U_S	424	Envelope glycoprotein (gI)
74	U_S	550	Envelope glycoprotein (gEI)
75	U_S	130	unknown
76	U_S	219	Tegument protein

Table 7. Envelope glycoproteins of EHV-1

Glycoprotein	Former/other name	Function
gB	gp14	Cell penetration and cell-to-cell spreading
gC	gp13	Attachment and egress
gD	gP17/18 or gp60	Cell penetration and cell-to-cell spreading
gE	None	Cell-to-cell spreading
gG	None	Unclear
gH	None	Unclear
gI	None	Cell-to-cell spreading
gK	None	Cell-to-cell spreading and virus egress
gL	None	Unclear
gM	gp21/22a or gp45	Cell penetration and cell-to-cell spreading
gN	UL49.5	Processing of gM/Immune evasion
gp2	Gp300	Unclear

The viral genome is contained in a nucleocapsid composed of six proteins [16]. All herpesviruses have a similar capsid structure composed of 162 capsomers (12 pentons and 150 hexons). Twelve portal proteins form a ring in the nucleocapsid, which is used by viral DNA to enter into the capsid [17, 18].

Cell Infection and Virus Replication

As for other alpha herpesviruses, EHV-1 can infect a large range of cell types in the respiratory tract, lymphoid organs and the nervous system [19]. Cells are infected by direct contact with EHV-1 or by cell-to-cell contact with infected cells.

Envelope glycoproteins of EHV-1 have been shown to play key roles in the entry of the virus into host cells. EHV-1 uses the same glycoproteins as other alpha herpesviruses (e.g. HSV, bovine herpes virus (BHV) and pseudorabies virus (PRV)) to bind to permissive cells. EHV-1 glycoprotein C (gC) binds to heparan sulphate-containing glycosaminoglycans on the cell surface [20, 21]. Glycoproteins D and M (gD and gM) are required for virus entry [22, 23], but another unique receptor, still unknown and distinct from virus-receptors previously described for alpha herpesviruses is also involved [21]. Once attached, the virus penetrates the cell by either fusion of the virus envelope and cell membrane or by non classical endocytosis/phagocytosis [24], which release the nucleocapsid and tegument proteins of EHV-1 into the cell (Figure 2). Like other herpesvirus, it is believed that most of the tegument proteins dissociate from the capsid, which associates with microtubules via dynein, a minus-end-director motor protein. The capsid is therefore transported along microtubules to the microtubules organising centre, near the nucleus. This mechanism of capsid transport is important in the infection of cells such as neurones, when the site of infection can be far from the nucleus. The nucleocapsid binds directly to the nucleopore complex (NPC) and the viral DNA is translocated into the nucleus while the nucleocapsid remains in the cytoplasm [25].

The transcription of the EHV-1 genome is sequentially ordered. The tegument VP16 (HSV) homologue protein of EHV-1, brought into the cell by the virus, is a strong activator of immediate early (IE) gene expression [26]. The IE protein is encoded by ORF 64 and synthesised by cellular RNA polymerase II [27, 28]. This gene is required for the transcription of the adjacent early and late genes [29]. Early genes encode the proteins involved in stimulating virus replication. Late genes encode the viral structural proteins (Figure 2).

Herpesvirus nucleocapsids are assembled in the nucleus around scaffolding proteins prior to viral DNA encapsidation. The nucleocapsid, surrounded by tegument proteins, leaves the nucleus by envelopment at the inner nuclear membrane that contains glycoproteins. This primary envelope is lost when the virus buds through the outer nuclear membrane. A second envelopment occurs at the cytoplasmic membranes (ER or exocytotic vesicles), which contain all the viral glycoproteins, before the migration of the mature virus through the secretory pathway (via the Golgi apparatus). The infectious virus can be released into the extracellular space [25] or infect other cells via virus-induced cell fusion. *In vitro*, gB is absolutely essential for direct cell-to-cell spread of virions [30]. EHV-1 gD, gB and gK are involved in the cell-cell fusion process [22, 31, 32].

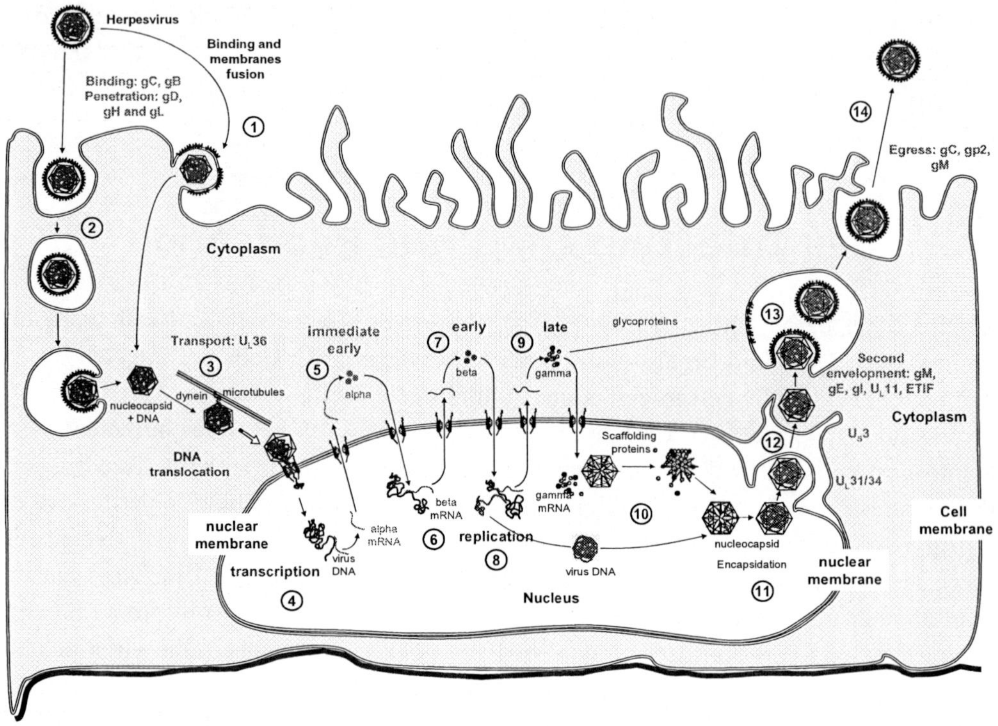

Figure 2. The reproductive cycle of herpesvirus. The virus enters susceptible cells by binding to cell surface receptors and fusing with the cell membrane (1) or/and by non classical endocytosis/phagocytosis (2). The nucleocapsid is subsequently released into the cytoplasm. The nucleocapsid reaches the nucleus via microtubules (3) and the viral DNA passes through NPC (nucleopore complex) into the nucleus (4) where transcription of immediate early gene takes place. Immediate early/alpha proteins synthesised in the cytoplasm (5) migrate into the nucleus to initiate transcription of early/beta mRNA (6). Early/beta proteins (7) migrate through NPC into the nucleus to start replication of the virus (8). Late/gamma proteins synthesised in the cytoplasm (9) migrate into the nucleus to form the nucleocapsid. Nucleocapsid proteins assemble themselves around scaffolding proteins (10) that degrade by autoproteolysis before encapsidation of new viral DNA (11). The nucleocapsid and tegument proteins migrate through nucleus (12) and cytoplasmic membranes (13) to be relased (14). Some of the proteins or gene products involved in the reproductive cycle of herpesvirus have been indicated in red.

Propagation and Virus Disease

In the horse, EHV-1 is transmitted by inhalation or direct contact with infected fomites such as aborted foetuses or placental tissues. Spread of infection occurs by intercellular routes involving many cell types [33].

Infection of the Respiratory Tract

The pathogenesis of EHV-1 infection is well described after experimental infection with the EHV-1 strain Ab4. In the absence of mucosal antibody, nasal and nasopharyngeal epithelial cells are infected with EHV-1 (Figure 3) [34]. Subsequent erosions, due to epithelial cell necrosis and an acute inflammatory response, occur during the first week after infection, resulting in infectious virus shedding. EHV-1 spreads quickly through the body. Leucocytes in adjacent lamina propria and endothelial cells of blood and lymphatic vessels are also infected due to a cell-to-cell spread of infectious virus from the respiratory epithelium. Progeny virus and viral antigens are detected in respiratory epithelium as soon as 12 hours post infection. Endothelium of local blood vessels is infected within 2-4 days of infection (Figue 3) [35].

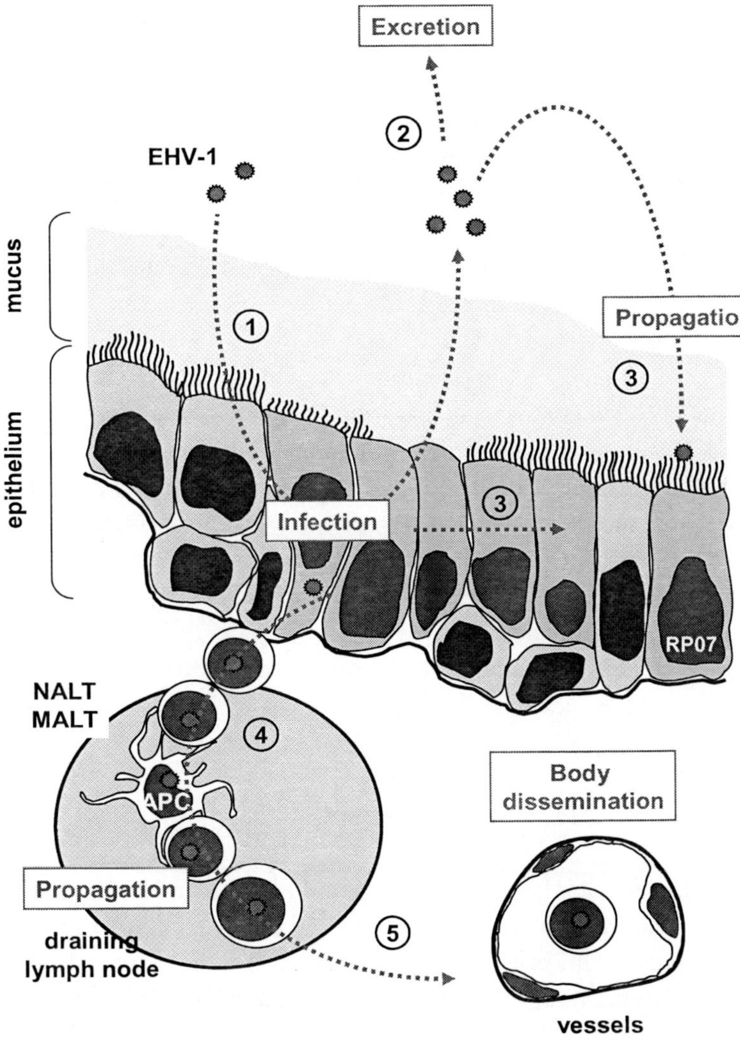

Figure 3. EHV-1 initially infects the epithelial cells of the upper respiratory tract (1). EHV-1 replicates and is shed (2), disseminates through the respiratory tract (3) or reaches the respiratory lymph nodes were PBMC will be infected (4). Circulation of infected leucocytes (5) during cell-associated viraemia disseminates EHV-1 to distant sites such as the central nervous system or the reproductive tract. MALT: mucosal associated lymphoid tissue; NALT: nasal associated lymphoid tissue [13].

In young horses, clinical signs of infection with EHV-1 consist of fever, serous to mucopurulent nasal discharge, occasional coughing, dyspnoea, lung sound and local lymphoadenopathy. Respiratory infection caused by EHV-1 in older horses is mild or subclinical. EHV-1 primarily infects the upper respiratory tract but infection of the lower respiratory tract may result from dissemination through airway surfaces or via blood vessels and cell-associated viraemia. EHV-1 may reach the lungs, inducing bronchopneumonia [6].

Before 1981, EHV-1 and EHV-4 were considered one and the same virus and the clinical signs of the respiratory disease induced by both viruses are indistinguishable [6, 7, 33]. EHV-4 can be detected in nasal swab extracts from day 1 to day 8 post infection [36-38].

Lymph Nodes of the Respiratory Tract and Cell Associated Viraemia

When lymphocytes have been infected and a cell-associated viraemia established, EHV-1 spreads rapidly through the host. Both infectious virus and viral antigens have been detected in submandibular, retropharyngeal and bronchial lymph nodes by 12-24 hours post infection. EHV-1 infection is likely to be amplified in lymph node cells (e.g. mononuclear leucocytes, macrophage and endothelial cells) [34]. Circulation of virus-infected leucocytes through the lymphatic and blood systems disseminates EHV-1 further to distant locations such as the pregnant uterus and central nervous system.

The identity of the leucocyte population in which EHV-1 replicates during cell-associated viraemia has been controversial. During the acute phase of viraemia, EHV-1 DNA has been detected in sub-populations of peripheral blood mononuclear cells (PBMC; i.e. CD4+, CD8+, monocytes and B cells) [39]. The expression of EHV-1 antigens has been detected on CD8+ cells, monocytes and CD4+ cells to a lesser extent, but not on B cells after *in vivo* infection [40]. However, EHV-1 antigen expression on B cells and all other PBMC populations has been shown after *in vitro* infection with EHV-1 [41, 42]. Dendritic cells (DC) are also sensitive to EHV-1 infection [43, 44].

EHV-4 induced a cell-associated viraemia detectable during the first 10 days post infection [36, 38].

Abortion, Neonatal and Perinatal Diseases

EHV-1 is a leading cause of infectious abortion in horses and was first recognised as the agent responsible for abortion in Kentucky in 1932 [45]. Infection of pregnant mares with EHV-1 can induce late-gestation abortion, stillbirth, and weak neonatal foals [33]. EHV-1 reaches the reproductive tract via cell-associated viraemia or by latent virus reactivation [19]. Mares can abort months or years after a primary infection that has led to latency [6]. Chorionic gonadotrophin (CG), which is one of the major hormones released by the placenta during early pregnancy (one to three months), is able to reactivate latent EHV-1 *in vitro*, and the endometrium has higher levels of CG than other tissues [46]. *In vivo*, the role of CG in latent EHV-1 reactivation during pregnancy is difficult to explain. CG is absent by 120 days of pregnancy, but abortions are rarely detected before 4 months gestation. EHV-1 infects endometrial endothelial cells inducing thrombosis and ischaemia in the microcotyledons of the placenta. These uterine pathologies lead to a premature separation of the placenta from the endometrium, with subsequent anoxic death of the foetus. EHV-1 can also be transferred to the foetus (Figure 4), inducing extensive multi-organ infection and a wide range of macroscopic and microscopic lesions. The mare's subsequent reproductive efficiency is not affected by abortion induced by EHV-1 infection [6]. When infection occurs during late gestation, the foetus may be born alive. However, the deterioration of the foal is rapid and almost all foals die. Infected foals show severe respiratory distress that amplifies the risk of viral pneumonia or secondary bacterial infection, which lead to respiratory failure within a few days [6, 19]. No treatment has been shown to prevent the fatal outcome of foetal infection with EHV-1[7].

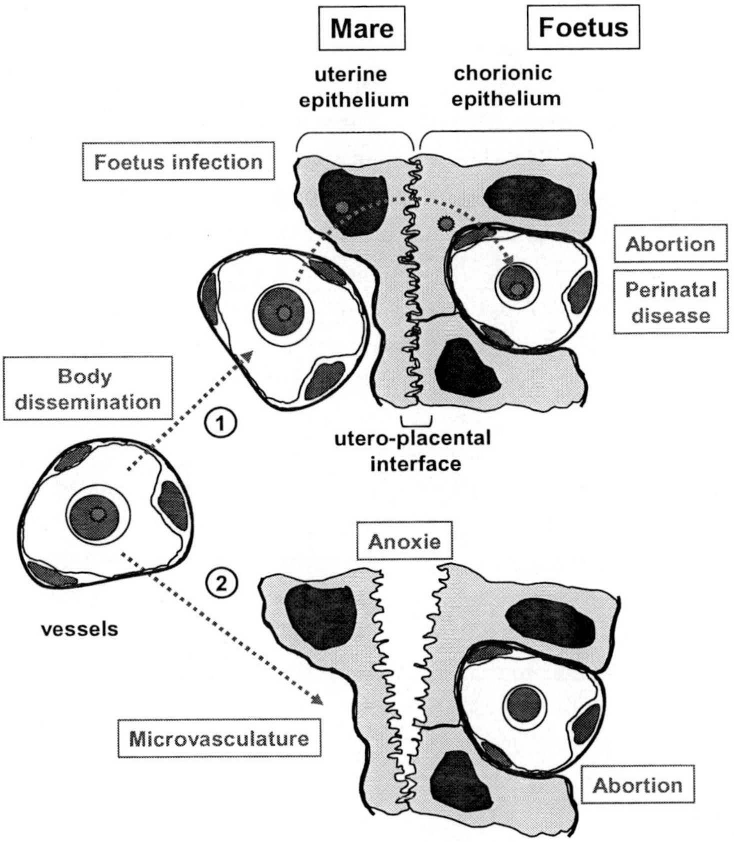

Figure 4. EHV-1 transmission from the infected pregnant mare to the foetus [13]. EHV-1-infected maternal lymphocytes reach the endometrial capillary during the cell-associated viraemia. EHV-1 spreads by cell-to-cell contact to the foetus through the endothelium of endometrial capillaries, the uterine epithelium, the chorionic epithelium and the endothelium of placental capillaries to finally infect foetal lymphocytes (1). EHV-1 can also infect endometrial endothelial cells inducing uterine pathologies leading to a premature placenta separation and foetus anoxy (2).

Neurological and Other Forms of the Disease

Neurological signs of disease, from a mild hind limb ataxia to quadraplegia, have been observed after EHV-1 infection (equine herpesvirus myeloencephalitis: EHM) [47].

Neurological signs are potential clinical sequels to EHV-1 respiratory tract infection and usually appear one week after infection [6]. The cell-associated viraemia brings EHV-1 to the vasculature of the central nervous system. Infection of endothelial cells can lead to vasculitis and thrombosis of small blood vessels in the brain or spinal cord. These lesions might be exacerbated by immunopathological mechanisms involving immune complex deposits, activation of the complement cascade, activation of polymorphonuclear leucocytes releasing cytotoxic agents, lysosomal enzymes and free radicals, and cell-mediated immunity [48]. From a pathologic point of view, EHV-1 myeloencephalitis is induced by a vascular compromise and a disease of endothelial cells (K. Smith, personal communication). The diagnosis of EHM is often difficult to achieve or questionable due to the absence of definite, objective or reliable markers of disease. The nature of the cerebro-spinal fluid (CSF) has been shown to change during EHM (aspect, content and cellularity). The development of new models to study the interaction between EHV-1 and the equine endothelial cells will be important to elucidate the biological mechanisms behind equine herpesvirus myeloencephalopathy (EHM). The development of a reliable animal model of EHM will also be essential. The use of a mouse model to understand EHM has not been successful so far.

A few cases of serious ocular disease have been reported in foals after infection with hypervirulent strains of EHV-1 [49]. Uveitis, and/or chorioretinitis have been observed and in some cases, extensive retinal destruction and blindness have been reported [50].

Latency

Infection of the respiratory epithelium and subsequent viral replication are followed by the development of a latent state of infection. Latency is a key element of EHV-1 biology as a survival strategy. Persisting within infected horses without clinical signs of diseases, virus shedding or cell-associated viraemia, EHV-1 can be shed and infect susceptible horses after reactivation. Reactivation of latent EHV-1 is likely to be one of the most important factors in precipitating outbreaks of neurological EHV-1. During latency, the expression of the EHV-1 genome is repressed and only a viral RNA transcribed from the IE gene, also named latent-associated transcript (LAT), is present.

The mechanisms that control latent EHV-1 infection and the precise function of RNA transcripts comprising EHV-1 LATs is not well understood. In HSV, LATs could promote latency but are not essential for the maintenance or reactivation of latent virus [51]. The alpha herpesvirus genome is in a transcriptionally repressed circular configuration associated with non-acetylated histone, which differs from the linear genome configuration after infection. In the case of HSV, latency can be explained by a defect in the initiation of IE gene activation by VP16 [51].

It has been proposed that reactivation of latent virus in trigeminal ganglion could lead to shedding of infectious EHV-1 into nasal secretions. Infectious virus can be reactivated by co-cultivation with susceptible cells [52]. The precise location of EHV-1 latency remains unclear [52-56]. Slater et al. [56] considered the latency in lymphoid cells and tissue to have little biological importance. Despite establishing latency in PBMC and lymph nodes, EHV-1 was not detected by co-cultivation of PBMC with susceptible cells during the reactivation of infection with immunosuppressive drugs (e.g. dexamethasone, cyclosporine A). Other studies report the presence of LAT mainly in lymphoid cells, with reactivation of EHV-1 by co-cultivation of PBMC with susceptible cells and only an occasional detection of LAT in the trigeminal ganglion [46, 54].

Recent studies by G. Allen (2006) detected latent infection in the submandibular lymph nodes of mares experimentally infected with EHV-1 as weanlings [57] and more recently in the Thoroughbred broodmare population in Kentucky [58]. The CD5+ CD8+ T lymphocytes have been defined as the predominant site of EHV-1 latency [46]. Reactivation of latent EHV-1 has been observed after treatment with corticosteroids or stressful events (e.g. castration, transport, weaning). Interleukin-2 (IL-2) has been shown to initiate the reactivation of EHV-1 in T lymphocytes by an indirect stimulation of possibly monocytes and the subsequent synthesis of secondary factors [46]. It is accepted that reactivation of HSV passes through the specific activation by cellular factors of ICP0 (infected cell polypeptide 0), which is an activator of gene expression. EHV-1 is likely to possess a similar mechanism of reactivation. It has been shown that a thymidine kinase negative (TK^-) EHV-1 mutant virus has impaired ability to reactivate following experimental infections, despite evidence that latency is established by these mutants [56]. Reactivation can be associated with all clinical signs of disease, including abortion, cell-associated viraemia and seroconversion. Between reactivation episodes, latently infected leukocytes are invisible to immune surveillance and elimination.

Diseases Induced by EHV-4

EHV-4 infects and replicates in the mucosal epithelial cells and induces primarily a mild disease of the upper respiratory tract (rhinopharyngitis and tracheobronchitis, also known as equine viral rhinopneumonitis). Clinical signs of disease are similar to those induced by EHV-1. EHV-4 rarely induces abortion when it infects pregnant mares. EHV-4 will establish latency after infection.

EHV-1 Strains and Origin of Clinical Signs Diversity

The nature and severity of disease induced by EHV-1 is likely to be dependent on numerous factors such as the age, the immune status and the health condition of the host. However, the pathogenic potential of the strain could also play a role in the development of different signs of disease (e.g. neurological signs and abortion). Thus, the existence of different strains or lineages of EHV-1 has been extensively investigated. EHV-1 strains were initially divided into different subgroups by the comparison of DNA fragment length after digestion of the genome with DNA restriction enzymes [59-61]. A study using 5 restriction enzymes conducted on isolates from 172 abortogenic and respiratory outbreaks in the US defined 16 strains of EHV-1 with significant differences in DNA fingerprint patterns. Two of these strains (EHV-1 P and EHV-1B, respectively), represented 90% of abortion-related isolates [59]. EHV-1 P has been identified as the main abortigenic strain in the US during the period 1960-1980. After 1981, abortion induced by EHV-1 involved principally the EHV-1 B strain [59]. Another study reported that all EHV-1 strains circulating in Japan were related to EHV-1 P until the recent isolation of EHV-1 B from a horse imported from Kentucky (USA). This study demonstrated that EHV-1 B could result from natural reassortant of EHV-1 P and EHV-4 progenitors and that EHV-1 isolates purified from horses with neurological disorders were type EHV-1 P only [62]. While such analysis may be used for tracing the genetic relatedness of strain, they allow identification only of those genetic changes resulting in restriction fragment variation, rather than the majority of changes that do not affect restriction cleavage sites.

A more recent study compared the sequence of two field isolates of EHV-1 that show consistent differences in pathogenicity: Ab4, a neuropathogenic EHV-1 strain [63], with V592, a non-neuropathogenic EHV-1 strain [64, 65]. Ab4 (EHV-1 P) infection results in severe clinical disease, including neurological signs and frequent abortion. Infection with V592 is largely restricted to a short-lived fever, moderate respiratory distress and a few cases of abortion. Comparison of the V592 sequence with that of Ab4 [14] showed a low sequence divergence of 0.1% with 50 regions of insertion or deletion of 1 or more nucleotides and 43 single nucleotide substitutions that resulted in amino acid coding changes. Notably, a single variable amino acid, causing a substitution of asparagine (N) by aspartic acid (D) at amino acid position 752 within the viral DNA polymerase (DNA pol), is significantly associated ($p<0.0001$) with outbreaks of neuropathogenic disease, when compared with outbreaks of abortion without neuropathogenic signs. More than 95% of non- neuropathogenic outbreaks are caused by virus strains encoding DNA pol N_{752}, and more than 86% of neuropathogenic outbreaks are caused by strains encoding D_{752} [66]. It is worthwhile noting that in neuropathogenic outbreaks that occurred in the UK in 2003-2004, were additional sampling was permitted, all infected and in-contact animals that were strain typed coded the neuropathogenic marker. By contrast, more recent research studies by G. Allen [67] and the Pusterla research group [68] have shown the co-circulation of both neuropathogenic and non-neuropathogenic marker in outbreaks associated with neuropathogenic disease in the USA. The DNA pol sequence variation (D/N_{752}) in ORF 30 has also been successfully applied to the development of diagnostic PCR tests to detect both active and latent infection in PBMC and tissue samples [57, 67]. Furthermore, the impact of this DNA pol sequence variation upon virus replication and pathogenicity has been determined [69]. A bacterial artificial chromosome (BAC) system [70] was used to produce two Ab4 EHV-1 recombinants that differed only at the DNA pol amino acid position 752 (D/N_{752}). *In vivo* studies in the natural host showed that the D752 virus showed increased levels of viraemia ($p=0.01$), which can be associated with greater virulence [57]. Three of the 12 animals in this group also showed clinical signs of ataxia whereas the N752 mutant virus caused no neuropathogenic signs in the natural host. Both viruses replicated with similar kinetics in fibroblasts and epithelial cells, but exhibited differences in leukocyte tropism with the non-neuropathogenic D752 viruses having a preference for CD4+ T lymphocytes. These cells play a role in the lytic and latent phase of infection and the inflammatory responses that result in EHV-1 disease. While field and experimental studies to date have demonstrated that this point mutation can influence neuropathogenic potential [66, 67, 69] there remains a lot of unanswered questions regarding the role this point mutation plays in the development of EHV-1 myeloencephalopathy and further research is required to glean a greater understanding of its role in EHV-1 pathogenesis.

Comparison of the V592 sequence with that of Ab4 also identified a polymorphic region of ORF68 that was found to be particularly useful for grouping isolates, since this locus displays several SNPs within a relatively short region (approx. 600bp). Phylogenetic analysis of ORF68 sequences from 104 field isolates (each from a different outbreak) identified 6 strain groups [66]. Analysis of the ORF68 strain distribution according to geographical origin of the isolates provided evidence for geographical restriction of certain strain groups. Seventeen of the 18 group 5 field isolates had been recovered from outbreaks in North America whereas the majority (36/42) of group 3 and 4 isolates had been recovered from outbreaks in Europe. Statistical analysis confirmed that there was a significant geographical clustering of the ORF68 groups, considering whether the isolates originated in North America or Europe (Fisher's exact test: $p<0.001$). Furthermore, fine-typing of these isolates have generated useful epidemiological data that strongly suggest that some oubreaks can be geographically linked over time and place ([66]; J. Nugent, unpublished data). For example, a large UK outbreak of EHV-1 respiratory disease in vaccinated Thoroughbreds in Suffolk (2004), which included some cases of ataxia, can be genetically linked via the detection of unique variant SNPs to two smaller outbreaks that included neurological cases in the same region with variant (J. Nugent, unpublished data). It has also been possible to link two outbreaks of neurological disease that occurred on different premises, linked by horse movement, in Yorkshire in 1999 and 2002. Isolates from these outbreaks typed strain group 2 and showed additional variant SNPs at ORF14: T_{1845}, ORF 29: A_{-11} and ORF34: C_{285} (J. Nugent, unpublished data). The epidemiological implications of these observations are far-reaching, supporting the long-held suspicion that horses recovering from an episode of EHV-1 neurological disease can present a subsequent risk, through re-activation of that isolate, to in-contact horses. Strain group 2 isolates were identified from an outbreak of neurological disease in hospitalized horses in Ohio (2003) and were suspected to have spread to three other premises via horse movement. Fine typing of the isolates from this outbreak showed an identical set of variant SNPs at ORF14: T_{1845}, ORF 29: A_{-11} and ORF34: C_{285} (J. Nugent and G. Allen, unpublished data). These data strongly suggest that the Ohio outbreaks were caused by the same strain of EHV-1 and furthermore, suggest a genetic linkage to paralytic outbreaks that occurred on premises in the UK in 1999 and 2002.

It has been hypothesised that neurological and non-neurological strains of EHV-1 may have different cell tropism influencing the type of disease developed after the initial infection. No correlation between the sensitivity of nervous endothelial cells to infection and the nature of EHV-1 (neurological and non-neurological strains) was reported after *in vitro* investigation [71].

Equine Gammaherpesviruses: EHV-2 and EHV-5

EHV-2 and EHV-5 are closely related gammaherpesviruses that are highly prevelant among equids. Isolation of EHV-2 was first documented in 1963 [72], when it was first classified as a betaherpesvirus by virtue of its slowly cytopathic and highly cell-associated biology. The existence of EHV-5 as a distinct species from EHV-2 was first proposed in 1987 on the basis of unique restriction enzyme profiles of several slow-growing equine herpesvirus isolates assumed to be EHV-2 [73], and later supported by the physical mapping of the EHV-5 genome, which revealed a genome structure quite different to EHV-2 [74]. Sequencing of random fragments of the genomes of EHV-2 and EHV-5 and analysis of the deduced amino acid sequence, demonstrated that EHV-2 and -5 were members of the gammaherpesvirus *Rhadinovirus* genus, and not members of the *Betaherpesvirinae* as previously held [75]. However, EHV-2 and EHV-5 appear to represent a distinct phylogenetic group within the *Rhadinovirus* genus, and it has since been reported that the International Committee on Taxonomy of Viruses (ICTV) plan to revise taxonomic arrangements so that the genus *Rhadinovirus* will become more tightly demarcated and the lineage containing *Equid herpesvirus-2* (EHV-2), *Equid herpesvirus-5* (EHV-5) and certain other perissodactyl and carnivore herpesviruses will form the genus *Percavirus*.

The entire genome sequence of one EHV-2 isolate (strain 86/67) was published in 1995 [76], but the genome sequence of closely related EHV-5 has yet to be determined. The 184 427bp EHV-2 genome (Genbank U20824) was found to contain 79 ORFs encoding 77 distinct proteins. Unusually for a herpesivirus, about a third of the sequence distributed in several large blocks appears not to encode proteins [76]. Several EHV-2 ORFs show striking homology to cellular genes. These include a homologue to the immunosuppressive cytokine, IL-10, encoded by ORF E7, and 3 homologues to seven-transmembrane receptors (7TMR) which are involved in signal transduction, encoded by ORFs E1, E6 and ORF74.

Prior to the development of specific PCR assays, EHV-5 was not readily distinguished from EHV-2, and so the results of many studies reported for EHV-2, may in fact apply to EHV-5 or both viruses. Even now, the validity of specific PCR developed to differentiate between EHV-2 and EHV-5 isolates, may be compromised by the large amount of strain variation that has been observed between isolates. Strain variation is a notable feature of EHV-2, and although sequence data for EHV-5 is limited, variation in EHV-5 glycoprotein B sequence has been observed [77]. Considerable biological, antigenic and genomic variability has been observed among EHV-2 field isolates [73, 77-79], with the very high level of heterogeneity observed in DNA fingerprints exceeding that recognised for other herpesviruses [73]. Such variability may reflect variations in strain pathogenicity, but although differences have been observed in tissue culture regarding growth rates and virus plaque sizes [79-81], correlations with different biological properties have not been ascertained. It is however clear that such heterogeneity leaves horses susceptible to multiple concurrent infections with genomically and antigenically distinct EHV-2 strains.

Recombination is thought to be an important source of genetic variation in herpesviruses, allowing the combination of genetic features shared by different strains. It has been demonstrated *in vitro* and/or *in vivo* between distinguishable strains of several alphaherpesviruses (collectively reviewed in [82]), has resulted in naturally occurring interspecies recombinants between EHV-1 and -4 [62] and has been noted as a major contributor to genetic diversity for clinical isolates of human herpesviruses [83-87]. It is likely that recombination between co-infecting EHV-2 isolate strains serves to broaden the scope of equine gammaherpesvirus heterogeneity, potentially with pathogenic implications.

Disease

The full extent of EHV-2 pathogenicity has yet to be determined. Studying EHV-2 pathogenicity is complicated by the fact the infection is ubiquitous among equine stock, and the virus can be isolated from clinically healthy horses. In addition, the disease process with which the virus is involved may vary a great deal between virus isolates. Since EHV-2 was first isolated [72] it has been associated with immunosuppression, inappetance, enlarged lymph nodes, general malaise and poor performance. Proposed to act as a predisposing factor for both viral and bacterial secondary infections, possibly through the impairment of local immune function, EHV-2 has also been associated with upper and lower respiratory tract disease, pneumonia and conjunctivitis [88-91], and has been suggested to act as a trans-activating factor to trigger EHV-1 and EHV-4 reactivation from latency [92, 93]. Foals are born without EHV-2 infection, but infection occurs soon after birth, often in the presence of maternal antibodies. Indeed where EHV-2 is endemic, virtually all foals can be expected to be infected by 3 months of age [90].

As for EHV-2, the pathogenic significance of EHV-5 is uncertain, however. There are relatively few descriptions of the isolation of EHV-5 [94-101], As for EHV-2, the pathogenic significance of EHV-5 is uncertain. EHV-5 was initially isolated from horses who had upper respiratory tract disease. It has recently been implicated in the pathogeneisis of multinodular equine pulmonary fibrosis [102].

About Other Equine Herpes Viruses

Asinine Herpes Virus (AsHV-1 to -6)

Asinine herpesvirus type 1 is the homologue of EHV-3 and they share some antigenic determinant [103]. Asinine herpesvirus type 2 (AsHV-2) was isolated from the blood of a healthy donkey and is a gamma herpesvirus [104]. Asinine herpesvirus type 3 (AsHV-3) is an alpha herpes virus that was isolated from healthy donkeys after steroid treatment and was genetically similar to EHV-1.

Asinine herpesvirus type 4, 5 and 6 were recently isolated from donkey's lung tissues and associated with fatal respiratory disease characterised by interstitial pneumonia lesions and syncytial cell formation. AsHV-4 and AsHV-5 are gamma herpes viruses most closely related to zebra herpesvirus (ZHV) and wildass herpesvirus (WAHV), respectively [4, 5]. ZHV and WAHV have not been associated with disease in their respective species of origins [105].

Equine Herpes Virus type 9 or Gazelle Herpes Virus

Equine herpes virus type 9 (EHV-9) is a neuropathogenic virus isolated from captive Thomson's gazelles (*Gazella Thomsoni*) in Japan and found to be pathogenic in horses [8]. EHV-9 infection in horses induced encephalitis and pneumonia, shedding of virus in nasal secretion and cell-associated viraemia. A recent serological survey in the Serenget National Park (Tanzania) revealed a high level of exposure of Burchell's zebras (*Equus burchelli*) to EHV-9 (60%). It was suggested that Burchell's zebras could be the natural host reservoir for EHV-9 [106]. EHV-9 has been shown to infect and induce a severe neurological disease in several mammals species such as Syrian hamsters[107], pigs [108], goats [109], cats [110], dogs [111] and marmosets [112].

Epidemiology of EHV

The lifecycles of the equid herpesviruses share four main features (i) early and widespread infection of young horses; (ii) widespread carrier of the virus in its latent state in the adult horse (iii) transmission from latently infected adults to new equine populations and (iv) widespread 'silent' / sub clinical infection from adult to adult, adult to foal and foal to foal [15].

Epidemiology of EHV-1/4

EHV-1 is ubiquitous in domestic and wild equid populations throughout the world, including zebras (*Equus grevyi* and *Equus burchelli*) and onager (*Equus hemionus onager*) [9-11]. It is estimated that 80 to 90% of horses have been exposed to EHV-1, or its closely relative EHV-4, by two years of age [12]. However, the exact annual incidence of either EHV-1 or EHV-4 infections is not defined. The seroprevalence of EHV-1 in the broodmare and racehorse population (in Australia) has been reported as approximately 30% (using a type specific ELISA to detect EHV-1 antibodies)[113]. The epidemiology of EHV-1 and EHV-4 is complicated by the fact that both EHV-1 and EHV-4 can establish lifelong latency within host tissues. The virus can be reactivated at any time during the life of the host resulting in viral shedding, with or without clinical signs of disease. Latent EHV-1 has been detected in 54% of central Kentucky brood mares evaluated at post mortem [58]. A study in the UK identified latent infection with EHV in greater than 60% of horses examined at an abattoir, however differentiation between EHV-1 and 4 was not performed in all cases [114]. A study in France identified that there was no difference in the prevalence of latent infection in vaccinated horses versus unvaccinated horses [115].

As previously described, EHV-1 can cause abortion (sporadic abortion and abortion storms), respiratory disease and neurological disease in horses. Respiratory disease associated with EHV-1 is most commonly seen in young animals, most frequently at weaning. This disease is generally self-limiting however affected animals are likely to develop life-long latency following infection. Clinical signs of disease at this time may be associated with new infection or recrudescence of latent infection. Virus is spread in respiratory secretions and can be transmitted between animals by direct and indirect contact [116]. Environmental contamination can result in indirect virus transmission, however the environment is not a particularly important maintenance reservoir of EHV-1 as the virus survives less than 35 days outside the horse, even in ideal conditions. Latently infected horses are the most significant reservoir of infection.

The incidence of abortion associated with EHV-1 infection has been well documented in central Kentucky. The highest incidence was reported as 17.3/1000 pregnant mares in 1963, but that had decreased to <2/1000 in 2002 (Dr. D. Powell, Gluck Equine Research Centre). It is likely that the widespread use of vaccination has contributed significantly to this decreased incidence. EHV-1 does remain an important cause of abortion despite its decreased incidence.

Extensive work was carried out on Australian stud farms to determine the transmission cycle of EHV-1 between mares and foals. This work showed that foals become infected with EHV-1 as young as 30 days old [117]. More recent work has identified EHV-1 shedding in foals as young as 22 days old [118]. Evidence suggests that infected brood mares act as a source of infection for foals through direct contact and that horizontal transmission between foals then occurs both before and after weaning. It is likely that brood mares undergo recrudescence of latent viral infection during pregnancy/parturition resulting in nasal shedding of virus and infection of foals. In one study of foals born to unvaccinated mares, 24% of foals had EHV-1 antibodies attributable to maternally derived antibodies. Of the remaining at-risk foals, 66.7% demonstrated seroconversion to EHV-1 prior to weaning [117]. Further work also identified new cases of EHV-1 in weaned foals, suggesting that ongoing horizontal transmission amongst foals occurs post weaning [119]. Despite the high rates of seroprevalence of EHV-1 among foals, no EHV associated abortions were identified on the farms in question during the study period. suggesting that the cycle of EHV-1 between mares and foals and subsequently between foals and between weanlings is a 'silent' cycle in many cases [120]. Thus the control of EHV-1 infection in very young foals is a key factor to manage the disease [117, 120]. When foals are infected early in life and establish latency, they may become sources of infection for their own offspring later in life.

EHV-1 associated abortion continues to be a threat to the equine industry despite rigorous vaccination protocols on many farms. The development of more accurate and sensitive diagnostic tools has aided in the identification of EHV associated abortion allowing better management of such cases. Diagnostic techniques such as PCR and immunohistochemistry have allowed the identification of cases of foetus-negative, placenta-positive EHV associated abortion. The abortion in such cases is likely due to placental compromise and subsequent foetal anoxia. It is believed that such abortions may be less of an infectious threat than foetus positive cases however all cases of herpes associated abortion should be treated as potentially highly contagious and appropriate precautions should be taken. In addition, during the course of a prospective cohort study, a placenta tested positive for EHV-1 in a case where a live, healthy foal was born that had no detectable EHV-1 antibodies [121]. This is the first case where EHV-1 has been identified in a placenta that did not result in abortion.

The incidence of neurological disease induced by EHV-1 appears to be increasing [57] and outbreaks have been described in Europe, North America and Australia. Not all animals exposed to, and infected with, neuropathogenic strains of EHV-1 will develop clinical signs of neurological disease. In four outbreaks in the USA for which records were kept, the neurologic attack rate ranged from 22%-50% (mean (33%) and the case fatality rate ranged from 20% - 50% (mean 40%) [66]. In addition, it should be remembered that the non-neuropathogenic strain of EHV-1 can cause neurologic disease, however it appears that the neurological attack rate in such cases is much lower [122].

Evaluation of the risk factors associated with the development of neurological disease have been performed in studies in Europe and in North America. A study in the Netherlands revealed a strong association between season and outbreaks of EHV neurological disease with all outbreaks occurring between mid-November and mid-May. This season specificity has not been mirrored in all countries but is an interesting phenomenon. Other identified risk factors included breed, sex, age and fever [123]. Neurological signs were seen at an increased frequency in Standardbreds, hispanic breeds and draught breeds. Interestingly, no cases of EHV-induced myeloencephalopathy were seen in archetypical ponies, Haflinger, Fjord and Icelandic horses. In addition, older horses, female horses and horses with fever were more at risk of developing severe neurological disease. Neurological signs were not seen in any horses less than 3 years old and the odds for severe neurological disease increased with age [123]. Retrospective analysis of a US outbreak also revealed a significant association between age and the development of neurological disease [124]. Neurological disease developed more frequently in horses older than 5 years and severe neurological deficits (i.e. grade 3 or above) were only observed in horses greater than 5 years old. There was no difference in EHV-1 morbidity in horses of different ages. Development of neurological disease and severity of neurological disease were negatively associated with survival. In the US study, horses that developed a temperature greater to or equal to 39.7°C were more likely to die although duration of fever was not associated with survival or development of neurological disease. The majority (96%) of horses in this outbreak were vaccinated against EHV. There appeared to be an association with vaccination 3 or 4 times in the year preceding neurological disease and development of neurological disease, however this must be interpreted with caution as older animals tended to have been vaccinated more frequently. During this outbreak, EHV-1 morbidity was 88% and 34% of horses developed neurological disease. Neurologic case fatality rate was 30% (overall mortality was 12%).

Much remains unknown about the epidemiology of neuropathogenic EHV and the factors that result in disease in some horses and not in others. Work is ongoing in this area to determine the best ways to prevent and control disease. At present no vaccinations are available that effectively decrease the risk of disease and there is some concern that vaccination in the face of exposure to the neuropathogenic strain of EHV-1 may exacerbate clinical signs.

Epidemiology of EHV-2

The prevalence of EHV-2 in equine populations has been assessed by serological surveys, by examining horses for the presence of EHV-2 DNA and by virus isolation. EHV-2 can be isolated from many sites including nasal swabs, leukocytes, conjunctiva, mammary glands, salivary glands, vagina, kidney, spleen and bone marrow, and EHV-2 DNA has been detected in both the peripheral and central nervous systems of ponies [125]. EHV-2 is highly prevalent in horse populations and previous serological surveys have suggested that approximately 100% of older horses carry antibodies to EHV-2 ([125] and references therein). EHV-2 establishes latency in B-lymphocytes, which themselves are not permissive for virus replication, but pass the virus or virus genome via direct cell to cell contact mechanisms to fully permissible epithelial cells [126]. The intermittent shedding of the virus from the nasal cavity of latently infected host animals is assumed to be associated with the natural spread of the virus.

Immunity, Immune Evasion and Vaccination

Herpesviruses are persistent virus. The acute disease resolves after a few weeks, but EHV establishes a persistent infection characterised by latency with chronic reactivations. Infection of primed animals with EHV-1 induced a fully protective immunity against re-infection lasting 4 to 8 months [127], although some reports demonstrate shorter periods of immunity lasting <3 months. The majority of infectious agents enter into the host via mucosal epithelium. The equine lung surface has been estimated to total around 2000 m^2 compared to around 400 m^2 in humans. Prevention of infection is likely to be facilitated by a strong mucosal immune response able to counteract the pathogen before its absorption into cells and tissue. This section will summarised conventional immune response to respiratory viruses, as presented in Figure 5, specific immunity to EHV-1 and mechanisms of immune evasion used by EHV.

EHV-1 Immunity

Immune Changes in the Respiratory Tract and Innate Immunity

In normal lungs, macrophages and lymphocytes predominate. A few days after infection with EHV-1, a transient modification of the percentage of neutrophils (increase), Mϕ and lymphocytes (decreases) has been observed [128]. These fluctuations of pulmonary cell populations were explained by a lysis of leucocytes and the recruitment of neutrophils subsequent to the tissue inflammation induced by the infection. During the 3 weeks after EHV-1 infection, bronchoalveolar CD8+ T lymphocytes increase significantly and could show a cytotoxic activity toward EHV-1 infected cells. Equine type 1 interferon (IFNα/β) has also been detected in nasal secretions and serum during the first and second week after experimental infection of ponies with EHV-1 [129]. IFNα/β shows a variety of immunomodulatory activities affecting both innate (e.g. enhancement of natural killer (NK) activity) and adaptive immunity (e.g. promotion of Th1 response). The secretion of such IFN was closely correlated with the duration of EHV-1 shedding and could be considered as a consequence of EHV-1 replication and epithelium damage [129].

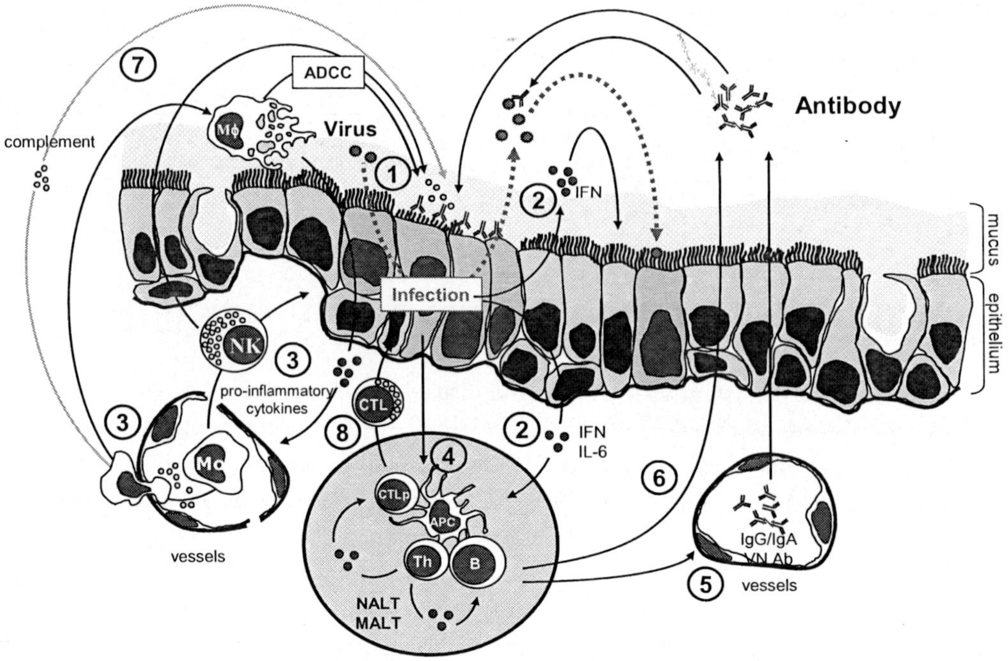

Figure 5. Immune response to respiratory virus infection [13]. Epithelial cells become infected (1) inducing the local synthesis of IFN and IL-6 that present a wide range of antiviral activities, inducing up-regulation of MHC class I molecules and antiviral resistance in uninfected cells (2). Alveolar Mϕ and neutrophils respond to the infection by releasing pro-inflammatory cytokines, leading to the containment of the infection, rise of body temperature and to the recruitment of further phagocytic and natural killer (NK) cells (3). NK cells are activated by IFNα and IL-12 synthesised by Mϕ, and are cytotoxic for virus-infected cells. Their activity is not major histocompatibility complex (MHC) restricted. NK cells synthesise IFNγ that drives the development of the adaptive immune response. The presentation of viral antigen (4) in lymphoid tissues induces the synthesis of serum (5) or mucosal antibodies (6) able to neutralise excreted virus and to stimulate antibody dependent cell cytotoxicity (ADCC; 7). Virus-specific CTL that lyse infected cells are also stimulated (8).

Adaptive Immune Response

Adaptive immune responses to EHV-1 are likely to be initiated in NALT (nasal associated lymphoid tissue) and MALT (mucosal associated lymphoid tissue). Studies have reported the presence of EHV-1 and viral antigens in the retropharyngeal and bronchial lymph nodes as early as 12h after infection with EHV-1 [34].

Humoral immune response: Natural immunity to EHV-1 is short-lived. Complement fixing (CF) and virus neutralising (VN) antibodies appear within 2 weeks after infection with EHV-1 [130] and IgGa, IgGb, IgGc, IgG(T) and IgM antibody serotypes can be detected [131]. However, CF antibodies are short lived and do not last over 3 months, whereas VN antibodies are more durable (>1 year). The local mucosal humoral response is composed predominantly by virus-specific IgA with virus neutralising activity. IgGa/b antibodies can be detected in the lumen during the acute phase of infection, but this could be the consequence of serum antibody diffusion induced by inflammation. The mucosal humoral immune response is believed to reduce virus shedding induced by subsequent infection with EHV-1 a few weeks after the initial infection [132]. As EHV-1 infects sub-epithelial cells, leucocytes, and is spread in the organism via the blood and lymphatic vessels, it is likely that EHV-1 specific immune responses also take place in the draining lymph nodes of the respiratory tract. The role of circulating antibodies is controversial. Some studies have reported that serum VN antibody does not correlate with either protection from infection or the level of virus shedding in nasal secretion [38]. Others have shown that the presence of VN antibody prior to EHV-1 infection reduces the amount and duration of nasopharyngeal virus shedding [130, 133]. These antibodies do not have any effect when EHV-1 is intracellular (i.e. during cell-associated viraemia).

IFNγ response: Virus-specific cell-mediated responses are crucial components of immunity to herpesviruses. IFNγ synthesis is one of the most widely used markers of cell-mediated immunity (CMI) to measure responses to herpesviruses in humans and it has now been applied to horses [134-136]. IFNγ promotes CMI by increasing viral peptides presentation by APC and promoting the development of T helper 1 (Th1) lymphocytes. IFNγ is a key factor in the development of a type-1 response involving cytotoxic T lymphocytes (CTL), which ultimately leads to the destruction of virus-infected cells (Figure 6).

The percentage of IFNγ synthesising cells that respond *in vitro* to EHV-1 stimulation is negligible or undetectable in foals or yearlings but this increases with age [134, 137]. This suggests that EHV-1-specific memory cells are likely to be re-stimulated throughout a horse's lifetime by reactivation of latent EHV-1, further infection or vaccination. This boosting of the immune response may explain why older ponies (28-years old), which were likely to have had numerous contacts with EHV-1 antigens throughout their lives, demonstrate the highest percentage of EHV-1 specific IFNγ+ cells [137]. A similar progression of increased frequencies of CTL precursors specific for EHV-1 induced by repeated exposures to EHV-1 has been described previously [138]. In humans, herpesvirus-specific immunity builds up with age and could be detrimental to the development of immune responses against pathogens by reducing the T-cell repertoire [139, 140]. The impact of high levels of EHV-1-specific PBL on the sensitivity of the horse to other pathogens is not known in old ponies but merits further investigation as infections with EHV-1 and the closely related EHV-4 are endemic in horses [9].

The kinetics of IFNγ synthesis has been investigated after experimental infection with EHV-1 in ponies of different ages [134, 135, 137]. The percentage of EHV-1 specific IFNγ+ cells increases during the second week after infection with EHV-1 and returns to a low level 3-4 weeks after infection. When measured several weeks after experimental infection, the percentage of EHV-1-specific IFNγ+ cells presents secondary peaks [134, 137]. This supports the hypothesis of frequent antigen stimulation. A similar virus-specific T cell response has been described in persistent herpesvirus infection in humans [141]. The importance of IFNγ for protection against experimental infection with EHV-1 has been recently illustrated in ponies. Protective immunity against EHV-1 was characterised in immune and protected ponies by stimulation of a polarised IFNγ mRNA expression response post challenge infection. In contrast, naive and EHV-1-sensitive ponies developed a bi-polar IFNγ and IL-4 mRNA expression response after experimental infection with EHV-1 [142].

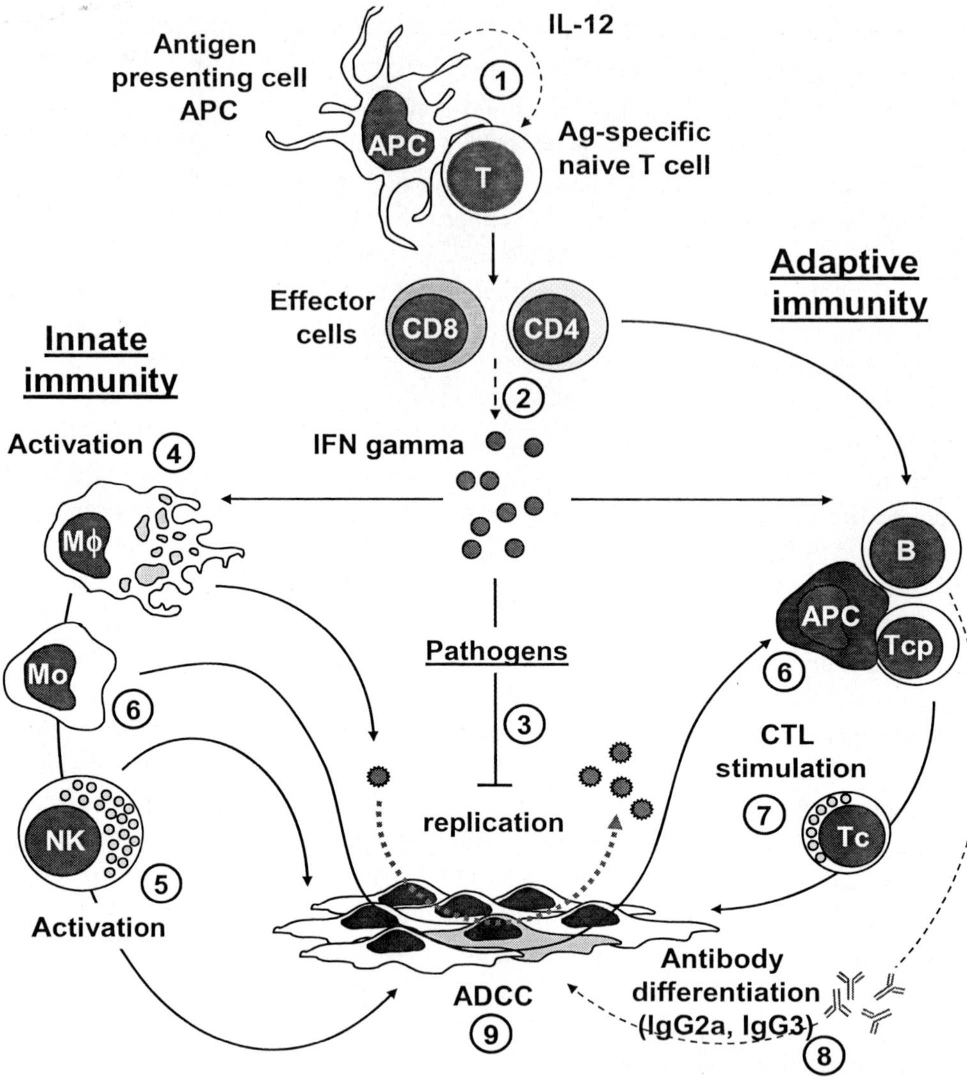

Figure 6. The effect of IFNγ on immune response and pathogens [13]. The presentation of an antigen to a naive antigen-specific T lymphocyte (1) may induce its derivation to a type 1 effector cell synthesising IFNγ (2). IFNγ can directly block pathogen replication (3), activate macrophages (Mϕ) for the pathogen elimination (4), and activate NK cells to lyse infected cells (5). IFNγ can up-regulate the expression of major histocompatibility complex (MHC) molecules on the monocyte (Mo) and Mϕ surface (6), increasing the efficiency of antigen presentation to cells of the adaptive immune response (6). IFNγ is a strong immunomodulator of the adaptive immune response leading to the activation of CTL (7) or driving the antibody isotype (8) to favour antibody-dependent cell mediated cytotoxicity (ADCC) (9).

The phenotype of IFNγ+ cells has been shown to be primarily CD5+CD8+ in ponies during the acute and convalescent phases after experimental infection. Increased percentages of CD8α+IFNγ+ cells were associated with elevated EHV-1-specific CTL activity [134, 135]. EHV-1-specific IFNγ synthesis by CD4+ T lymphocytes has also been described [136]. In 'healthy' adult ponies with no recent experimental infection, the majority of EHV-1 specific IFNγ+ cells were CD5+ and CD8-. These are likely to be CD4+ T cells, as a proportion of IFNγ synthesis was inhibited by chloroquine that inhibits cellular lysosomal function and subsequently blocks exogenous antigen processing and presentation by MHC class II molecules. In humans, CD4+ memory T cells specific for herpesviruses (i.e. varicella-zoster virus, herpes simplex virus and CMV) were efficiently detected by *ex vivo* virus stimulation, and IFNγ was identified as the main cytokine secreted by these cells [143, 144]. The reason behind a preferential CD5+CD8- population in adult ponies has not been determined. While the phenotype of PBMC responding to EHV-1 by synthesising IFNγ was mainly CD8+ in blood immediately after experimental infection, this appeared to evolve toward a CD8- type with time, as measured in 'healthy' adult horses with no recent exposure to EHV-1. This observation tends to indicate a potential maturation or evolution of the EHV-1 specific IFNγ response through repeated exposure to live virus or reactivation of latent virus. In conclusion, EHV-1 stimulates a complex IFNγ response, particularly in terms of memory responses, which requires further study.

CTL response: The rapid infection of epithelial cells and its dissemination by cell-to-cell contact allow EHV-1 to avoid the neutralising effect of circulating VN antibodies. Results suggest that neither antibody dependent cell cytotoxicity (ADCC) nor natural killer (NK) cytotoxicity have an impact on EHV-1 infection [145, 146]. In ponies infected experimentally with EHV-1, the percentage of lymphoblasts has been shown to increase in the peripheral blood during cell-associated viraemia [147] and populations of CD8+ T lymphocytes also increase in the blood and lungs after infection [128]. EHV-1-specific cytotoxicity has also been recently demonstrated in the upper respiratory tract and associated lymphoid tissues during the acute phase after EHV-1 infection [148]. EHV-1 specific cytotoxic activity has been associated with MHC class I restricted CD8+ T lymphocyte effectors, activated from precursor or memory cells [138, 149]. In adult ponies, the frequency of EHV-1 specific CTL depends principally on infection history, but increases after experimental infection with EHV-1 [149]. However, the degree of disease induced by infection depends on this frequency. Young ponies with a low level of circulating EHV-1 specific CTL develop clinical signs of disease, virus shedding and cell-associated viraemia after infection with EHV-1. In contrast, older ponies that have had several previous infections and have higher frequencies of EHV-1 specific CTL, show reduced or no signs of disease, virus shedding or cell-associated viraemia after experimental infection with EHV-1 [138]. In pregnant mares, a positive correlation between the frequency of EHV-1 CTL and the protection against the disease, including abortion, induced by experimental infection with EHV-1 has also been reported [150]. EHV-1 specific CTL can be detected 1 week after infection with EHV-1, with a maximum level reached by the second or third week, and remain detectable for a year after infection [149]. These results indicate that CTL activity is efficient in controlling the virus during its intracellular life and subsequently, to restrain cell-associated viraemia, which is a key element of the disease. Therefore, virus-specific CTL activity and frequency have been shown to correlate with the efficiency of cellular immunity against EHV-1.

Two very important points in the development of CMI specific for EHV-1 are the target proteins of EHV-1 and the genetic diversity of the equine MHC. Products of the single EHV-1 IE gene (ORF 64) have already been identified as CTL targets [151, 152]. Dendritic cells (DC) transfected with ORF 64 can induce a CTL response from cells purified from EHV-1 primed ponies that express the MHC class I A3 serological haplotype [152]. This haplotype is common in the Thoroughbred population [153], which is the primary market for commercial vaccines. However, the presentation of IE products by others haplotypes (e.g. A2, A5 and A9) is unknown. Approximately 18 haplotypes of equine MHC class I have been identified by serological typing [154]. Fifteen MHC class I genes and pseudogenes have been sequenced from the A3 haplotype (e.g. the B2 gene) and seven are transcribed [155, 156]. Presentation of IE by the MHC class I gene B2 has been recently demonstrated [157]. The identification of immunodominant EHV-1 peptides broadly recognised and presented by a broad range of equine MHC class I molecules is crucial for vaccine development [157].

Evasion and Transparency to Immunity Displayed by EHV-1

In the early phase of infection, a virus-specific adaptive immune response is not always available to oppose the pathogen. In such conditions, the immediate protection of the host against infectious agents is based on the innate immunity. As a result, the outcome of infection depends primarily on virus ability to avoid the mechanisms of the 'non-specific' immune response. The alternative complement pathway (antibody independent) is one of the primary lines of defence against infectious agents characterised by the binding of the complement protein C3b to the pathogen envelope or the infected cell membrane. This helps phagocytosis by Mϕ or leads to the complement pathway activation and the subsequent generation of a membrane-attack complex. Glycoprotein C of EHV-1 has been shown to bind the C3b component of complement [158]. Thus, gC prevents the complement proteins C5 and properdin from interacting with C3b and activating the alternative complement pathway. This ability to evade complement pathway activation could be one factor of herpesvirus pathogenicity. It has been reported that gC antibodies can reduce HSV-1 virulence and prevent disease by abolishing the fixation of C3b by gC [159-161]. The humoral response stimulated by immunisation with a vaccinia vector encoding the EHV-1 gC/gp13 gene has been shown to confer protection in rodents experimentally infected with EHV-1. This activity is associated with the presence of virus-specific VN antibodies but the restoration of the alternative complement pathway may also be involved [162, 163].

Glycoprotein G of EHV-1 has been identified as a chemokine binding protein (vCKBP). Chemokines are chemotactic cytokines that guide cells from both innate and adaptive immunity. Chemokines are produced at sites of infection and form chemotactic gradient by interacting wit glycosamnoglycans molecules at the surface of endotheliales cells. Glycoprotein G binds a broad range of chemokines (e.g. XCL1/lymphotactin; CXCL1/growth-related oncogene-α; CXCL8/IL-8) with high affinity when secreted or expressed on the infected cell surface, and blocks chemokine activity by preventing their interaction with specific receptors [164]. Interleukin-8 dependent chemotaxism of equine neutrophils has been shown to be inhibited by EHV-1-infected cell culture supernatant or increasing concentration of recombinant EHV-1 gG molecules [165]. Recently, gG has been shown to inhibit CCL3-mediated chemotaxis *in vivo* in mice experimentally infected with EHV-1, leading to an increased virus load in lungs of infected animals [166].

EHV-1, as with other herpesviruses, uses several mechanisms to escape the 'specific' immune response. This is clearly illustrated by the development of EHV-1 cell-associated viraemia despite the presence of high levels of systemic EHV-1 specific antibodies or CTL precursor (CTLp). This indicates that the recognition of EHV-1 infected PBMC by the immune system is incomplete. EHV-1 avoids the VN antibody response by becoming intracellular a few hours after infection of epithelial cells and by disseminating via cell-to-cell contact. HSV-1 glycoproteins gE and gI (homologous glycoproteins are expressed by EHV-1) form a complex that functions as an IgG Fc receptor, blocking IgG Fc-mediated function such as complement activation (classical pathway) or ADCC [161]. It has also been reported that EHV-1 infected PBMC do not present EHV-1 glycoproteins on their surface, after *in vitro* infection [167] or during cell-associated viraemia induced by experimental infection of ponies [168]. This absence of surface glycoproteins has been shown to protect infected cells from complement-mediated lysis [167]. However, expression of EHV-1 antigens has been detected on the surface of PBMC in another study during the acute phase of viraemia, therefore this method of immune evasion by EHV-1 remains controversial [40]. EHV-1 infection *in vitro* also results in the loss of MHC class I expression on infected cells, both through the inhibition of the peptide transport activity of TAP (transporter associated with antigen processing) and enhanced endocytosis of MHC class I molecules [169, 170] (Figure 7).

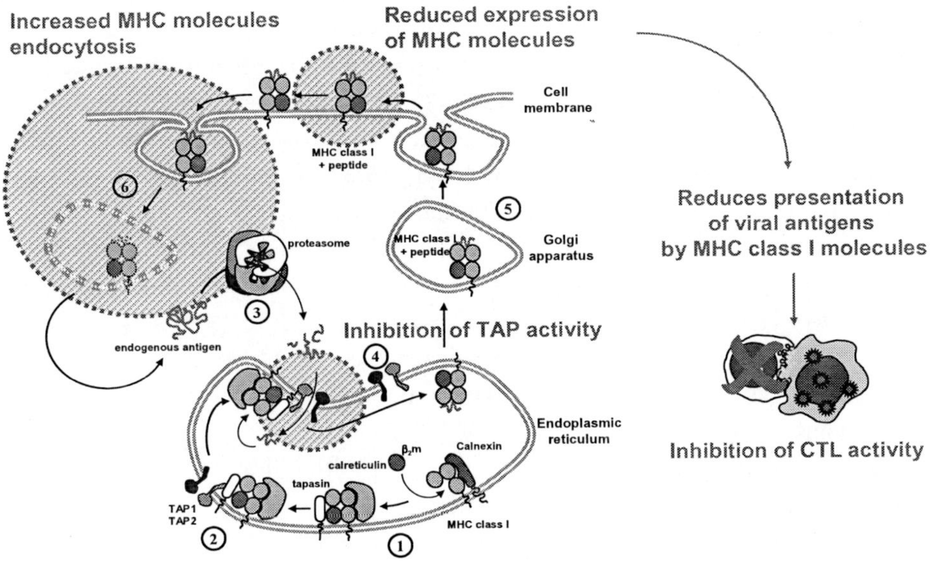

Figure 7. Disregulation of MHC class I pathway by EHV-1. Newly synthesised MHC class I molecules are bound to the calnexin in the endoplasmic reticulum. Binding of MHC class I molecules to β2 microglobulin (β2m) displaces calnexin and allows binding of chaperone proteins (calreticulin and tapasin)(1). The MHC class I-β2m complex binds TAP complex (TAP1-TAP2)(2). Cytosolic proteins are degraded by proteasomes into short peptides that are transported into the endoplasmic reticulum through the TAP complex (3). The peptide binding the antigenic groove of the MHC class I-β2m complex stabilises the structure and induces the release of the TAP complex (4). The complex MHC class I-β2m-peptide is transported to the cell surface via the golgi apparatus (5) and is later internalised and recycled (6). EHV-1 has been shown to reduce expression of the complex MHC class I-β2m peptide on the surface of infected cells, by increasing the turn-over of MHC class I molecules and by targeting the TAP complex.

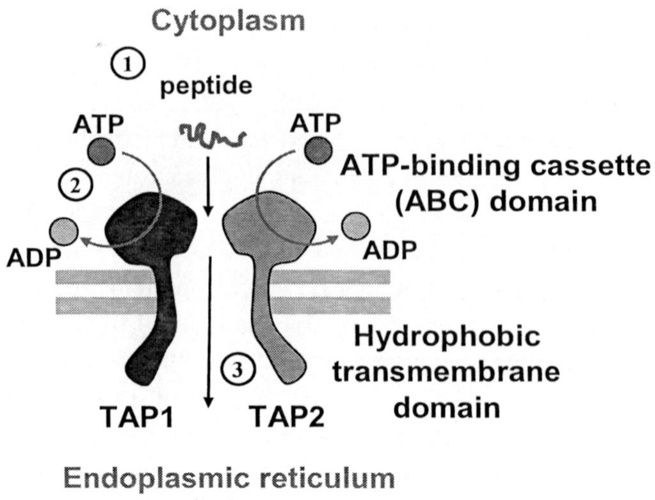

Figure 8. Translocation of peptides through TAP molecules. Peptide binding (1) stimulates ATP binding and hydrolysis (2) that energises peptide translocation (3).

It has been recently demonstrated that the UL49.5 protein (ORF10/gN) of EHV-1/4 inhibited the recruitment of ATP by TAP molecules. Peptide binding by TAP molecules stimulates ATP binding and hydrolysis, which presumably energises peptide translocation (Figure 8). UL49.5 potentially arrests TAP in a translocation incompetent state [171]. The maximum level of MHC class I down-regulation has been measured by 24 hrs post infection. However, after *in vivo* infection with EHV-1 and during cell-associated viraemia, MHC class I expression on the surface of EHV-1 infected PBMC is equivalent to the expression measured in PBMC purified from uninfected ponies [168].

Another aspect of immune evasion activity of herpesviruses is their ability to inhibit T cell responses. The immunosuppression of T cell activity has been reported after EHV-1 infection *in vivo* [172]. The serum from a pony exposed to live or ultraviolet (UV)-inactivated EHV-1 was shown to inhibit a T cell response to antigen or mitogens *in vitro* and this immunosuppressive activity was associated with the presence of soluble TGFβ1 [173]. In mice and humans, closely related members of the TGFβ family (β1, β2 and β3) have been shown to inhibit T cell activation, differentiation and proliferation. CD8+ T cells activated in the presence of TGFβ do not acquire CTL function and CD4+ T cells fail to become Th1 or Th2 cells. Furthermore, TGFβ has been shown to prevent DC maturation and is one major factor expressed by Treg (regulatory) cells [174]. The expression of TGFβ was reported after *in vitro* infection of human PBMC with HSV-1 [175], and in rat after *in vivo* infection with CMV (betaherpesvirus) [176]. In the horse, another study has described the immunosuppression of T cell function by contact with PBMC isolated one week after experimental infection with EHV-1, but not with serum purified at the same time [177]. This result is not absolutely in contradiction to the TGFβ hypothesis previously described [173] as TGFβ can be expressed on the cell surface, allowing Treg cells to inhibit APC and self-reactive T cells by cell-to-cell contact in humans [174].

To date, a few studies have investigated immune evasion strategies of EHV-1, however, the results have sometimes been contradictory. Further investigation is necessary to understand more clearly the factors and mechanisms surrounding this aspect of EHV-1 biology, which are certainly related to its pathogenicity and should be kept in mind for the design of new strategies to protect against EHV-1 infection and disease.

Immunity to EHV-4 and Cross-Immunity to EHV-1

Experimental infection with EHV-4 has been shown to stimulate CF and VN antibody, which were detected from 2 to 7 weeks post infection [36-38, 178]. It has been shown previously that EHV-4 can induce effectors that lyse EHV-1 infected target cells [151]. This observation of potential cross-priming of CMI by EHV-1 and EHV-4 was also noted for antibody responses [45, 179] but this is still controversial. A foal immunised with an inactivated EHV-1 vaccine has been shown to develop a type-specific VN antibody response, whereas this response was cross-reactive after immunisation with inactivated EHV-4 [180]. In terms of CMI, foals vaccinated with a modified live EHV-1 developed a cytolytic activity against both EHV-1 and EHV-4 infected target cells [181]. Therefore, it is important to know, if possible, the status of EHV-4 infection prior to any investigation involving EHV-1.

EHV-2 Immune Evasion

Immunity to EHV-2 and EHV-5 has been rarely investigated. EHV-2-specific VN antibody has been successfully detected in foals newly infected with EHV-2 [182]. However, EHV-2 potential to evade and subvert host immune responses has been well documented. Firstly, by establishing latency in cells that are integral to the immune system, the immune functions of these cells may be impaired. Secondly, examination of the EHV-2 genome reveals the presence of several genes that show striking homology to cellular genes that have immunomodulatory potential. These include an IL-10 homologue and three 7-transmembrane receptors (encoded by ORFs E1, E6 and ORF74) that show homology to the chemokine receptor family of G protein-coupled receptors (GPCR). Thirdly, it was reported that infection of PBMC with EHV-2 resulted in the down-regulation of the chemokine monocyte chemoattractant protein-1 (CCL2) [183]. The potential of EHV-2 infection to down-regulate cellular chemokines and the presence of chemokine receptor homologues in the EHV-2 genome would suggest that modulation of the chemokine environment in the vicinity of infected cells is likely to be one of the strategies by which the virus avoids the host immune system, and is likely to be an important factor in the pathogenesis of EHV-2 infections.

Virally encoded homologues of cytokines, chemokines and their receptors are found almost exclusively in herpesviruses and another family of large DNA viruses, the Poxviruses, with only a few exceptions to this rule (for examples, see [184] and [185]). However, while herpesviruses are specialised for the production of homologues of cellular cytokines and chemokines along with a large repertoire of homologues to the chemokine receptor group of GPCR (Table 8) [186-188] and references therein], poxviruses are more specialised in the secretion of soluble cytokine receptors and secreted vCKBP, which lack any sequence conservation with chemokine receptors.

Amongst herpesviruses, homologues of GPCR are only found among members of the *Beta-* and *Gammaherpesvirinae*. While some appear to be unique to a particular herpesvirus and are therefore likely to be relatively recently acquired, most are members of conserved gene families (Table 8), consistent with their descent from a common gene precursor captured by an ancient herpesvirus. Although the majority of herpesvirus GPCR are currently orphan receptors for which the cognate ligand is not yet known, they show highest homology to cellular chemokine receptors. Indeed, all those for which ligands have been identified have been found to be functional receptors of chemokines.

Table 8. Summary of GPCR homologues currently identified among members of the *Gamma-* and *Betaherpesvirinae*

Gammaherpesvirus GPCR homologues				
Gammaherpesvirus genus	Abbreviated virus name (see Table 2-4)	Gammaherpesvirus-conserved GPCR gene families		Other‡
		Lymphocryptovirus and Rhadinovirus-conserved BILF1 family*	Rhadinovirus-conserved ORF74 family†	
Lymphocryptovirus	EBV	EBV BILF1		
	RhEBV	RhEBV BILF1		
	CHV-3	ORF6		
Rhadinovirus	AlHV-1	A5		
	PLHV-1/2/3	A5		
	EHV-2	E6	ORF74	E1
	HVS		ORF74 (ECRF3)	
	HHV-8		ORF74	
	RRV		ORF74	
	MHV-68		ORF74	
	HVA		ORF74	
Betaherpesvirus GPCR homologues				
Beta-herpesvirus genus	Abbreviated virus name (see Table-1.3)	Betaherpesvirus-conserved GPCR gene families‡		
		UL33 family	UL78 family	US28 family
Cytomegalovirus	HCMV	UL33	UL78	US28 US27
	RhCMV	UL33	UL78	US28.1-US28.5 gene cluster
	CCMV	UL33	UL78	US28 US27
	SCMV			ORF3-7 gene cluster
Muramegalovirus	MCMV	M33	M78	
	RCMV	R33	R78	
Roseolovirus	HHV-6	U12	U51	
	HHV-7	U12	U51	

*Low homology to chemokine receptors; †, homology to CXCR; ‡, homology to CCR.

Characterisation of viral GPCR (vGPCR) has revealed the presence of several characteristics largely absent from most cellular counterparts. Many have been shown to signal constitutively in the absence of ligand binding, and many vGPCR exhibit promiscuous ligand binding to chemokines of a particular subclass, or even to chemokines from different subclasses [188] and references therein].

EHV-2 is unusual in that it encodes three very different GPCR homologues that are likely to have been acquired through ancient acts of 'molecular piracy' from host genomes, at distinctly different stages during its evolution. E6 is believed to be the most anciently acquired GPCR of EHV-2 and is poorly conserved with cellular GPCR. E6 shares homology with member of the BILF1 gene family, which includes GPCR homologues encoded by rhadinoviruses and lymphocryptoviruses [189-191], and presumably evolved from a GPCR homologue which was incorporated into the genome of a progenitor gammaherpesvirus prior to the division into the genera *Rhadinovirus* and *Lymphocryptovirus*. ORF74 is conserved with many members of the genus *Rhadinovirus*, but absent from members of the genus *Lymphocryptovirus*, and was presumably acquired after the division of these two genera. ORF74 receptors exhibit sequence similarity with cellular CXCR2. They exhibit constitutive signalling activity and promiscuous affinity for CXC chemokines [192-196], and have been associated with triggering of cell-proliferation and transformation [197-199].A highly conserved feature of Rhodopsin-like GPCR is a 'DRY' motif on the intracellular face of the third transmembrane region, the Arg of which is one of the most conserved residues and has generally been considered to be essential for coupling of the receptors to intracellular G proteins. The ORF74 family members encode variants of the 'DRY' motif, namely VRY (HHV-8), LRC (HVS), HRC (MHV-68) and IRC (RRV). EHV-2 ORF74 is the only family member encoding a variant motif (DTW) that lacks the central Arg. A recent study of the molecular pharmacology of EHV-2 ORF74 highlighted the novelty of this receptor, which was functional and exhibited both constitutive and ligand-induced G protein mediated signalling [200]. Furthermore, EHV2-ORF74 contrasted with other ORF74 receptors via a comparatively narrow ligand-binding spectrum, restricted to granulocyte chemotactic protein-2 (CXCL6), and a limited, rather than promiscuous, activation of G proteins. With 47% amino acid identity to CCR3, E1 has the highest reported similarity to cellular chemokine receptors of any vGPCR [201], and lacks sequence homologues in other gammaherpesviruses. This, and its position within the genome, within the two direct terminal repeats, indicates that E1 was relatively recently acquired. Like CCR3, E1 has been shown to be a functional receptor for the chemokine eotaxin (CCL11) [201].

A recent study investigating the genetic variability of the EHV-2 GPCR among virus isolates revealed striking differences in the level of conservation of the different GPCR ORFs, with an inverse relationship between the sequence diversity and the order that the EHV-2 GPCR were likely to have been acquired from the host [77]. Phylogenetic analysis revealed six 'genogroups' for E1 and four for ORF74, which exhibited approximately 10-38% and 11-27% amino acid difference between groups, respectively. Despite the high level of variation, structural and functional hallmarks of GCPR were conserved, and the majority of the variation confined to the extracellular domains of the protein. In contranst E6 was highly conserved. 2 genogroups were identified for E6, which differed by <6% amino acid non-identities, with all variation confined to the N-terminal domain [77]. Interestingly, studies of genetic vartiation of GPCR encoded by other herpesviruses have found them to be highly conserved among isolates [202].

Although many vGPCR appear not to be essential for virus replication in cell culture, several gene deletion experiments have demonstrated that some receptors facilitate viral replication and/or dissemination *in vivo* (e.g. M33, R33, M78 and R78 [203-207]), whereas others (e.g. ORF74 of MHV-68 [208, 209]) contribute to the reactivation of virus from latency. While the precise roles that vGPCR play in the herpesvirus lifecycle have yet to be fully elucidated, current evidence suggests they may be involved in several strategies to compromise immune surveillance mechanisms. Incorporation of vGPCR into the virion envelope may facilitate their deposition into cell plasma membranes upon viral entry, thus enabling changes in infected cell signalling immediately following infection [210]. Receptor expression may modify the response of infected cells to certain ligands allowing the establishment of an intracellular environment favourable for virus replication or the proliferation of the infected cell [199]. Alternatively, receptor expression at the cell surface and rapid internalisation may facilitate chemokine sequestration from the extracellular environment and potentially prevent lymphocyte recruitment and stimulation of lymphocyte effector mechanisms in the vicinity of infected cells [211]. vGPCR cell surface expression may also assist viral dissemination by modifying the chemotactic behaviour of infected cells along gradients of soluble or membrane bound chemokines [212, 213]. The potential of EHV-2 infection to down-regulate cellular chemokines and the presence of chemokine receptor homologues in the EHV-2 genome would suggest that modulation of the chemokine environment in the vicinity of infected cells is likely to be one of the strategies by which the virus avoids the host immune system, and is likely to be an important factor in the pathogenesis of EHV-2 infections.

Vaccines against EHV-1

Vaccination remains today an important strategy to fight EHV-1 infection, in combination with management measures. Whole inactivated EHV-1 vaccines, which provide variable levels of protection against the disease through the induction of antibodies, have been the main type of vaccine commercially available. However, new strategies of vaccination that aim to mimic more closely the stimulation of the immune system induced by EHV-1 have been investigated (i.e. vaccines composed of live attenuated virus or poxvirus-vector coding for virus proteins). Current commercialised or experimental vaccination strategies can be divided into the administration of either inert or live vaccines. Inert vaccines contain killed whole virus, subunit proteins or DNA, in contrast with live vaccines that include attenuated virus or living virus-based vector vaccines.

It is believed that successful vaccination against EHV-1 requires stimulation of both antibody and cellular immune responses. High titres of virus neutralising antibodies will protect against epithelial infection with EHV-1, reduce the development of respiratory disease, subsequent virus shedding from the nasopharynx and spread of the disease to other horses. EHV-1 myeloencephalopathy and abortion are consequences of EHV-1 systemic dissemination through a cell-associated viraemia. During this phase of the disease, antibodies are usually inefficient but EHV-1-infected cells can be controlled by cell-mediated immunity, which will also limit the impact of EHV-1 reactivation. Thus different immune responses have to be stimulated by vaccines to treat the different aspects of the disease induced by EHV-1. Envelope glycoproteins of EHV-1 are essential for the entry of the virus into cells and contain antibody epitopes. As targets of the humoral immune reponses, they act as strong candidates and have been widely studied and used for vaccine development. The cellular immune response is essential to tackle EHV-1 during its intracellular cycle of life and CTL target proteins have to be identified and included in vaccines when possible.

Many studies have attempted to determine the CTL target proteins of EHV-1. However, such targets are often MHC class I restricted as has been observed with herpesviruses of other species. Murine MHC-restricted CTL epitopes from Herpes Simplex virus (HSV) have been identified and HSV disease severity is related to MHC haplotype in both mice and humans. In the horse it is also clear that activation of CTL by viruses is influenced by MHC class I haplotype [149, 214] and the IE early gene of EHV-1 has been shown to be an effective CTL activator only in certain MHC class I haplotypes [152, 157]. In addition, sub-typic variation within MHC class I haplotypes can also effect the stimulation of a CTL immune response, as seen with antigens from both EHV-1 and EIAV [152, 215]. Therefore, a CTL target antigen must be effective across a broad range of MHC class I haplotypes for it to be used in a vaccine that will provide widespread protection across the equine population in question.

Markers of Protection

Markers of protection afforded by vaccination are generally defined according to the goals that must be achieved. In assessing vaccine efficacy in horses, clinical protection against diseases induced by EHV-1 is defined by the absence of pyrexia and of other clinical signs induced by infection with a respiratory virus such as nasal discharge, cough, anorexia and depression. Neurological pathology (e.g. paralysis) and abortion are also clinical signs of disease associated with EHV-1 infection that may be considered. Virological protection is defined by the absence of EHV-1 in mucosal secretions as detected by titration of virus in nasal swab extracts. Virological protection also includes the absence of cell-associated viraemia. The humoral response stimulated by vaccination is generally quantified by the titration of CF and/or VN antibodies for EHV-1. Seroconversion is defined as a significant increase (4-fold) of antibody titres. The cellular immune response can be assessed by measurement of antigen-specific T cell proliferation, EHV-1 specific CTL activity, up regulation of cytokine mRNA or EHV-1-specific IFNγ synthesis.

Strain Selection

EHV-1 is considered to be genetically and antigenically stable. No definitive regulation exists concerning the selection of specific strains for vaccine design. The combination of both EHV-1B and P strains is sometimes present in vaccines. Other pharmaceutical companies have based their selection on circulating EHV-1 strains. One may argue that the recent identification of neurological and non-neurological strains may be taken in count for the future selection of vaccine strain.

Schedule of Vaccination

It is generally recommended to vaccinate foals over 3-5 months of age, with a second immunisation within 4 to 6 weeks. The immune system has to be boosted by a single vaccination every 3 or 6 months, depending of vaccines. To avoid EHV-1 induced abortion, it is recommended to vaccinate pregnant mares at the 5th, 7th and 9th months of pregnancy.

Inert Vaccines

Inactivated whole EHV-1 Vaccines and Sub-Unit Vaccines

Since the introduction of EHV-1 vaccines in the 1960s, the majority of vaccines commercially available have been inactivated whole virus or subunit vaccines (Figure 9). The main advantages of these vaccines are the absence of pathogenicity, virus replication and subsequent spread between hosts. Viruses are usually inactivated by formaldehyde or β-propriolactone. However, several issues are associated with this type of vaccine, such as local tolerance, pyrexia due to high antigenic load, risk of incomplete inactivation and manipulation of high pathogenic organisms in production.

The first killed EHV-1 vaccines introduced in the 1950-60s were prepared from the tissue of infected foals or hamsters. These preparations were inappropriate for vaccination due to a weak immunogenicity and high incidence of adverse reactions [216, 217]. A partially purified, formaldehyde inactivated EHV-1 vaccine was reported later to provide a good humoral response in horses and partial protection against clinical signs of disease and virus shedding after experimental infection with EHV-1 [218]. Today, inactivated whole EHV-1 vaccines are widely used. For example, Duvaxyn EHV1/4 is an inactivated whole EHV-1 and EHV-4 vaccine, adjuvanted with carbomer.

Carbomer, an emulsifying agent, is a polyacrylic acid with an extremely high molecular weight [219]. Duvaxyn EHV1/4 has been shown to induce or increase both VN and CF antibody responses in foals and pregnant mares after 1 or 2 vaccinations. In foals, vaccination significantly reduced clinical signs of disease and the duration of both cell-associated viraemia and virus shedding after experimental infection. Virus shedding after experimental infection with EHV-1 was reduced in vaccinated mares when compared with control ponies, although all animals developed a cell-associated viraemia. In addition the incidence of abortion in the vaccinated pregnant mares was significantly lower (1 out of 5) than in the unvaccinated mares (4 out of 4). Clinical signs of disease induced by EHV-4 challenge were also reduced in vaccinated ponies [37]. In a recent study, ponies vaccinated twice with a conventional whole EHV-1 inactivated vaccine adjuvanted with carbomer developed a strong humoral response (both CF and VN antibodies) after both immunisations [220]. No mucosal humoral immune response has been directly induced by intramuscular immunisations with an inactivated EHV-1 vaccine [132]. However, intramuscular vaccination primed horses efficiently to mount a mucosal immune response during challenge infection with EHV-1. A 6-month duration of immunity against clinical signs of disease was reported after immunisation with an inactivated whole EHV-1/4 vaccine adjuvanted with carbomer [221, 222].

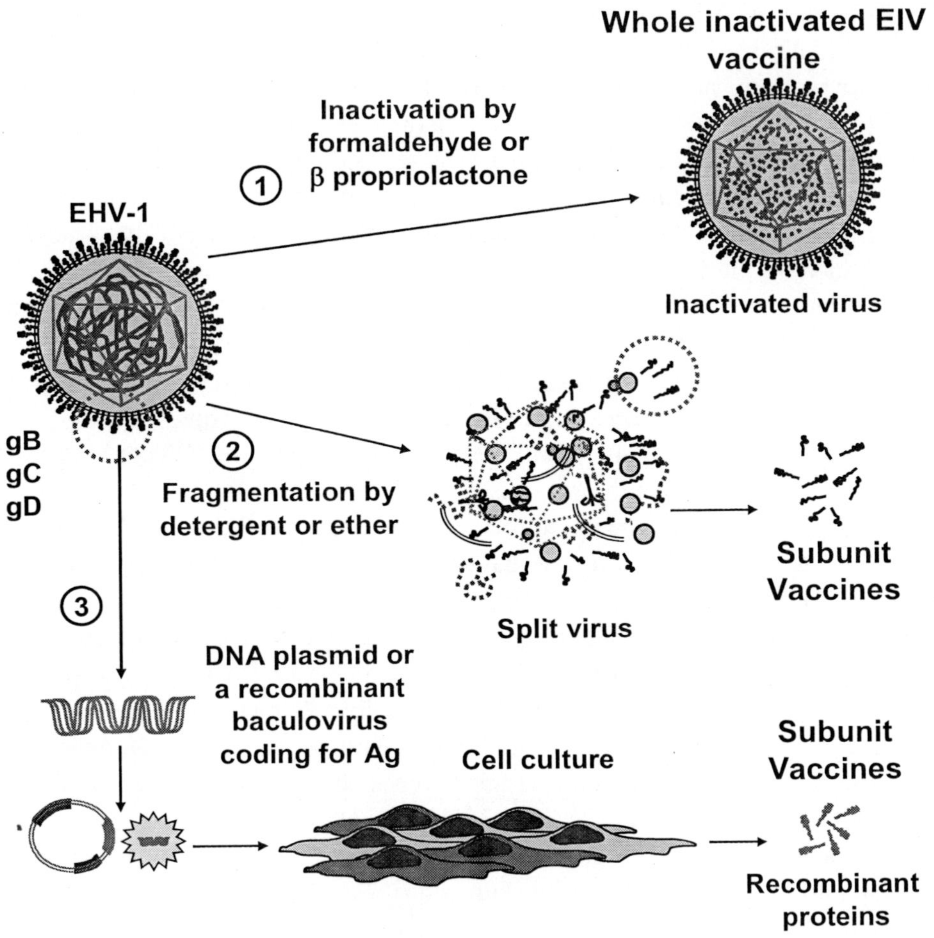

Figure 9. Inactivated and subunit vaccines [13]. EHV-1 is either inactivated to produce a vaccine (1) or fragmented to produce split virus or subunit vaccines (2). Recombinant viral proteins can also be used in subunit vaccines (3). Genes encoding proteins of interest are cloned into a plasmid or viral vector, which are used to transfect or infect cultured cells. The generated recombinant viral proteins are then purified for use in the vaccine.

Responses to inactivated EHV-1 vaccines in the field however are different. A study carried out in Australia has measured the seroconversion of 159 mares and 101 foals after 3 vaccinations with an inactivated whole EHV-1/4 vaccine. Less than 30% of mares and 50% of foals responded to vaccination [223]. Australian studies have also shown infection of foals in the early weeks of life continues to occur despite vaccination of mares during pregnancy [118, 224]. Indeed these studies have shown that the introduction of vaccination has not changed the number of mares seropositive for EHV-1 in the pre-weaning period and does not appear to have affected the rate of new infection of foals pre-weaning [225]. These studies show that the presence of maternal antibodies alone is not enough to prevent EHV-1 seroconversion associated with EHV infection. Thus, despite vaccination, the silent cycle of EHV continues. These findings are supported by a study in the Northern hemisphere where 3 foals born to EHV vaccinated dams seroconverted to EHV-1 during the first month of life [121]. Despite an extensive use of inactivated virus vaccines in many countries over decades, abortion storms are still being reported [226].

Numerous split or subunit vaccines have been developed to replace whole inactivated virus vaccines. A split vaccine is obtained by the disintegration of purified virions using detergents (e.g. triton) or ether, which are afterwards removed. Split vaccines contain the same elements as inactivated whole virus vaccines and generally induce similar adverse reactions. Subunit vaccines contain one or more pure or semi-pure antigens, purified from the pathogen or produced by a baculovirus-expression systems using insect cells. Therefore, it is important to identify the proteins or glycoproteins that are involved in inducing protection. Since only a few proteins are included in subunit vaccines, less antigenic competition is expected.

Due to the large number of proteins expressed by EHV-1, the selection of relevant proteins for subunit EHV-1 vaccines tends to be difficult. Glycoproteins of EHV-1 are essential for cell receptor recognition and the entry into target cells. Glycoproteins B and C contain antibody epitopes strongly recognised by the immune system of horses infected or vaccinated with EHV-1, and are therefore candidates for inclusion in sub-unit vaccines against EHV-1 [227, 228]. Such vaccines have been tested for antigenicity in a rodent model. Insect cells (Sf9) infected with baculoviruses coding for gB, gC, gD or gH of EHV-1, have been inoculated into mice, either individually or in combination. Recombinant gD and gH baculoviruses induce serum antibodies to EHV-1. Immunisation with gD also produces VN antibody and increases EHV-1 clearance from the respiratory tract of mice after experimental infection [229]. Similar results have been obtained with baculovirus recombinant gC [228] and gB [230, 231]. In other studies, 3 or 4 repeated immunisations with recombinant glycoproteins (gB, gC or gD, alone or in combination), at 2-week intervals, have been shown to induce a humoral immune response composed of VN antibodies, which protects mice against respiratory disease induced by infection with EHV-1, 2 weeks after the last immunisations [232, 233].

Immunostimulating Complex-Based Vaccines

Immunisations with proteins generally require the presence of strong adjuvants to stimulate an immune response. Membrane protein/antigens are generally adjuvanted with *Quillaia* saponin (Quil A), integrated in immuno-stimulating complexes (ISCOM™) or mixed with Iscomatrix™ to improve their antigenicity. ISCOMs™ and Iscomatrix™ are formed from a matrix (i.e. a combination of Quil A, phospholipids and cholesterol), which incorporates or binds membrane proteins to give stable, self adjuvanting particles held together by hydrophobic interactions (Figure 10). In other species, ISCOM™ or Iscomatrix™-based vaccines have shown successful protection against numerous pathogens [234] and are successfully used against EIV in the horse [235-237]. ISCOMs and Iscomatrix™ are not fusogenic but can associate with intracellular lipid membranes in the cytoplasm and vesicular compartments after up-take by APC [238].

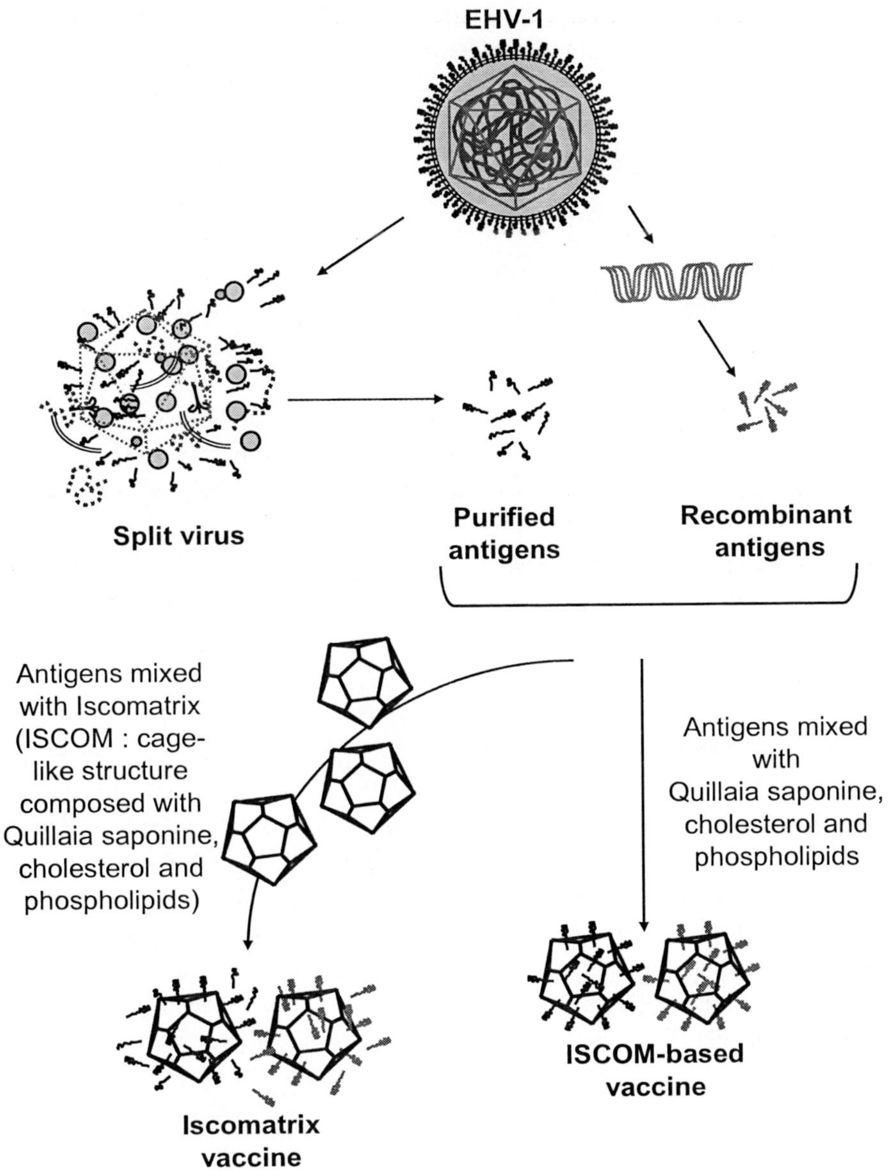

Figure 10. ISCOM/Iscomatrix™ vaccines [13]. Antigens are either split virus products or purified/recombinant proteins.

An experimental sub-unit vaccine containing glycoproteins gp2, gp10, gB, gC, gD and gM, purified by gradient density from the EHV-1 strain V592 (isolated from an abortion outbreak in England in 1985) and formulated with the adjuvant Iscomatrix™ has been shown to induce a VN antibody response and protect hamsters from a live EHV-1 challenge [239]. When tested in ponies, two intramuscular immunisations with this sub-unit vaccine stimulated a strong humoral immune response composed mainly of VN and, to a lesser extent, CF antibodies. In ponies vaccinated three times and subsequently infected with an homologous strain of EHV-1 a few weeks after the third immunisation, the clinical signs of disease, virus shedding in nasal secretions and the amount of virus isolated from PBMC were markedly reduced when compared with control unvaccinated ponies [130]. It is likely that antigens delivered by immunostimulating complex-based sub-unit vaccines were processed through both exogenous and endogenous routes, stimulating VN antibody and CMI that resulted in the modulation of the disease. A good correlation between the amount of VN antibody prior to the challenge infection with EHV-1 and a reduction in the duration and amount of virus excretion has been observed. More recently, a similar vaccine composed of inactivated Sf9 insect cells infected by a recombinant baculovirus coding for EHV-1 gD and mixed with the adjuvant Iscomatrix™ was administered to ponies, pregnant mares and foals via the intramuscular route [240]. EHV-1 gD was shown to possess a neutralising epitope [241]. Vaccinated ponies developed a mixed virus-specific antibody response with neutralising activity and composed of IgGa, IgGb, IgG(T) and IgA antibodies [240, 242]. Interestingly, this antibody response was similar to the response induced by vaccination with an inactivated whole EHV-1 vaccine, which confirms the importance of gD in containing antibody epitopes and justifies its inclusion in sub-unit vaccines. Mares and foals vaccinated twice with a sub-unit vaccine containing both gB and gD mixed with the Iscomatrix™ adjuvant have shown reduced virus shedding after experimental infection with EHV-1. However, EHV-1 cell-associated viraemia was not affected by vaccination [243].

DNA Vaccines against EHV-1

DNA vaccination is the administration of DNA plasmids expressing genes from a specific pathogen, encoding whole antigenic proteins or simply epitopes of these proteins. These antigens are directly expressed in the target host cell and result in the *in vivo* expression of antigenic proteins leading to their presentation by both exogenous and endogenous antigen processing routes and ultimately to the stimulation of both humoral and cellular immune responses. This approach is therefore advantageous compared with inactivated whole virus or sub-unit vaccines. DNA vaccines can also be adjuvanted by the insertion of genes coding for costimulatory molecules (e.g. cytokines), which in theory allow a more controlled modulation of the immune response than the one induced by conventional adjuvants. DNA vaccines have good stability and can be lyophilised for long-term storage.

Within the last decade, several studies in mice have evaluated the antigenicity and efficacy of DNA vaccination against EHV-1 infection. A DNA vaccine encoding gD has been shown to elicit both humoral and cell-mediated immune responses after two intramuscular immunisations, and to reduce respiratory lesions, the amount and duration of virus shedding [244, 245], and abortion [246] induced by challenge infection. The protection was improved by modifying the scheme of vaccination and including a protein booster immunisation with gD, 4 weeks after a DNA priming [247].

The immunogenicity of a DNA vaccine encoding gD was therefore verified in horses after intramuscular administration. An increased level of gD-specific antibody was measured after immunisation [248]. However, in a more recent study, immunisation of horses with DNA coding for gD failed to induce a detectable antibody response [240]. The protection against EHV-1 infection stimulated by a DNA vaccine coding for gB, gC and gD glycoproteins of EHV-1 has been investigated. DNA constructs were administrated alone, in combination with adjuvants (i.e. aluminium phosphate or carbopol), or complexed with the cationic lipid DMRIE-DOPE in the presence of a DNA plasmid coding for granulocyte-macrophage colony stimulating factor (GM-CSF).

The expression of GM-CSF under these conditions is expected to stimulate the proliferation of monocytes, Mϕ and monocyte-derived dendritic cells and subsequently to increase antigen presentation. The amount of VN antibody was increased in ponies vaccinated with the DNA/DMRIE-DOPE vaccine, and the duration of nasopharyngeal virus excretion after experimental infection with EHV-1 was reduced following immunisation with a DNA vaccine adjuvanted with aluminium phosphate. Cell-associated viraemia was not affected by vaccination [220]. Another study investigated the protective effects of particle-mediated DNA immunisation with combinations of gB/gCand gD or of the immediate early (IE) and early (UL5) genes [249]. However, although there was a slight increase in gD and gC antibody titre, vaccination did not effect EHV-1 lymphoprliferative or CTL responses and again limited protection against clinical signs of disease was observed. It is clear that DNA vaccination efficiently stimulates an EHV-1 specific antibody response in the horse but so far there is no evidence that cellular immune responses are stimulated. Therefore, the protection afforded by this type of vaccine needs further investigation.

Non infectious EHV-1 L-Particles

Generation of non-infectious virion-related particles shortly after cell infection with EHV-1 has been described [250]. These particles are formed by tegument proteins surrounded by an envelope but lack the internal capsid and viral DNA. They have been name light-particles (L-particles) for their ability to be separated into a low density band on Ficoll gradients [251]. The exact role of L-particles during infection has not been determined and needs further investigation. It has been suggested that L-particles could support successful initiation of viral replication at the early stage of infection and/or may serve as decoys for the immune response [251]. L-particles possess an intact envelope membrane with all immunogenic glycoproteins allowing virus entry into the cell. Therefore, they are expected to stimulate an immune response towards the viral glycoproteins similar to that during the natural viral infection. As a result, they have been identified has potential immunising agents. In mice, immunisation with non replicative EHV-1 L-particles induced protective CMI and an antibody response. However, the level of immunity induced by immunisation was dependent of the inoculation route [252]. In specific-pathogen-free (spf) foals, immunisation with EHV-1 L-particles induced a CF antibody response. Clinical signs of disease, virus shedding and cell-associated viraemia subsequent to an experimental infection with the EHV-1 strain Ab4 were milder in immunised ponies when compared with unvaccinated controls [253]. However, some concern remains around the safety of such vaccinal preparation, which needs to be free from any residual infectious particles. The use of pre-viral DNA replication particles (PREP), generated in conditions where viral DNA synthesis is blocked, instead of L-particles, could solve the problem of contaminating infectious virus in vaccinal preparation [254]. Another concern is the ability of L-particles to induce a lytic cycle from a non replicative transfected EHV-1 DNA or heterologous alpha herpesviruses DNA (i.e. HSV-1 and PRV) [251]. This activity could lead to the enhancement of latent virus reactivation by L-particles and would be detrimental to their use as immunising agent in horses that have been previously in contact with EHV-1 and potentially harbour latent virus.

Live EHV-1 Vaccines

A live vaccine is defined as a vaccinal preparation containing live organisms. These organisms can be an attenuated or a modified form of the pathogen itself, or a heterologous organism used as a carrier or vector of the pathogen's antigens (live recombinant vector vaccines).

Live Attenuated Vaccines

Immunisation with a live attenuated virus closely mimics natural infection. Antigens are presented to the immune system via both exogenous and endogenous antigen presentation pathways, and vaccines are therefore expected to stimulate an immune response similar to those induced by infection.

The intranasal or intramuscular inoculation of a live attenuated/modified EHV-1 is an attractive approach for the vaccination against EHV-1. However, the risk of reversion to virulence remains a concern for this strategy of vaccination. Two principal types of EHV-1 mutants have been derived and used as live attenuated EHV-1 vaccines, namely thymidine kinase negative (TK-) and temperature sensitive (Ts) mutants.

The use of mutagenic agents such as bromodeoxyuridine (BrdUrd) or 1-B-D arabinofuranosylthymine (araT) has led to the derivation of thymidine kinase negative (TK-) mutants of the Army 183 EHV-1 strain. Their virulence and ability to establish latency is reduced in the horse while immunogenicity and stability is retained. Immunisation of EHV-1 unprimed ponies with TK- EHV-1 by intramuscular or intravenous injection did not induce any clinical signs of disease. After challenge infection with EHV-1, an anamnestic VN antibody response was measured in vaccinated ponies. Clinical signs of disease and virus shedding were also reduced in TK- EHV-1 immunised ponies [255]. Another TK- EHV-1 mutant was evaluated in specific pathogen free foals. While it was able to replicate in foals, it was found less pathogenic than the wild type EHV-1. Vaccination with the TK- mutant partially reduced the clinical signs of disease induced by challenge infection with the wild type virus but did not prevent cell-associated viraemia [256].

A temperature sensitive (Ts) mutant of EHV-1 (clone 147) has been derived from a German abortion isolate of EHV-1 (strain M8) by culture with BrdUrd and does not grow at ≥38.5°C. This Ts clone has been used as a live intranasal attenuated vaccine in the horse. Ponies developed mild or no clinical signs of disease after intranasal inoculation of the Ts virus, but 11 out of 15 vaccinated ponies shed virus for one week and 10 ponies showed a cell-associated viraemia. All vaccinates had an increased level of VN antibody six weeks after the inoculation. After challenge infection, vaccinated ponies developed only mild clinical signs of disease and although the majority shed virus but none of them developed a cell-associated viraemia [38]. Another study reported the intranasal immunisation of 11 pregnant mares (vaccination at 3 to 6 months of gestation). The majority of them shed virus after challenge infection with the virulent EHV-1 strain Ab4 and 5 out of 11 developed a cell-associated viraemia. However, 9 out of 11 mares were protected against abortion when infected with EHV-1, 4 to 6 months after the inoculation of the Ts virus [257]. When used in young foals (1.4-3.5 months old), the live EHV-1 vaccine (Ts mutant clone 147) induced a partial but significant protection against clinical signs of disease, virus shedding and cell-associated viraemia, despite the presence of maternal antibodies [258]. However, there are safety concerns due to the nasopharyngeal shedding and cell-associated viraemia detected after vaccination with this Ts mutant and its derivation from an abortigenic isolate.

Two vaccinations of foals with a modified live EHV-1 cultivated on an equine cell line (Rhino-Flu; SmithKline Animal Health; this vaccine has been withdrawn from the market) have been shown to increase the cell-mediated cytotoxicity against EHV-1 infected homologous target cells when compared with pre-vaccination cytotoxic activity. However, the cytolysis has not been fully characterised [181]. In another study, the intranasal administration of a live attenuated EHV-1 vaccine (Rhinomune, Pfizer) failed to induce mucosal antibodies, which could explain the failure of attenuated EHV-1 vaccines to prevent virus shedding. It was speculated that the attenuation may have reduced the virus's mucosal immunogenicity. However, the lack of mucosal antibodies could also be due to a lack of systemic prime to EHV-1 prior to mucosal immunisation [132].

Poxvirus-Based Vector Vaccine for EHV-1

Live recombinant vector vaccines are constructed by inserting selected genes from the pathogen of interest into live, infectious, but non-disease-causing viruses, which may have been genetically modified. With virus-based vector vaccines, viral antigens are expressed and synthesised *de novo* within the infected cell. Thus, because they are presented via MHC class I (endogenous) and class II (exogenous) antigen-processing routes, the selected viral antigens will stimulate both humoral and cellular immune responses (Figure 11). Recombinant poxviruses have been widely used for vaccination [259, 260]. Poxviruses are genetically stable and allow the insertion of a large segment of foreign DNA coding for selected antigens. Recombinant poxviruses derived from vaccinia or avipoxvirus (i.e. canarypox or fowlpox virus) are commercially available and several recombinant canarypox-based vaccines have been developed for the horse [134, 220].

The first experiment using a poxvirus as a vaccine vector for EHV-1 proteins was tested in rodents. The immunisation of hamsters with recombinant vaccinia viruses (Copenhagen strain) expressing EHV-1 gB and gC glycoproteins elicited a VN antibody response and protected from a lethal EHV-1 challenge [163, 261]. More recently, a MVA-based (modified vaccinia Ankara) vaccine coding for EHV-1 gC (priming) was evaluated in hamsters in combination with a DNA vaccination coding for the same protein (boost). This scheme of vaccination induced both humoral and cellular immune responses, including proliferation and CTL activity [262]. MVA virus is a highly attenuated strain of vaccinia virus presenting with replication defects, which is frequently used in prime-boost vaccination protocols. Following extensive *in vitro* culture passage, the parental vaccinia virus becomes replication-deficient in virtually all mammalian cells [260]. These promising results in rodents has supported the evaluation of poxvirus as vaccine vectors in the horse. Two intramuscular immunisations of canarypox-based constructs coding for gB, gC and gD glycoproteins of the Kentucky strain of EHV-1, have been administered to ponies a few weeks apart, with and without adjuvant (carbopol/carbomer 974P). Challenge infection was carried out three weeks after second vaccination with the highly pathogenic Ab4 strain of EHV-1. A marked reduction of virus excretion in the vaccinates was noted when compared to ponies vaccinated without the carbopol adjuvant or control unvaccinated ponies experimentally infected with EHV-1.

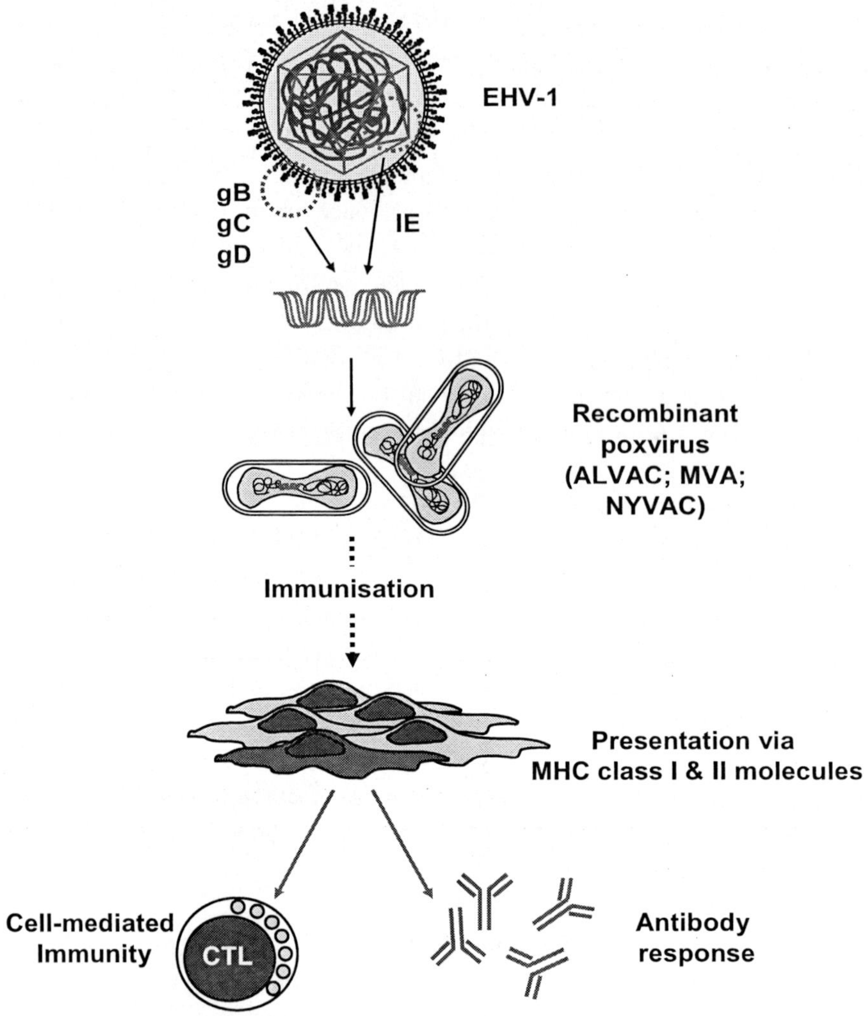

Figure 11. Poxvirus as vaccine vector for EHV-1 [13]. The virus proteins of interest are selected and genes coding for these proteins are inserted into the poxvirus genome. The recombinant poxvirus is used for immunisation, which stimulates both humoral and cellular immune responses.

However, vaccination did not affect the prevalence and duration of cell-associated viraemia [220, 263]. It was speculated that none of the EHV-1 glycoproteins chosen contained CTL epitopes, which could be a potential explanation for the lack of control of cell-associated viraemia. This study nevertheless highlights the potential of immunisation with a canarypox-based vectors for the immunological control of EHV-1 infection in the horse. In addition it emphasises the importance of carbopol as an adjuvant.

Recently, a recombinant poxvirus vector (vaccinia-derived NYVAC strain) coding for the IE protein, a known CTL target protein, has been used for vaccination in horses. Multiple immunisations with NYVAC-IE increased CTL activity and IFNγ synthesis specific for EHV-1 compared with unvaccinated or single-vaccinated ponies. Furthermore, multiple-vaccinated ponies demonstrated an increased proportion of CD8α- T cells synthesising IFNγ when compared with the unvaccinated pony. This demonstrates a predominant CD8α+ T lymphocyte population synthesising IFNγ after EHV-1 stimulation. The results showed that vaccination with a NYVAC-based construct coding for the EHV-1 IE protein stimulated CMI. This immune response alone did not protect against challenge infection. However, the study does illustrate that vaccinia-based vaccines can stimulate CMI in the horse and may therefore contribute to protection against disease caused by EHV-1 [135].

Only a few CTL target proteins have been identified in EHV-1 [152]. The most promising of all, the IE protein, has been shown to induce a strong Type 1 immunity composed of both CTL and IFNγ [135, 157]. However, inclusion of a CTL target proteins in EHV-1 vaccines will face another difficulty. CTL response is MHC class I restricted and the diversity and complexity of the equine MHC class I genes will make difficult selection of CTL target proteins or epitopes suitable for vaccine development [156]. The IE protein of EHV-1 has been shown to be a target for effector CTL expressing the MHC class I B2 molecules of horses from the ELA-A3 haplotype. Its presentation by other MHC class I haplotypes is either limited or unknown, which may limit the benefit of incorporating the IE protein in EHV-1 vaccines intended to be used in horse populations of diverse haplotype origins.

Effect of Maternal Antibodies and Age on EHV-1 Vaccination

One strategy used to protect young foals against EHV-1 is to increase the amount of maternal antibodies in foals by vaccinating the pregnant mare against EHV-1 [240], however, the impact of maternal antibodies upon EHV-1 infection (if any) is not completely understood. The control of EHV-1 infection in young animals is crucial. Yet the vaccination of foals at less than 5 months of age with inactivated whole EHV-1/EHV-4 [223, 264] or sub-unit vaccines is not successful in mounting an immune response [240]. A factor that influences vaccine efficacy in young animals is the foal's weak immune response to primary vaccination. In the context of *Rhodococcus equi* vaccination, the absence of immune responses after DNA vaccinations has been associated with a potential immature antigen presenting cell function compared with adult horses [265]. It has also been reported that pre-existing antibodies to EHV-4 may interfere and be detrimental to EHV-1 immunisation [223]. Vaccination with live attenuated EHV-1 vaccines has shown some degree of protection in foals (>5 months old) against signs of disease, virus shedding and cell-associated viraemia induced by challenge infection with EHV-1 [258]. In the current conditions, vaccinations have little effect on the early infection of foals with EHV-1 or the formation of the latently infected pool of ponies in the horse population. The poor reactivity of the foal immune system to vaccination is a crucial question that needs to be resolved.

About the use of EHV-1 as Vaccine Vector

The use of replication-incompetent herpesviruses as vectors is a new strategy for gene delivery and vaccination in humans. It is worth mentioning that EHV-1 has been evaluated as a potential vector candidate for gene delivery and vaccination in human and veterinary species. EHV-1 possesses a high capacity for packaging foreign DNA (i.e. more than 100kb of foreign DNA encoding proteins of vaccination interest). In comparison, poxvirus can harbour approximately 25kb of foreign DNA. EHV-1 shows a broad cell and species tropism and has been shown to efficiently express transgenes in porcine, bovine and human PBMC as well as in cell lines of avian, canine and feline origin. It can also be used in humans without being affected by pre-existing immunity directed against human herpesviruses (human sera do not neutralise EHV-1) [266]. Several strains of EHV-1 have been cloned as infectious BACs [70] to provide vaccine strains. In this context, the vaccine strain RacH that is attenuated by the absence of gene 67 (IR6) and other alterations of the genome has been recently used to deliver several structural proteins of Bovine viral diarrhea virus (BVDV) in cattle. Intramuscular vaccination with this recombinant vaccine stimulated a BVDV-specific antibody response and reduced viraemia and virus shedding post experimental infection when compared with unvaccinated animals [267]. A similar experiment has been carried out in the horse using a recombinant EHV-1 coding for West Nile virus (WNV) protein. Vaccinated horses developed a WNV-specific neutralising antibody response [268].

Vaccines against EHV-2

Vaccination against EHV-2 is not commonplace, although vaccination experiments have been conducted in attempts to define EHV-2 as a predisposing factor for secondary bacterial infections. Although there are conflicting data regarding the pathogenicity of EHV-2, the role of EHV-2 as a predisposing factor for the invasion of the lungs by *Rhodococcus equi* pneumonia and the developement of a two-phase respiratory disease complex in foals, was indicated by a protective effect of EHV-2 hyperimmune serum [269]. EHV-2 hyperimmune serum treatment was subsequently put into practice in Hungarian studs in 1980 with protection continually reported in the treated group of foals, and two-phase respiratory disease in the untreated control groups [91].

To obtain further evidence for the predisposing role of EHV-2, a novel strategy of active immunization was tested, utilising immunostimulatory complexes (iscoms) containing EHV-2 envelope components [270, 271]. In a pilot study, immunization of foals with an iscom-based EHV-2 vaccine provided protection against the entire respiratory disease complex, including the development of *R. equi* pneumonia [91], thus strongly supporting the hypothesis that EHV-2 is a predisposing factor for the *R. equi* invasion of the respiratory tract.

Therapeutics

During the 1980s and early 1990s, several acyclic nucleoside analogues, antiherpetic drugs that target nucleic acid synthesis, have been studied *in vitro* against EHV-1 for a potential use in the horse [272-274]. The interest for these drugs has been recently reniewed following the epidemic of EHM outbreaks in the recent years. Acyclic nucleoside analogues regroup a large family of molecules such as penciclovir, acyclovir, ganciclovir, cidofovir and foscarnet. When tested *in vitro* against different abortigenic or neuropathogenic strains of EHV-1, ganciclovir has been found to be the most potent acyclic nucleoside analogues to inhibit EHV-1 replication and plaque formation [275]. To be efficient *in vivo*, a fine balance has to be achieved. Concentration of antiherpetic drugs has to be maintained high and long enough to inhibit viral replication while keeping cytotoxicity acceptable. The pharmacokinetics of acyclovir and its prodrug valacyclovir have been measured in the horse [276-278]. Acyclovir has been used with potential benefit to the horse during several outbreaks of EHV-1 displaying neurological signs disease [124, 279, 280]. Efficacy of valacyclovir against neurological strain of EHV-1 is currently under investigation [281]. Results about the efficiency of acyclic nucleoside analogues in monitored experimental infection of horses with EHV-1 have not been reported yet.

There is no report of therapeutic drugs used to treat EHV-2/EHV-5 infections, probably because the disease associations with these viruses are equivocal.

Conclusion

Compared to other equine herpesviruses, EHV-1 is the most studied. EHV-1 is very common, induces severe clinical signs of disease, and represents an economic cost to all sectors of the equine industry. Future researche is essentially for the development of new management and vaccine programs. The relationship EHV-1 might have with other viral/bacterial infections and its implication for disease severity needs to be further investigated. Better understanding of the host factors, such as the individual genetic makeup (e.g. MHC), that influence all aspects of EHV life cycle and associated diseases is absolutely necessary.

Considering their high prevelance among equids, and lack of a clearly-defined association with clinical disease, research on the equine gammaherpesviruses is not regarded as a priority, and is likely to be conducted in only a few laboratories. Nevertheless, given EHV-2's potential to modulate, and hence potentially lower host immune responses, EHV-2 may prove to be an important factor in the outcome of disease of co-infecting pathogens. Thus it is important that efforts to learn more about equine gammaherpesviruses are continued.

References

[1] McGeoch, DJ; Dolan, A; Ralph, AC. Toward a comprehensive phylogeny for mammalian and avian herpesviruses. *J. Virol.* 2000;74(22):10401-10406.

[2] Davison, AJ. Evolution of the herpesviruses. *Vet. Microbiol.* 2002;86(1-2):69-88.

[3] McGeoch, DJ; Rixon, FJ; Davison, AJ. Topics in herpesvirus genomics and evolution. *Virus Res.* 2006;117(1):90-104.

[4] Kleiboeker, SB; Schommer, SK; Johnson, PJ; Ehlers, B; Turnquist, SE; Boucher, M; Kreeger, JM. Association of two newly recognized herpesviruses with interstitial pneumonia in donkeys (Equus asinus). *J. Vet. Diagn. Invest* 2002;14(4):273-80.

[5] Kleiboeker, SB; Turnquist, SE; Johnson, PJ; Kreeger, JM. Detection and nucleotide sequencing of a DNA-packaging protein gene of equine gammaherpesviruses. *J Vet Diagn. Invest* 2004;16(1):67-74.

[6] Crabb, BS; Studdert, MJ. Equine rhinopneumonitis (equine herpesvirus 4) and equine abortion (equine herpesvirus 1). In: Studdert MJ, editor. Virus infections of equines: Elsevier Sciences; 1996. p. 11-37.

[7] Ostlund, EN. The equine herpesviruses. *Vet. Clin. North Am. Equine Pract.* 1993;9(2):283-294.

[8] Taniguchi, A; Fukushi, H; Matsumura, T; Yanai, T; Masegi, T; Hirai, K. Pathogenicity of a new neurotropic equine herpesvirus 9 (gazelle herpesvirus 1) in horses. *J. Vet. Med. Sci.* 2000;62(2):215-218.

[9] Patel, JR; Heldens, J. Equine herpesviruses 1 (EHV-1) and 4 (EHV-4)--epidemiology, disease and immunoprophylaxis: a brief review. *Vet. J.* 2005;170(1):14-23.

[10] Borchers, K; Wiik, H; Frolich, K; Ludwig, H; East, ML. Antibodies against equine herpesviruses and equine arteritis virus in Burchell's zebras (Equus burchelli) from the Serengeti ecosystem. *J. Wildl Dis.* 2005;41(1):80-86.

[11] Fischer-Tenhagen, C; Hamblin, C; Quandt, S; Frolich, K. Serosurvey for selected infectious disease agents in free-ranging black and white rhinoceros in Africa. *J. Wildl Dis.* 2000;36(2):316-323.

[12] Allen, G. Respiratory infections by equine herpesvirus types 1 and 4. In: Lekeux P, editor. Equine respiratory diseases. Ithaca: International Veterinary Information Service (www.ivis.org); 2002.

[13] Paillot, R; Case, R; Ross, J; Newton, JR; Nugent, J. Equine Herpes Virus-1: Virus, Immunity and Vaccines. *The Open Veterinary Science Journal* 2008;2:68-91.

[14] Telford, EA; Watson, MS; McBride, K; Davison, AJ. The DNA sequence of equine herpesvirus-1. *Virology* 1992;189(1):304-316.

[15] Slater, J. Equine Herpesviruses. In: Sellon DC, Long MT, editors. Equine Infectious Diseases: Saunders Elseiver; 2007. p. pp 134-153.

[16] Perdue, ML; Kemp, MC; Randall, CC; O'Callaghan, DJ. Studies of the molecular anatomy of the L-M cell strain of equine herpes virus type 1: proteins of the nucleocapsid and intact virion. *Virology* 1974;59(1):201-216.

[17] Newcomb, WW; Brown, JC; Booy, FP; Steven, AC. Nucleocapsid mass and capsomer protein stoichiometry in equine herpesvirus 1: scanning transmission electron microscopic study. *J. Virol.* 1989;63(9):3777-3783.

[18] Baker, TS; Newcomb, WW; Booy, FP; Brown, JC; Steven, AC. Three-dimensional structures of maturable and abortive capsids of equine herpesvirus 1 from cryoelectron microscopy. *J. Virol.* 1990;64(2):563-573.

[19] Allen, G; Kydd, JH; Slater, J; Smith, KC. Advances in understanding of the pathogenesis, epidemiology and immunological control of equine herpesvirus abortion. In: U. Wernery JFW, J.A. Mumford and O-R. Kaaden, editor. Equine Infectious Diseases VIII: Proceedings of the 8th International Conference on Equine Infectious Diseases. Newmarket, UK: RandW Publications (Newmarket); 1999. p. 129-146.

[20] Osterrieder, N. Construction and characterization of an equine herpesvirus 1 glycoprotein C negative mutant. *Virus Res.* 1999;59(2):165-177.

[21] Frampton, AR, Jr.; Goins, WF; Cohen, JB; von Einem, J; Osterrieder, N; O'Callaghan, DJ; Glorioso, JC. Equine herpesvirus 1 utilizes a novel herpesvirus entry receptor. *J. Virol.* 2005;79(5):3169-3173.

[22] Csellner, H; Walker, C; Wellington, JE; McLure, LE; Love, DN; Whalley, JM. EHV-1 glycoprotein D (EHV-1 gD) is required for virus entry and cell-cell fusion, and an EHV-1 gD deletion mutant induces a protective immune response in mice. *Arch. Virol.* 2000;145(11):2371-2385.

[23] Osterrieder, N; Neubauer, A; Brandmuller, C; Braun, B; Kaaden, OR; Baines, JD. The equine herpesvirus 1 glycoprotein gp21/22a, the herpes simplex virus type 1 gM homolog, is involved in virus penetration and cell-to-cell spread of virions. *J. Virol.* 1996;70(6):4110-4115.

[24] Frampton, AR, Jr.; Stolz, DB; Uchida, H; Goins, WF; Cohen, JB; Glorioso, JC. Equine herpesvirus 1 enters cells by two different pathways, and infection requires the activation of the cellular kinase ROCK1. *J. Virol.* 2007;81(20):10879-10889.

[25] Whittaker, GR; Helenius, A. Nuclear import and export of viruses and virus genomes. *Virology* 1998;246(1):1-23.

[26] Purewal, AS; Allsopp, R; Riggio, M; Telford, EA; Azam, S; Davison, AJ; Edington, N. Equid herpesviruses 1 and 4 encode functional homologs of the herpes simplex virus type 1 virion transactivator protein, VP16. *Virology* 1994;198(1):385-389.

[27] Gray, WL; Baumann, RP; Robertson, AT; Caughman, GB; O'Callaghan, DJ; Staczek, J. Regulation of equine herpesvirus type 1 gene expression: characterization of immediate early, early, and late transcription. *Virology* 1987;158(1):79-87.

[28] Gray, WL; Baumann, RP; Robertson, AT; O'Callaghan, DJ; Staczek, J. Characterization and mapping of equine herpesvirus type 1 immediate early, early, and late transcripts. *Virus Res.* 1987;8(3):233-244.

[29] Garko-Buczynski, KA; Smith, RH; Kim, SK; O'Callaghan, DJ. Complementation of a replication-defective mutant of equine herpesvirus type 1 by a cell line expressing the immediate-early protein. *Virology* 1998;248(1):83-94.

[30] Neubauer, A; Braun, B; Brandmuller, C; Kaaden, OR; Osterrieder, N. Analysis of the contributions of the equine herpesvirus 1 glycoprotein gB homolog to virus entry and direct cell-to-cell spread. *Virology* 1997;227(2):281-294.

[31] Wellington, JE; Love, DN; Whalley, JM. Evidence for involvement of equine herpesvirus 1 glycoprotein B in cell-cell fusion. *Arch. Virol.* 1996;141(1):167-175.

[32] Neubauer, A; Osterrieder, N. Equine herpesvirus type 1 (EHV-1) glycoprotein K is required for efficient cell-to-cell spread and virus egress. *Virology* 2004;329(1):18-32.

[33] Reed, SM; Toribio, RE. Equine herpesvirus 1 and 4. *Vet. Clin. North Am. Equine Pract* 2004;20(3):631-642.

[34] Kydd, JH; Smith, KC; Hannant, D; Livesay, GJ; Mumford, JA. Distribution of equid herpesvirus-1 (EHV-1) in respiratory tract associated lymphoid tissue: implications for cellular immunity. *Equine Vet. J.* 1994;26(6):470-473.

[35] Kydd, JH; Smith, KC; Hannant, D; Livesay, GJ; Mumford, JA. Distribution of equid herpesvirus-1 (EHV-1) in the respiratory tract of ponies: implications for vaccination strategies. *Equine Vet. J.* 1994;26(6):466-469.

[36] Damiani, AM; Matsumura, T; Yokoyama, N; Mikami, T; Takahashi, E. A deletion in the gI and gE genes of equine herpesvirus type 4 reduces viral virulence in the natural host and affects virus transmission during cell-to-cell spread. *Virus Res.* 2000;67(2):189-202.

[37] Heldens, JG; Hannant, D; Cullinane, AA; Prendergast, MJ; Mumford, JA; Nelly, M; Kydd, JH; Weststrate, MW; van den Hoven, R. Clinical and virological evaluation of the efficacy of an inactivated EHV1 and EHV4 whole virus vaccine (Duvaxyn EHV1,4). Vaccination/challenge experiments in foals and pregnant mares. *Vaccine* 2001;19(30):4307-4317.

[38] Patel, JR; Foldi, J; Bateman, H; Williams, J; Didlick, S; Stark, R. Equid herpesvirus (EHV-1) live vaccine strain C147: efficacy against respiratory diseases following EHV types 1 and 4 challenges. *Vet. Microbiol.* 2003;92(1-2):1-17.

[39] Edington, N; Chester, P; Azam, S; Welch, H; McGladdery, AJ; Purewal, AS. Profiles of α-herpesviruses in circulating leucocytes from thoroughbred mares and foals using PCR and co-cultivation. In: H. Nakajima and W. Plowright, editor. Equine Infectious Diseases VII: *Proceedings of Seventh International Conference on Equine Infectious Diseases.* Newmarket, UK: R and W Publications Ltd; 1994. p. 251-254.

[40] Slater, J; Baxi, M; Tewari, D; Gibson, JS; Field, HJ; Ludwig, H; Steinbach, F; Borchers, K. Experimental infection of specific pathogen-free ponies with Equid herpesvirus-1: detection of infectious virus and viral DNA. In: H. Nakajima and W. Plowright, editor. Equine Infectious Diseases VII: *Proceedings of Seventh International Conference on Equine Infectious Diseases.* Newmarket, UK: R and W Publications Ltd; 1994. p. 255-260.

[41] van Der Meulen, KM; Nauwynck, HJ; Buddaert, W; Pensaert, MB. Replication of equine herpesvirus type 1 in freshly isolated equine peripheral blood mononuclear cells and changes in susceptibility following mitogen stimulation. *J. Gen. Virol.* 2000;81(Pt 1):21-25.

[42] van der Meulen, KM; Nauwynck, HJ; Pensaert, MB. Mitogen stimulation favours replication of equine herpesvirus-1 in equine blood mononuclear cells by inducing cell proliferation and formation of close intercellular contacts. *J. Gen. Virol.* 2001;82(Pt 8):1951-1957.

[43] Siedek, EM; Edington, N; Hamblin, A. Equine dendritic cell infection with equid herpesvirus type 1 reduces their ability to support mitogenic T cell proliferation. *Biochem. Soc. Trans* 1997;25(2):283S.

[44] Siedek, EM; Whelan, M; Edington, N; Hamblin, A. Equine herpesvirus type 1 infects dendritic cells in vitro: stimulation of T lymphocyte proliferation and cytotoxicity by infected dendritic cells. *Vet. Immunol. Immunopathol.* 1999;67:17-32.

[45] Allen, GP; Bryans, JT. Molecular epizootiology, pathogenesis, and prophylaxis of equine herpesvirus-1 infections. *Prog. Vet Microbiol. Immunol.* 1986;2:78-144.

[46] Smith, DJ; Iqbal, J; Purewal, A; Hamblin, AS; Edington, N. In vitro reactivation of latent equid herpesvirus-1 from CD5+/CD8+ leukocytes indirectly by IL-2 or chorionic gonadotrophin. *J. Gen. Virol.* 1998;79 (Pt 12):2997-3004.

[47] Timoney, PJ. Rhinopneumonitis and viral abortion. In: Castro AEH, W.P., editor. *Veterinary diagnostic virology*. St Louis: Mosby Year Book Inc.; 1992. p. 173-177.

[48] Borchers, K; Thein, R; Sterner-Kock, A. Pathogenesis of equine herpesvirus-associated neurological disease: a revised explanation. *Equine Vet. J.* 2006;38(3):283-287.

[49] McCartan, CG; Russell, MM; Wood, JL; Mumford, JA. Clinical, serological and virological characteristics of an outbreak of paresis and neonatal foal disease due to equine herpesvirus-1 on a stud farm. *Vet. Rec.* 1995;136(1):7-12.

[50] Slater, JD; Gibson, JS; Barnett, KC; Field, HJ. Chorioretinopathy associated with neuropathology following infection with equine herpesvirus-1. *Vet. Rec.* 1992;131(11):237-239.

[51] Efstathiou, S; Preston, CM. Towards an understanding of the molecular basis of herpes simplex virus latency. *Virus Res.* 2005;111(2):108-119.

[52] Welch, HM; Bridges, CG; Lyon, AM; Griffiths, L; Edington, N. Latent equid herpesviruses 1 and 4: detection and distinction using the polymerase chain reaction and co-cultivation from lymphoid tissues. *J. Gen. Virol.* 1992;73 (Pt 2):261-268.

[53] Baxi, MK; Efstathiou, S; Lawrence, G; Whalley, JM; Slater, JD; Field, HJ. The detection of latency-associated transcripts of equine herpesvirus 1 in ganglionic neurons. *J. Gen. Virol.* 1995;76 (Pt 12):3113-3118.

[54] Chesters, PM; Allsop, R; Purewal, A; Edington, N. Detection of latency-associated transcripts of equid herpesvirus 1 in equine leukocytes but not in trigeminal ganglia. *J. Virol.* 1997;71(5):3437-3443.

[55] Borchers, K; Wolfinger, U; Ludwig, H. Latency-associated transcripts of equine herpesvirus type 4 in trigeminal ganglia of naturally infected horses. *J. Gen. Virol.* 1999;80 (Pt 8):2165-2171.

[56] Slater, JD; Borchers, K; Thackray, AM; Field, HJ. The trigeminal ganglion is a location for equine herpesvirus 1 latency and reactivation in the horse. *J. Gen. Virol.* 1994;75 (Pt 8):2007-2016.

[57] Allen, GP. Antemortem detection of latent infection with neuropathogenic strains of equine herpesvirus-1 in horses. *Am. J. Vet. Res.* 2006;67(8):1401-1405.

[58] Allen, GP; Bolin, DC; Bryant, U; Carter, CN; Giles, RC; Harrison, LR; Hong, CB; Jackson, CB; Poonacha, K; Wharton, R; Williams, NM. Prevalence of latent, neuropathogenic equine herpesvirus-1 in the Thoroughbred broodmare population of central Kentucky. *Equine Vet. J.* 2008;40(2):105-110.

[59] Allen, GP; Yeargan, MR; Turtinen, LW; Bryans, JT. A new field strain of equine abortion virus (equine herpesvirus-1) among Kentucky horses. *Am. J. Vet. Res.* 1985;46(1):138-140.

[60] Binns, MM; McCann, S; zhang, L; Wood, J; Mumford, JA. Molecular epidemiology of EHV-1 and EHV-4: a search for variable restriction sites. In: H. Nakajima and W. Plowright, editor. Equine Infectious Diseases VII: Proceedings of Seventh International Conference on Equine Infectious Diseases. Newmarket, UK: R and W Publications Ltd; 1994. p. 237-241.

[61] Galosi, CM; Norimine, J; Echeverria, MG; Oliva, GA; Nosetto, EO; Etcheverrigaray, ME; Tohya, Y; Mikami, T. Diversity of genomic electropherotypes of naturally occurring equine herpesvirus 1 isolates in Argentina. *Braz. J. Med. Biol. Res.* 1998;31(6):771-774.

[62] Pagamjav, O; Sakata, T; Matsumura, T; Yamaguchi, T; Fukushi, H. Natural recombinant between equine herpesviruses 1 and 4 in the ICP4 gene. *Microbiol. Immunol.* 2005;49(2):167-179.

[63] Crowhurst, FA; Dickinson, G; Burrows, R. An outbreak of paresis in mares and geldings associated with equid herpesvirus 1. *Vet. Rec.* 1981;109(24):527-528.

[64] Mumford, JA; Hannant, D; Jessett, DM; O'Neill, T; Smith, KC; Ostlund, EN. Abortigenic and neurological disease caused by experimental infection with Equid herpesvirus-1. In: H. Nakajima and W. Plowright, editor. Equine Infectious Diseases VII: Proceedings of Seventh International Conference on Equine Infectious Diseases. Newmarket, UK: R and W Publications Ltd; 1994. p. 261-275.

[65] Smith, KC; Whitwell, KE; Mumford, JA; Hannant, D; Blunden, AS; Tearle, JP. Virulence of the V592 isolate of equid herpesvirus-1 in ponies. *J. Comp. Pathol.* 2000;122(4):288-297.

[66] Nugent, J; Birch-Machin, I; Smith, KC; Mumford, JA; Swann, Z; Newton, JR; Bowden, RJ; Allen, GP; Davis-Poynter, N. Analysis of equid herpesvirus 1 strain variation reveals a point mutation of the DNA polymerase strongly associated with neuropathogenic versus nonneuropathogenic disease outbreaks. *J. Virol.* 2006;80(8):4047-4060.

[67] Allen, GP. Development of a real-time polymerase chain reaction assay for rapid diagnosis of neuropathogenic strains of equine herpesvirus-1. *J. Vet. Diagn Invest.* 2007;19(1):69-72.

[68] Pusterla, N; Mapes, S; Wilson, WD. Use of viral loads in blood and nasopharyngeal secretions for the diagnosis of EHV-1 infection in field cases. *Vet Rec* 2008;162(22):728-9.

[69] Goodman, LB; Loregian, A; Perkins, GA; Nugent, J; Buckles, EL; Mercorelli, B; Kydd, JH; Palu, G; Smith, KC; Osterrieder, N; Davis-Poynter, N. A point mutation in a herpesvirus polymerase determines neuropathogenicity. *PLoS Pathog* 2007;3(11):e160.

[70] Rudolph, J; O'Callaghan, DJ; Osterrieder, N. Cloning of the genomes of equine herpesvirus type 1 (EHV-1) strains KyA and racL11 as bacterial artificial chromosomes (BAC). *J. Vet. Med. B Infect Dis. Vet. Public Health* 2002;49(1):31-36.

[71] Yamada, S; Matsumura, T; Tsujimura, K; Yamaguchi, T; Ohya, K; Fukushi, H. Comparison of the growth kinetics of neuropathogenic and nonneuropathogenic equid herpesvirus type 1 (EHV-1) strains in cultured murine neuronal cells and the relevance of the D/N(752) coding change in DNA polymerase gene (ORF30). *J. Vet. Med. Sci.* 2008;70(5):505-11.

[72] Plummer, G; Waterson, AP. Equine herpes viruses. *Virology* 1963;19:412-6.

[73] Browning, GF; Studdert, MJ. Genomic heterogeneity of equine betaherpesviruses. *J. Gen. Virol.* 1987;68 (Pt 5):1441-7.

[74] Agius, CT; Nagesha, HS; Studdert, MJ. Equine herpesvirus 5: comparisons with EHV2 (equine cytomegalovirus), cloning, and mapping of a new equine herpesvirus with a novel genome structure. *Virology* 1992;191(1):176-86.

[75] Telford, EA; Studdert, MJ; Agius, CT; Watson, MS; Aird, HC; Davison, AJ. Equine herpesviruses 2 and 5 are gamma-herpesviruses. *Virology* 1993;195(2):492-9.

[76] Telford, EA; Watson, MS; Aird, HC; Perry, J; Davison, AJ. The DNA sequence of equine herpesvirus 2. *J. Mol. Biol.* 1995;249(3):520-8.

[77] Sharp, EL; Farrell, HE; Borchers, K; Holmes, EC; Davis-Poynter, NJ. Sequence analysis of the equid herpesvirus 2 chemokine receptor homologues E1, ORF74 and E6 demonstrates high sequence divergence between field isolates. *J. Gen. Virol.* 2007;88(Pt 9):2450-62.

[78] Browning, GF; Studdert, MJ. Physical mapping of the genomic heterogeneity of isolates of equine herpesvirus 2 (equine cytomegalovirus). *Arch. Virol.* 1989;104(1-2):87-94.

[79] Plummer, G; Goodheart, CR; Studdert, MJ. Equine herpesviruses: antigenic relationships and deoxyribonucleic acid densities. *Infect Immun.* 1973;8(4):621-7.

[80] Plummer, G; Bowling, CP; Goodheart, CR. Comparison of four horse herpesviruses. *J Virol.* 1969;4(5):738-41.

[81] Studdert, MJ; Turner, AJ; Peterson, JE. Equine herpesviruses. I. Isolation and characterisation of equine rhinopneumonitis virus and other equine herpesviruses from horses. *Aust. Vet. J.* 1970;46(3):83-9.

[82] Schynts, F; Meurens, F; Detry, B; Vanderplasschen, A; Thiry, E. Rise and survival of bovine herpesvirus 1 recombinants after primary infection and reactivation from latency. *J. Virol.* 2003;77(23):12535-42.

[83] Kakoola, DN; Sheldon, J; Byabazaire, N; Bowden, RJ; Katongole-Mbidde, E; Schulz, TF; Davison, AJ. Recombination in human herpesvirus-8 strains from Uganda and evolution of the K15 gene. *J. Gen. Virol.* 2001;82(Pt 10):2393-404.

[84] Norberg, P; Bergstrom, T; Rekabdar, E; Lindh, M; Liljeqvist, JA. Phylogenetic analysis of clinical herpes simplex virus type 1 isolates identified three genetic groups and recombinant viruses. *J. Virol.* 2004;78(19):10755-64.

[85] Poole, LJ; Zong, JC; Ciufo, DM; Alcendor, DJ; Cannon, JS; Ambinder, R; Orenstein, JM; Reitz, MS; Hayward, GS. Comparison of genetic variability at multiple loci across the genomes of the major subtypes of Kaposi's sarcoma-associated herpesvirus reveals evidence for recombination and for two distinct types of open reading frame K15 alleles at the right-hand end. *J. Virol.* 1999;73(8):6646-60.

[86] Rasmussen, L; Geissler, A; Cowan, C; Chase, A; Winters, M. The genes encoding the gCIII complex of human cytomegalovirus exist in highly diverse combinations in clinical isolates. *J. Virol.* 2002;76(21):10841-8.

[87] Zong, J; Ciufo, DM; Viscidi, R; Alagiozoglou, L; Tyring, S; Rady, P; Orenstein, J; Boto, W; Kalumbuja, H; Romano, N; Melbye, M; Kang, GH; Boshoff, C; Hayward, GS. Genotypic analysis at multiple loci across Kaposi's sarcoma herpesvirus (KSHV) DNA molecules: clustering patterns, novel variants and chimerism. *J. Clin. Virol.* 2002;23(3):119-48.

[88] Collinson, P; O'Rielly, JL; Ficorilli, N; Studdert, MJ. Isolation of equine herpesvirus type 2 (equine gammaherpesvirus 2) from foals with keratoconjunctivitis. *J. Am. Vet. Med. Assoc.* 1994;205(2):329-31.

[89] Kershaw, O; von Oppen, T; Glitz, F; Deegen, E; Ludwig, H; Borchers, K. Detection of equine herpesvirus type 2 (EHV-2) in horses with keratoconjunctivitis. *Virus Res.* 2001;80(1-2):93-9.

[90] Murray, MJ; Eichorn, ES; Dubovi, EJ; Ley, WB; Cavey, DM. Equine herpesvirus type 2: prevalence and seroepidemiology in foals. *Equine Vet. J.* 1996;28(6):432-6.

[91] Nordengrahn, A; Rusvai, M; Merza, M; Ekstrom, J; Morein, B; Belak, S. Equine herpesvirus type 2 (EHV-2) as a predisposing factor for Rhodococcus equi pneumonia in foals: prevention of the bifactorial disease with EHV-2 immunostimulating complexes. *Vet. Microbiol.* 1996;51(1-2):55-68.

[92] Purewal, AS; Smallwood, AV; Kaushal, A; Adegboye, D; Edington, N. Identification and control of the cis-acting elements of the immediate early gene of equid herpesvirus type 1. *J. Gen. Virol.* 1992;73 (Pt 3):513-9.

[93] Welch, HM; Bridges, CG; Lyon, AM; Griffiths, L; Edington, N. Latent equid herpesviruses 1 and 4: detection and distinction using the polymerase chain reaction and co-cultivation from lymphoid tissues. *J. Gen. Virol.* 1992;73 (Pt 2):261-8.

[94] Franchini, M; Akens, M; Bracher, V; von Fellenberg, R. Characterisation of gamma herpesviruses in the horse by PCR. *Virology* 1997;238(1):8-13.

[95] Dunowska, M; Meers, J; Wilks, CR. Isolation of equine herpesvirus type 5 in New Zealand. *N Z Vet. J.* 1999;47(2):44-6.

[96] Dunowska, M; Holloway, SA; Wilks, CR; Meers, J. Genomic variability of equine herpesvirus-5. *Arch. Virol.* 2000;145(7):1359-71.

[97] Nordengrahn, A; Merza, M; Ros, C; Lindholmc, A; Palfl, V; Hannant, D; Belak, S. Prevalence of equine herpesvirus types 2 and 5 in horse populations by using type-specific PCR assays. *Vet. Res.* 2002;33(3):251-9.

[98] Bell, SA; Balasuriya, UB; Nordhausen, RW; MacLachlan, NJ. Isolation of equine herpesvirus-5 from blood mononuclear cells of a gelding. *J. Vet. Diagn. Invest.* 2006;18(5):472-5.

[99] Agius, CT; Studdert, MJ. Equine herpesviruses 2 and 5: comparisons with other members of the subfamily gammaherpesvirinae. *Adv. Virus Res.* 1994;44:357-79.

[100] Borchers, K; Frolich, K; Ludwig, H. Detection of equine herpesvirus types 2 and 5 (EHV-2 and EHV-5) in Przewalski's wild horses. *Arch. Virol.* 1999;144(4):771-80.

[101] Agius, CT; Crabb, BS; Telford, EA; Davison, AJ; Studdert, MJ. Comparative studies of the structural proteins and glycoproteins of equine herpesviruses 2 and 5. *J. Gen. Virol.* 1994;75 (Pt 10):2707-17.

[102] Williams, KJ; Maes, R; Del Piero, F; Lim, A; Wise, A; Bolin, DC; Caswell, J; Jackson, C; Robinson, NE; Derksen, F; Scott, MA; Uhal, BD; Li, X; Youssef, SA; Bolin, SR. Equine multinodular pulmonary fibrosis: a newly recognized herpesvirus-associated fibrotic lung disease. *Vet. Pathol.* 2007;44(6):849-62.

[103] Crabb, BS; Studdert, MJ. Equine herpesviruses 4 (equine rhinopneumonitis virus) and 1 (equine abortion virus). *Adv. Virus Res.* 1995;45:153-90.

[104] Browning, GF; Ficorilli, N; Studdert, MJ. Asinine herpesvirus genomes: comparison with those of the equine herpesviruses. *Arch. Virol.* 1988;101(3-4):183-90.

[105] Ehlers, B; Borchers, K; Grund, C; Frolich, K; Ludwig, H; Buhk, HJ. Detection of new DNA polymerase genes of known and potentially novel herpesviruses by PCR with degenerate and deoxyinosine-substituted primers. *Virus Genes* 1999;18(3):211-20.

[106] Borchers, K; Wiik, H; Frolich, K; Ludwig, H; East, ML. Antibodies against equine herpesviruses and equine arteritis virus in Burchell's zebras (Equus burchelli) from the Serengeti ecosystem. *J. Wildl Dis.* 2005;41(1):80-6.
[107] Fukushi, H; Taniguchi, A; Yasuda, K; Yanai, T; Masegi, T; Yamaguchi, T; Hirai, K. A hamster model of equine herpesvirus 9 induced encephalitis. *J. Neurovirol.* 2000;6(4):314-9.
[108] Narita, M; Uchimura, A; Kimura, K; Tanimura, N; Yanai, T; Masegi, T; Fukushi, H; Hirai, K. Brain lesions and transmission of experimental equine herpesvirus type 9 in pigs. *Vet. Pathol.* 2000;37(5):476-9.
[109] Taniguchi, A; Fukushi, H; Yanai, T; Masegi, T; Yamaguchi, T; Hirai, K. Equine herpesvirus 9 induced lethal encephalomyelitis in experimentally infected goats. *Arch. Virol.* 2000;145(12):2619-27.
[110] Yanai, T; Tujioka, S; Sakai, H; Fukushi, H; Hirai, K; Masegi, T. Experimental infection with equine herpesvirus 9 (EHV-9) in cats. *J. Comp. Pathol.* 2003;128(2-3):113-8.
[111] Yanai, T; Fujishima, N; Fukushi, H; Hirata, A; Sakai, H; Masegi, T. Experimental infection of equine herpesvirus 9 in dogs. *Vet. Pathol.* 2003;40(3):263-7.
[112] Kodama, A; Yanai, T; Yomemaru, K; Sakai, H; Masegi, T; Yamada, S; Fukushi, H; Kuraishi, T; Hattori, S; Kai, C. Acute neuropathogenicity with experimental infection of equine herpesvirus 9 in common marmosets (Callithrix jacchus). *J. Med. Primatol.* 2007;36(6):335-42.
[113] Crabb, BS; MacPherson, CM; Reubel, GH; Browning, GF; Studdert, MJ; Drummer, HE. A type-specific serological test to distinguish antibodies to equine herpesviruses 4 and 1. *Arch. Virol.* 1995;140(2):245-258.
[114] Edington, N; Welch, HM; Griffiths, L. The prevalence of latent Equid herpesviruses in the tissues of 40 abattoir horses. *Equine Vet. J.* 1994;26(2):140-142.
[115] Taouji, S; Collobert, C; Gicquel, B; Sailleau, C; Brisseau, N; Moussu, C; Breuil, MF; Pronost, S; Borchers, K; Zientara, S. Detection and isolation of equine herpesviruses 1 and 4 from horses in Normandy: an autopsy study of tissue distribution in relation to vaccination status. *J. Vet. Med. B Infect Dis. Vet. Public Health* 2002;49(8):394-399.
[116] Slater, J. *Epidemiology and control of EHV-1 infections*. In: ACVIM Forum; 2006; 2006.
[117] Gilkerson, JR; Whalley, JM; Drummer, HE; Studdert, MJ; Love, DN. Epidemiological studies of equine herpesvirus 1 (EHV-1) in Thoroughbred foals: a review of studies conducted in the Hunter Valley of New South Wales between 1995 and 1997. *Vet. Microbiol.* 1999;68(1-2):15-25.
[118] Foote, CE; Love, DN; Gilkerson, JR; Whalley, JM. Detection of EHV-1 and EHV-4 DNA in unweaned Thoroughbred foals from vaccinated mares on a large stud farm. *Equine Vet. J.* 2004;36(4):341-345.
[119] Gilkerson, JR; Love, DN; Drummer, HE; Studdert, MJ; Whalley, JM. Seroprevalence of equine herpesvirus 1 in thoroughbred foals before and after weaning. *Aust. Vet. J.* 1998;76(10):677-682.

[120] Gilkerson, JR; Whalley, JM; Drummer, HE; Studdert, MJ; Love, DN. Epidemiology of EHV-1 and EHV-4 in the mare and foal populations on a Hunter Valley stud farm: are mares the source of EHV-1 for unweaned foals. *Vet. Microbiol.* 1999;68(1-2):27-34.

[121] Brown, JA; Mapes, S; Ball, BA; Hodder, AD; Liu, IK; Pusterla, N. Prevalence of equine herpesvirus-1 infection among Thoroughbreds residing on a farm on which the virus was endemic. *J. Am. Vet Med. Assoc.* 2007;231(4):577-580.

[122] Reed, SM; Allen, G; Henninger, RW. Equine herpes virus 1 myeloencephalopathy. In: CL Davis Foundation-AAEP pre meeting symposium; 2007; Orlando (US); 2007.

[123] Goehring, LS; van Winden, SC; van Maanen, C; Sloet van Oldruitenborgh-Oosterbaan, MM. Equine herpesvirus type 1-associated myeloencephalopathy in The Netherlands: a four-year retrospective study (1999-2003). *J. Vet. Intern. Med.* 2006;20(3):601-607.

[124] Henninger, RW; Reed, SM; Saville, WJ; Allen, GP; Hass, GF; Kohn, CW; Sofaly, C. Outbreak of neurologic disease caused by equine herpesvirus-1 at a university equestrian center. *J. Vet. Intern. Med.* 2007;21(1):157-165.

[125] Rizvi, SM; Slater, JD; Wolfinger, U; Borchers, K; Field, HJ; Slade, AJ. Detection and distribution of equine herpesvirus 2 DNA in the central and peripheral nervous systems of ponies. *J. Gen. Virol.* 1997;78 (Pt 5):1115-8.

[126] Drummer, HE; Reubel, GH; Studdert, MJ. Equine gammaherpesvirus 2 (EHV2) is latent in B lymphocytes. *Arch. Virol.* 1996;141(3-4):495-504.

[127] Doll, ER; Crowe, ME; Bryans, JT; Mc, CW. Infection immunity in equine virus abortion. *Cornell Vet.* 1955;45(3):387-410.

[128] Kydd, JH; Hannant, D; Mumford, JA. Residence and recruitment of leucocytes to the equine lung after EHV-1 infection. *Vet. Immunol Immunopathol.* 1996;52(1-2):15-26.

[129] Edington, N; Bridges, CG; Griffiths, L. Equine interferons following exposure to equid herpesvirus-1 or -4. *J. Interferon Res.* 1989;9(4):389-392.

[130] Hannant, D; Jessett, DM; O'Neill, T; Dolby, CA; Cook, RF; Mumford, JA. Responses of ponies to equid herpesvirus-1 ISCOM vaccination and challenge with virus of the homologous strain. *Res. Vet. Sci.* 1993;54(3):299-305.

[131] Sugiura, T; Kondo, T; Matsumura, T; Kamada, M. IgG subclass responses in equind herpesvirus-1 infected horses. In: H. Nakajima and W. Plowright, editor. Equine Infectious Diseases VII: *Proceedings of Seventh International Conference on Equine Infectious Diseases*. Newmarket, UK: R and W Publications Ltd; 1994. p. 350.

[132] Breathnach, CC; Yeargan, MR; Sheoran, AS; Allen, GP. The mucosal humoral immune response of the horse to infective challenge and vaccination with equine herpesvirus-1 antigens. *Equine Vet. J.* 2001;33(7):651-657.

[133] Mumford, JA; Rossdale, PD; Jessett, DM; Gann, SJ; Ousey, J; Cook, RF. Serological and virological investigations of an equid herpesvirus 1 (EHV-1) abortion storm on a stud farm in 1985. *J. Reprod Fertil Suppl.* 1987;35:509-518.

[134] Paillot, R; Daly, J; Juillard, V; Minke, JM; Hannant, D; Kydd, JH. Equine interferon gamma synthesis in lymphocytes after in vivo infection and in vitro stimulation with EHV-1. *Vaccine* 2005;23(36):4541-4551.

[135] Paillot, R; Ellis, SA; Daly, JM; Audonnet, JC; Minke, JM; Davis-Poynter, N; D., H; Kydd, JH. Characterisation of CTL and IFN-γ synthesis in ponies following

vaccination with a NYVAC-based construct coding for EHV-1 immediate early gene, followed by challenge infection. *Vaccine* 2006;24(10):1490-1500.

[136] Breathnach, CC; Soboll, G; Suresh, M; Lunn, DP. Equine herpesvirus-1 infection induces IFN-gamma production by equine T lymphocyte subsets. *Vet. Immunol. Immunopathol.* 2005;103(3-4):207-215.

[137] Paillot, R; Daly, JM; Luce, R; Montesso, F; Davis-Poynter, N; Hannant, D; Kydd, JH. Frequency and phenotype of EHV-1 specific, IFN-gamma synthesising lymphocytes in ponies: The effects of age, pregnancy and infection. *Dev. Comp. Immunol.* 2007;31(2):202-214.

[138] O'Neill, T; Kydd, JH; Allen, GP; Wattrang, E; Mumford, JA; Hannant, D. Determination of equid herpesvirus 1-specific, CD8+, cytotoxic T lymphocyte precursor frequencies in ponies. *Vet. Immunol. Immunopathol.* 1999;70(1-2):43-54.

[139] Darji, A; Beschin, A; Sileghem, M; Heremans, H; Brys, L; De Baetselier, P. In vitro simulation of immunosuppression caused by Trypanosoma brucei: active involvement of gamma interferon and tumor necrosis factor in the pathway of suppression. *Infect Immun.* 1996;64(6):1937-1943.

[140] Wherry, EJ; Blattman, JN; Murali-Krishna, K; van der Most, R; Ahmed, R. Viral persistence alters CD8 T-cell immunodominance and tissue distribution and results in distinct stages of functional impairment. *J. Virol.* 2003;77(8):4911-4927.

[141] Crough, T; Burrows, JM; Fazou, C; Walker, S; Davenport, MP; Khanna, R. Contemporaneous fluctuations in T cell responses to persistent herpes virus infections. *Eur. J. Immunol.* 2005;35(1):139-149.

[142] Coombs, DK; Patton, T; Kohler, AK; Soboll, G; Breathnach, C; Townsend, HG; Lunn, DP. Cytokine responses to EHV-1 infection in immune and non-immune ponies. *Vet. Immunol. Immunopathol.* 2006;111(1-2):109-116.

[143] Asanuma, H; Sharp, M; Maecker, HT; Maino, VC; Arvin, AM. Frequencies of memory T cells specific for varicella-zoster virus, herpes simplex virus, and cytomegalovirus by intracellular detection of cytokine expression. *J. Infect. Dis.* 2000;181(3):859-866.

[144] Waldrop, SL; Pitcher, CJ; Peterson, DM; Maino, VC; Picker, LJ. Determination of antigen-specific memory/effector CD4+ T cell frequencies by flow cytometry: evidence for a novel, antigen-specific homeostatic mechanism in HIV-associated immunodeficiency. *J. Clin. Invest.* 1997;99(7):1739-1750.

[145] Bridges, CG; Edington, N. The proteins of equid herpesvirus 1 (EHV 1) recognised by equine antisera and their ability to promote antibody-dependent cell-mediated cytotoxicity. *Tierarztl Prax Suppl.* 1987;2:47-49.

[146] Chong, YC; Duffus, WP; Hannant, D. Natural killer cells in normal horses and specific-pathogen-free foals infected with equine herpesvirus. *Vet. Immunol. Immunopathol.* 1992;33(1-2):103-113.

[147] McCulloch, J; Williamson, SA; Powis, SJ; Edington, N. The effect of EHV-1 infection upon circulating leucocyte populations in the natural equine host. *Vet Microbiol* 1993;37(1-2):147-161.

[148] Breathnach, CC; Yeargan, MR; Timoney, JF; Allen, GP. Detection of equine herpesvirus-specific effector and memory cytotoxic immunity in the equine upper respiratory tract. *Vet. Immunol. Immunopathol.* 2006;111(1-2):117-125.

[149] Allen, G; Yeargan, M; Costa, LR; Cross, R. Major histocompatibility complex class I-restricted cytotoxic T-lymphocyte responses in horses infected with equine herpesvirus 1. *J. Virol.* 1995;69(1):606-612.
[150] Kydd, JH; Wattrang, E; Hannant, D. Pre-infection frequencies of equine herpesvirus-1 specific, cytotoxic T lymphocytes correlate with protection against abortion following experimental infection of pregnant mares. *Vet. Immunol. Immunopathol.* 2003;96(3-4):207-217.
[151] O'Neill, T. T Lymphocyte Responses to Equid Herpesvirus 1 and 4 in Horses. PhD Thesis: OPEN University; 1995.
[152] Soboll, G; Whalley, JM; Koen, MT; Allen, GP; Fraser, DG; Macklin, MD; Swain, WF; Lunn, DP. Identification of equine herpesvirus-1 antigens recognized by cytotoxic T lymphocytes. *J. Gen. Virol.* 2003;84(Pt 10):2625-2634.
[153] Bodo, G; Marti, E; Gaillard, M; Weiss, M; Bruckner, L; Gerber, H; Lazary, S. Association of the immune response with the major histocompatibility complex in the horse. In: H. Nakajima and W. Plowright, editor. Equine Infectious Diseases VII: Proceedings of Seventh International Conference on Equine Infectious Diseases. Newmarket, UK: R and W Publications Ltd; 1994. p. 143-151.
[154] Antczak, DF. The major histocompatibility complex of the horse. In: Plowright W, Rossdale, P.D. and Wade, J.F., editor. Equine Infectious Diseases VI, *Proceedings of the Sixth International Conference*. Newmarket: R and W Publications Ltd; 1992. p. 99-112.
[155] Ellis, SA; Martin, AJ; Holmes, EC; Morrison, WI. At least four MHC class I genes are transcribed in the horse: phylogenetic analysis suggests an unusual evolutionary history for the MHC in this species. *Eur. J. Immunogenet* 1995;22(3):249-260.
[156] Tallmadge, RL; Lear, TL; Antczak, DF. Genomic characterization of MHC class I genes of the horse. *Immunogenetics* 2005;57(10):763-774.
[157] Kydd, JH; Davis-Poynter, NJ; Birch, J; Hannant, D; Minke, J; Audonnet, JC; Antczak, DF; Ellis, SA. A molecular approach to the identification of cytotoxic T-lymphocyte epitopes within equine herpesvirus 1. *J. Gen. Virol.* 2006;87(Pt 9):2507-2515.
[158] Huemer, HP; Nowotny, N; Crabb, BS; Meyer, H; Hubert, PH. gp13 (EHV-gC): a complement receptor induced by equine herpesviruses. *Virus Res.* 1995;37(2):113-126.
[159] Lubinski, J; Wang, L; Mastellos, D; Sahu, A; Lambris, JD; Friedman, HM. In vivo role of complement-interacting domains of herpes simplex virus type 1 glycoprotein gC. *J. Exp. Med.* 1999;190(11):1637-1646.
[160] Judson, KA; Lubinski, JM; Jiang, M; Chang, Y; Eisenberg, RJ; Cohen, GH; Friedman, HM. Blocking immune evasion as a novel approach for prevention and treatment of herpes simplex virus infection. *J. Virol.* 2003;77(23):12639-12645.
[161] Lubinski, JM; Jiang, M; Hook, L; Chang, Y; Sarver, C; Mastellos, D; Lambris, JD; Cohen, GH; Eisenberg, RJ; Friedman, HM. Herpes simplex virus type 1 evades the effects of antibody and complement in vivo. *J. Virol.* 2002;76(18):9232-9241.
[162] Stokes, A; Corteyn, AH; Pullen, LA; Doel, TR; Meredith, DM; Killington, RA; Halliburton, IW; Whittaker, GR; Wheldon, LA; Nicolson, L; et al. Studies on glycoprotein 13 (gp13) of equid herpesvirus 1 using affinity-purified gp13,

glycoprotein-specific monoclonal antibodies and synthetic peptides in a hamster model. *J. Gen. Virol.* 1991;72 (Pt 4):923-931.

[163] Guo, PX; Goebel, S; Davis, S; Perkus, ME; Languet, B; Desmettre, P; Allen, G; Paoletti, E. Expression in recombinant vaccinia virus of the equine herpesvirus 1 gene encoding glycoprotein gp13 and protection of immunized animals. *J. Virol.* 1989;63(10):4189-4198.

[164] Bryant, NA; Davis-Poynter, N; Vanderplasschen, A; Alcami, A. Glycoprotein G isoforms from some alphaherpesviruses function as broad-spectrum chemokine binding proteins. *Embo. J.* 2003;22(4):833-846.

[165] Van de Walle, GR; May, ML; Sukhumavasi, W; von Einem, J; Osterrieder, N. Herpesvirus chemokine-binding glycoprotein G (gG) efficiently inhibits neutrophil chemotaxis in vitro and in vivo. *J. Immunol.* 2007;179(6):4161-9.

[166] Van de Walle, GR; Sakamoto, K; Osterrieder, N. CCL3 and viral chemokine-binding protein gg modulate pulmonary inflammation and virus replication during equine herpesvirus 1 infection. *J. Virol.* 2008;82(4):1714-1722.

[167] van der Meulen, KM; Nauwynck, HJ; Pensaert, MB. Absence of viral antigens on the surface of equine herpesvirus-1-infected peripheral blood mononuclear cells: a strategy to avoid complement-mediated lysis. *J. Gen. Virol.* 2003;84(Pt 1):93-97.

[168] van der Meulen, K; Caij, B; Pensaert, M; Nauwynck, H. Absence of viral envelope proteins in equine herpesvirus 1-infected blood mononuclear cells during cell-associated viremia. *Vet. Microbiol.* 2006;113(3-4):265-273.

[169] Rappocciolo, G; Birch, J; Ellis, SA. Down-regulation of MHC class I expression by equine herpesvirus-1. *J. Gen. Virol.* 2003;84(Pt 2):293-300.

[170] Ambagala, AP; Gopinath, RS; Srikumaran, S. Peptide transport activity of the transporter associated with antigen processing (TAP) is inhibited by an early protein of equine herpesvirus-1. *J. Gen. Virol.* 2004;85(Pt 2):349-353.

[171] Koppers-Lalic, D; Verweij, MC; Lipinska, AD; Wang, Y; Quinten, E; Reits, EA; Koch, J; Loch, S; Rezende, MM; Daus, F; Bienkowska-Szewczyk, K; Osterrieder, N; Mettenleiter, TC; Heemskerk, MH; Tampe, R; Neefjes, JJ; Chowdhury, SI; Ressing, ME; Rijsewijk, FA; Wiertz, EJ. Varicellovirus UL 49.5 proteins differentially affect the function of the transporter associated with antigen processing, TAP. *PLoS Pathog* 2008;4(5):e1000080.

[172] Hannant, D; O'Neill, T; Jessett, D; Mumford, JA. Evidence for non-specific immunosuppression during the development of immune responses to equid herpesvirus-1. *Equine Vet. J.* 1991;Suppl 12:41-45.

[173] Charan, S; Palmer, K; Chester, P; Mire-Sluis, AR; Meager, A; Edington, N. Transforming growth factor-beta induced by live or ultraviolet-inactivated equid herpes virus type-1 mediates immunosuppression in the horse. *Immunology* 1997;90(4):586-591.

[174] Gorelik, L; Flavell, RA. Transforming growth factor-beta in T-cell biology. *Nat. Rev. Immunol.* 2002;2(1):46-53.

[175] Mendez-Samperio, P; Hernandez, M; Ayala, HE. Induction of transforming growth factor-beta 1 production in human cells by herpes simplex virus. *J. Interferon Cytokine Res.* 2000;20(3):273-280.

[176] Haagmans, BL; Teerds, KJ; van den Eijnden-van Raaij, AJ; Horzinek, MC; Schijns, VE. Transforming growth factor beta production during rat cytomegalovirus infection. *J. Gen. Virol.* 1997;78 (Pt 1):205-213.

[177] Hannant, D; O'Neill, T; Ostlund, EN; Kydd, JH; Hopkin, PJ; Mumford, JA. Equid herpesvirus-induced immunosuppression is associated with lymphoid cells and not soluble circulating factors. *Viral. Immunol.* 1999;12(4):313-321.

[178] Mizukoshi, F; Maeda, K; Hamano, M; Iwata, H; Matsumura, T; Kondo, T; Sugiura, T. IgG antibody subclass response against equine herpesvirus type 4 in horses. *Vet. Immunol. Immunopathol.* 2002;88(1-2):97-101.

[179] Crabb, BS; Studdert, MJ. Comparative studies of the proteins of equine herpesviruses 4 and 1 and asinine herpesvirus 3: antibody response of the natural hosts. *J. Gen. Virol.* 1990;71 (Pt 9):2033-41.

[180] Fitzpatrick, DR; Studdert, MJ. Immunologic relationships between equine herpesvirus type 1 (equine abortion virus) and type 4 (equine rhinopneumonitis virus). *Am. J. Vet. Res.* 1984;45(10):1947-52.

[181] Ellis, JA; Steeves, E; Wright, AK; Bogdan, JR; Davis, WC; Kanara, EW; Haines, DM. Cell-mediated cytolysis of equine herpesvirus-infected cells by leukocytes from young vaccinated horses. *Vet. Immunol. Immunopathol.* 1997;57(3-4):201-214.

[182] Nordengrahn, A; Klingeborn, B; Lindholm, A; Merza, M. The use of a neutralizing monoclonal antibody to detect infections of equine herpesvirus type 2 (EHV-2). *J. Vet. Diagn. Invest* 2001;13(5):389-93.

[183] Dunowska, M; Meers, J; Johnson, RD; Wilks, CR. Influence of equine herpesvirus type 2 infection on monocyte chemoattractant protein 1 gene transcription in equine blood mononuclear cells. *Res. Vet. Sci.* 2001;71(2):111-3.

[184] Albini, A; Ferrini, S; Benelli, R; Sforzini, S; Giunciuglio, D; Aluigi, MG; Proudfoot, AE; Alouani, S; Wells, TN; Mariani, G; Rabin, RL; Farber, JM; Noonan, DM. HIV-1 Tat protein mimicry of chemokines. *Proc. Natl. Acad. Sci. USA* 1998;95(22):13153-8.

[185] Tripp, RA; Jones, LP; Haynes, LM; Zheng, H; Murphy, PM; Anderson, LJ. CX3C chemokine mimicry by respiratory syncytial virus G glycoprotein. *Nat. Immunol.* 2001;2(8):732-8.

[186] Murphy, PM. Viral exploitation and subversion of the immune system through chemokine mimicry. *Nat. Immunol.* 2001;2(2):116-22.

[187] Alcami, A. Viral mimicry of cytokines, chemokines and their receptors. *Nat. Rev. Immunol.* 2003;3(1):36-50.

[188] Rosenkilde, MM; Kledal, TN. Targeting herpesvirus reliance of the chemokine system. *Curr. Drug Targets* 2006;7(1):103-18.

[189] Beisser, PS; Verzijl, D; Gruijthuijsen, YK; Beuken, E; Smit, MJ; Leurs, R; Bruggeman, CA; Vink, C. The Epstein-Barr virus BILF1 gene encodes a G protein-coupled receptor that inhibits phosphorylation of RNA-dependent protein kinase. *J. Virol.* 2005;79(1):441-9.

[190] Davis-Poynter, NJ; Degli-Esposti, M; Farrell, HE. Murine cytomegalovirus homologues of cellular immunomodulatory genes. *Intervirology* 1999;42(5-6):331-41.

[191] Paulsen, SJ; Rosenkilde, MM; Eugen-Olsen, J; Kledal, TN. Epstein-Barr virus-encoded BILF1 is a constitutively active G protein-coupled receptor. *J. Virol.* 2005;79(1):536-46.

[192] Ahuja, SK; Murphy, PM. Molecular piracy of mammalian interleukin-8 receptor type B by herpesvirus saimiri. *J. Biol. Chem.* 1993;268(28):20691-4.

[193] Arvanitakis, L; Geras-Raaka, E; Varma, A; Gershengorn, MC; Cesarman, E. Human herpesvirus KSHV encodes a constitutively active G-protein-coupled receptor linked to cell proliferation. *Nature* 1997;385(6614):347-50.

[194] Couty, JP; Geras-Raaka, E; Weksler, BB; Gershengorn, MC. Kaposi's sarcoma-associated herpesvirus G protein-coupled receptor signals through multiple pathways in endothelial cells. *J Biol Chem* 2001;276(36):33805-11.

[195] Rosenkilde, MM; Kledal, TN; Holst, PJ; Schwartz, TW. Selective elimination of high constitutive activity or chemokine binding in the human herpesvirus 8 encoded seven transmembrane oncogene ORF74. *J. Biol. Chem.* 2000;275(34):26309-15.

[196] Rosenkilde, MM; McLean, KA; Holst, PJ; Schwartz, TW. The CXC chemokine receptor encoded by herpesvirus saimiri, ECRF3, shows ligand-regulated signaling through Gi, Gq, and G12/13 proteins but constitutive signaling only through Gi and G12/13 proteins. *J. Biol. Chem.* 2004;279(31):32524-33.

[197] Estep, RD; Axthelm, MK; Wong, SW. A G protein-coupled receptor encoded by rhesus rhadinovirus is similar to ORF74 of Kaposi's sarcoma-associated herpesvirus. *J. Virol.* 2003;77(3):1738-46.

[198] Wakeling, MN; Roy, DJ; Nash, AA; Stewart, JP. Characterization of the murine gammaherpesvirus 68 ORF74 product: a novel oncogenic G protein-coupled receptor. *J. Gen. Virol.* 2001;82(Pt 5):1187-97.

[199] Yang, TY; Chen, SC; Leach, MW; Manfra, D; Homey, B; Wiekowski, M; Sullivan, L; Jenh, CH; Narula, SK; Chensue, SW; Lira, SA. Transgenic expression of the chemokine receptor encoded by human herpesvirus 8 induces an angioproliferative disease resembling Kaposi's sarcoma. *J. Exp. Med.* 2000;191(3):445-54.

[200] Rosenkilde, MM; Kledal, TN; Schwartz, TW. High Constitutive Activity of a Virus-Encoded Seven Transmembrane Receptor in the Absence of the Conserved DRY Motif (Asp-Arg-Tyr) in Transmembrane Helix 3. *Mol. Pharmacol.* 2005;68(1):11-9.

[201] Camarda, G; Spinetti, G; Bernardini, G; Mair, C; Davis-Poynter, N; Capogrossi, MC; Napolitano, M. The equine herpesvirus 2 E1 open reading frame encodes a functional chemokine receptor. *J. Virol.* 1999;73(12):9843-8.

[202] Michel, D; Milotic, I; Wagner, M; Vaida, B; Holl, J; Ansorge, R; Mertens, T. The human cytomegalovirus UL78 gene is highly conserved among clinical isolates, but is dispensable for replication in fibroblasts and a renal artery organ-culture system. *J. Gen. Virol.* 2005;86(Pt 2):297-306.

[203] Davis-Poynter, NJ; Lynch, DM; Vally, H; Shellam, GR; Rawlinson, WD; Barrell, BG; Farrell, HE. Identification and characterization of a G protein-coupled receptor homolog encoded by murine cytomegalovirus. *J. Virol.* 1997;71(2):1521-9.

[204] Beisser, PS; Vink, C; Van Dam, JG; Grauls, G; Vanherle, SJ; Bruggeman, CA. The R33 G protein-coupled receptor gene of rat cytomegalovirus plays an essential role in the pathogenesis of viral infection. *J. Virol.* 1998;72(3):2352-63.

[205] Oliveira, SA; Shenk, TE. Murine cytomegalovirus M78 protein, a G protein-coupled receptor homologue, is a constituent of the virion and facilitates accumulation of immediate-early viral mRNA. *Proc. Natl. Acad. Sci. USA* 2001;98(6):3237-42.

[206] Beisser, PS; Grauls, G; Bruggeman, CA; Vink, C. Deletion of the R78 G protein-coupled receptor gene from rat cytomegalovirus results in an attenuated, syncytium-inducing mutant strain. *J. Virol.* 1999;73(9):7218-30.

[207] Streblow, DN; Vomaske, J; Smith, P; Melnychuk, R; Hall, LA; Pancheva, D; Smit, M; Casarosa, P; Schlaepfer, DD; Nelson, JA. Human cytomegalovirus chemokine US28 induced SMC migration is mediated by focal adhesion kinase and Src. *J. Biol. Chem.* 2003.

[208] Lee, BJ; Koszinowski, UH; Sarawar, SR; Adler, H. A gammaherpesvirus G protein-coupled receptor homologue is required for increased viral replication in response to chemokines and efficient reactivation from latency. *J. Immunol.* 2003;170(1):243-51.

[209] Moorman, NJ; Willer, DO; Speck, SH. The gammaherpesvirus 68 latency-associated nuclear antigen homolog is critical for the establishment of splenic latency. *J. Virol.* 2003;77(19):10295-303.

[210] Margulies, BJ; Browne, H; Gibson, W. Identification of the human cytomegalovirus G protein-coupled receptor homologue encoded by UL33 in infected cells and enveloped virus particles. *Virology* 1996;225(1):111-25.

[211] Bodaghi, B; Jones, TR; Zipeto, D; Vita, C; Sun, L; Laurent, L; Arenzana-Seisdedos, F; Virelizier, JL; Michelson, S. Chemokine sequestration by viral chemoreceptors as a novel viral escape strategy: withdrawal of chemokines from the environment of cytomegalovirus-infected cells. *J. Exp. Med.* 1998;188(5):855-66.

[212] Streblow, DN; Soderberg-Naucler, C; Vieira, J; Smith, P; Wakabayashi, E; Ruchti, F; Mattison, K; Altschuler, Y; Nelson, JA. The human cytomegalovirus chemokine receptor US28 mediates vascular smooth muscle cell migration. *Cell* 1999;99(5):511-20.

[213] Melnychuk, RM; Smith, P; Kreklywich, CN; Ruchti, F; Vomaske, J; Hall, L; Loh, L; Nelson, JA; Orloff, SL; Streblow, DN. Mouse cytomegalovirus M33 is necessary and sufficient in virus-induced vascular smooth muscle cell migration. *J. Virol.* 2005;79(16):10788-95.

[214] McGuire, TC; Fraser, DG; Mealey, RH. Cytotoxic T lymphocytes in protection against equine infectious anemia virus. *Anim. Health Res. Rev.* 2004;5(2):271-6.

[215] Zhang, W; Lonning, SM; McGuire, TC. Gag protein epitopes recognized by ELA-A-restricted cytotoxic T lymphocytes from horses with long-term equine infectious anemia virus infection. *J. Virol.* 1998;72(12):9612-20.

[216] Doll, ER; Bryans, JT. Immunization of young horses against viral rhinopneumonitis. *Cornell Vet.* 1963;53:24-41.

[217] Doll, ER; Bryans, JT; Mc, CW. A procedure for evaluating the antigenicity of killed virus vaccines for equine rhinopneumonitis. *Cornell Vet.* 1959;49(2):212-220.

[218] Thomson, GR; Mumford, JA; Smith, IM. Experimental immunisation against respiratory disease due to equine herpesvirus 1 infection (rhinopneumonitis) using formalin-inactivated virus with various adjuvants. *Veterinary Microbiology* 1979;4(3):255-259.

[219] ChemIDplus. Polyacrylic acid, RN 9003-01-4. In.

[220] Minke, JM; Fischer, L; Baudu, P; Guigal, PM; Sindle, T; Mumford, JA; Audonnet, JC. Use of DNA and recombinant canarypox viral (ALVAC) vectors for equine herpes virus vaccination. *Vet. Immunol. Immunopathol.* 2006;111(1-2):47-57.

[221] Minke, JM; Flore, PH; Vaarten, J; Vandehoek, J; Weststrate, MW. An inactivated EHV-1 and EHV-4 containing vaccine reduces clinical signs in horses infected experimentally with EHV-1 or EHV-4 six months after a single vaccination. In: U.Wernery JFW, J.A.Mumford and O-R.Kaaden., editor. Equine Infectious Diseases VIII: *Proceedings of the 8th International Conference on Equine Infectious Diseases.* Newmarket, UK: RandW Publications (Newmarket); 1998. p. 564-565.

[222] Heldens, JG; Kersten, AJ; Weststrate, MW; van den Hoven, R. Duration of immunity induced by an adjuvanted and inactivated equine influenza, tetanus and equine herpesvirus 1 and 4 combination vaccine. *Vet Q* 2001;23(4):210-217.

[223] Foote, CE; Love, DN; Gilkerson, JR; Whalley, JM. Serological responses of mares and weanlings following vaccination with an inactivated whole virus equine herpesvirus 1 and equine herpesvirus 4 vaccine. *Vet. Microbiol.* 2002;88(1):13-25.

[224] Foote, CE; Love, DN; Gilkerson, JR; Wellington, JE; Whalley, JM. EHV-1 and EHV-4 infection in vaccinated mares and their foals. *Vet. Immunol. Immunopathol.* 2006;111(1-2):41-46.

[225] Foote, CE; Gilkerson, JR; Whalley, JM; Love, DN. Seroprevalence of equine herpesvirus 1 in mares and foals on a large Hunter Valley stud farm in years pre- and postvaccination. *Aust. Vet. J.* 2003;81(5):283-288.

[226] van Maanen, C; Willink, DL; Smeenk, LA; Brinkhof, J; Terpstra, C. An equine herpesvirus 1 (EHV1) abortion storm at a riding school. *Vet Q* 2000;22(2):83-87.

[227] Allen, G; Coogle, LD; Ostlund, EN; Yeargan, M. Molecular dissection of two major equid herpesvirus-1 glycoprotein antigens (gB and gC) that elicit humoral immune response in the horse. In: Plowright W, Rossdale, P.D. and Wade, J.F., editor. Equine Infectious Diseases VI, *Proceedings of the Sixth International Conference.* Newmarket: R and W Publications Ltd; 1992. p. 181-193.

[228] Tewari, D; Nair, SV; De Ungria, MC; Lawrence, GL; Hayden, M; Love, DN; Field, HJ; Whalley, JM. Immunization with glycoprotein C of equine herpesvirus-1 is associated with accelerated virus clearance in a murine model. *Arch. Virol.* 1995;140(4):789-797.

[229] Tewari, D; Whalley, JM; Love, DN; Field, HJ. Characterization of immune responses to baculovirus-expressed equine herpesvirus type 1 glycoproteins D and H in a murine model. *J. Gen. Virol.* 1994;75 (Pt 7):1735-1741.

[230] Osterrieder, N; Wagner, R; Brandmuller, C; Schmidt, P; Wolf, H; Kaaden, OR. Protection against EHV-1 challenge infection in the murine model after vaccination with various formulations of recombinant glycoprotein gp14 (gB). *Virology* 1995;208(2):500-510.

[231] Kukreja, A; Walker, C; Fitzmaurice, T; Awan, A; Love, DN; Whalley, JM; Field, HJ. Protective effects of equine herpesvirus-1 (EHV-1) glycoprotein B in a murine model of EHV-1-induced abortion. *Vet Microbiol* 1998;62(4):303-311.

[232] Stokes, A; Alber, DG; Cameron, RS; Marshall, RN; Allen, GP; Killington, RA. The production of a truncated form of baculovirus expressed EHV-1 glycoprotein C and its

role in protection of C3H (H-2Kk) mice against virus challenge. *Virus Res.* 1996;44(2):97-109.

[233] Packiarajah, P; Walker, C; Gilkerson, J; Whalley, JM; Love, DN. Immune responses and protective efficacy of recombinant baculovirus-expressed glycoproteins of equine herpesvirus 1 (EHV-1) gB, gC and gD alone or in combinations in BALB/c mice. *Vet Microbiol.* 1998;61(4):261-278.

[234] Sanders, MT; Brown, LE; Deliyannis, G; Pearse, MJ. ISCOM-based vaccines: the second decade. *Immunol. Cell Biol.* 2005;83(2):119-128.

[235] Crouch, CF; Daly, J; Hannant, D; Wilkins, J; Francis, MJ. Immune responses and protective efficacy in ponies immunised with an equine influenza ISCOM vaccine containing an 'American lineage' H3N8 virus. *Vaccine* 2004;23(3):418-425.

[236] Crouch, CF; Daly, J; Henley, W; Hannant, D; Wilkins, J; Francis, MJ. The use of a systemic prime/mucosal boost strategy with an equine influenza ISCOM vaccine to induce protective immunity in horses. *Vet Immunol. Immunopathol.* 2005;108(3-4):345-355.

[237] Paillot, R; Grimmett, H; Elton, D; Daly, JM. Protection, systemic IFN and antibody responses induced by an ISCOM-based vaccine against a recent equine influenza virus in its natural host. *Vet Res.* 2008;39:21.

[238] Bungener, L; Huckriede, A; Wilschut, J; Daemen, T. Delivery of protein antigens to the immune system by fusion-active virosomes: a comparison with liposomes and ISCOMs. *Biosci. Rep.* 2002;22(2):323-338.

[239] Cook, RF; O'Neill, T; Strachan, E; Sundquist, B; Mumford, JA. Protection against lethal equine herpes virus type 1 (subtype 1) infection in hamsters by immune stimulating complexes (ISCOMs) containing the major viral glycoproteins. *Vaccine* 1990;8(5):491-496.

[240] Foote, CE; Love, DN; Gilkerson, JR; Rota, J; Trevor-Jones, P; Ruitenberg, KM; Wellington, JE; Whalley, JM. Serum antibody responses to equine herpesvirus 1 glycoprotein D in horses, pregnant mares and young foals. *Vet. Immunol Immunopathol* 2005;105(1-2):47-57.

[241] Flowers, CC; O'Callaghan, DJ. Equine herpesvirus 1 glycoprotein D: mapping of the transcript and a neutralization epitope. *J. Virol.* 1992;66(11):6451-6460.

[242] Weerasinghe, CU; Learmonth, GS; Gilkerson, JR; Foote, CE; Wellington, JE; Whalley, JM. Equine herpesvirus 1 glycoprotein D expressed in E. coli provides partial protection against equine herpesvirus infection in mice and elicits virus-neutralizing antibodies in the horse. *Vet. Immunol Immunopathol.* 2006;111(1-2):59-66.

[243] Foote, CE; Raidal, SL; Pecenpetelovska, G; Wellington, JE; Whalley, JM. Inoculation of mares and very young foals with EHV-1 glycoproteins D and B reduces virus shedding following respiratory challenge with EHV-1. *Vet. Immunol Immunopathol* 2006;111(1-2):97-108.

[244] Ruitenberg, KM; Walker, C; Wellington, JE; Love, DN; Whalley, JM. Potential of DNA-mediated vaccination for equine herpesvirus 1. *Vet. Microbiol.* 1999;68(1-2):35-48.

[245] Ruitenberg, KM; Walker, C; Wellington, JE; Love, DN; Whalley, JM. DNA-mediated immunization with glycoprotein D of equine herpesvirus 1 (EHV-1) in a murine model of EHV-1 respiratory infection. *Vaccine* 1999;17(3):237-244.

[246] Walker, C; Ruitenberg, KM; Love, DN; Millar Whalley, J. Immunization of BALB/c mice with DNA encoding equine herpesvirus 1 (EHV-1) glycoprotein D affords partial protection in a model of EHV-1-induced abortion. *Vet. Microbiol.* 2000;76(3):211-220.

[247] Ruitenberg, KM; Walker, C; Love, DN; Wellington, JE; Whalley, JM. A prime-boost immunization strategy with DNA and recombinant baculovirus-expressed protein enhances protective immunogenicity of glycoprotein D of equine herpesvirus 1 in naive and infection-primed mice. *Vaccine* 2000;18(14):1367-1373.

[248] Ruitenberg, KM; Love, DN; Gilkerson, JR; Wellington, JE; Whalley, JM. Equine herpesvirus 1 (EHV-1) glycoprotein D DNA inoculation in horses with pre-existing EHV-1/EHV-4 antibody. *Vet. Microbiol.* 2000;76(2):117-127.

[249] Soboll, G; Hussey, SB; Whalley, JM; Allen, GP; Koen, MT; Santucci, N; Fraser, DG; Macklin, MD; Swain, WF; Lunn, DP. Antibody and cellular immune responses following DNA vaccination and EHV-1 infection of ponies. *Vet Immunol Immunopathol.* 2006;111(1-2):81-95.

[250] McLauchlan, J; Rixon, FJ. Characterization of enveloped tegument structures (L particles) produced by alphaherpesviruses: integrity of the tegument does not depend on the presence of capsid or envelope. *J. Gen. Virol.* 1992;73 (Pt 2):269-276.

[251] Dargan, DJ; Subak-Sharpe, JH. The effect of herpes simplex virus type 1 L-particles on virus entry, replication, and the infectivity of naked herpesvirus DNA. *Virology* 1997;239(2):378-388.

[252] Mohd-Azmi, ML; Field, HJ; Rixon, FJ; McLauchlan, J. Protective immun responses induced by non-infectious L-particles of equine herpesvirus type-1: Implication of cellular immunity. *The Journal of Microbiology* 2002;40(1):11-19.

[253] Mohd-Azmi, ML; Gibson, JS; Rixon, FJ; McLauchlan, J; Field, HJ. Protection of specific pathogen free (Spf) Foals from severe equine herpesvirus type-1 (EHV-1) infection following immunization with non-infectious L-particles. *The Journal of Microbiology* 2002;40(3):183-192.

[254] Dargan, DJ; Patel, AH; Subak-Sharpe, JH. PREPs: herpes simplex virus type 1-specific particles produced by infected cells when viral DNA replication is blocked. *J Virol* 1995;69(8):4924-4932.

[255] Cornick, J; Martens, J; Martens, R; Crandell, R; McConnell, S; Kit, S. Safety and efficacy of a thymidine kinase negative equine herpesvirus-1 vaccine in young horses. *Can J. Vet Res* 1990;54(2):260-266.

[256] Slater, JD; Gibson, JS; Field, HJ. Pathogenicity of a thymidine kinase-deficient mutant of equine herpesvirus 1 in mice and specific pathogen-free foals. *J. Gen. Virol.* 1993;74 (Pt 5):819-828.

[257] Patel, JR; Bateman, H; Williams, J; Didlick, S. Derivation and characterisation of a live equid herpes virus-1 (EHV-1) vaccine to protect against abortion and respiratory disease due to EHV-1. *Vet. Microbiol.* 2003;91(1):23-39.

[258] Patel, JR; Didlick, S; Bateman, H. Efficacy of a live equine herpesvirus-1 (EHV-1) strain C147 vaccine in foals with maternally-derived antibody: protection against EHV-1 infection. *Equine Vet. J.* 2004;36(5):447-451.

[259] Paoletti, E. Applications of pox virus vectors to vaccination: an update. *Proc. Natl. Acad Sci. USA* 1996;93(21):11349-11353.

[260] Moss, B. Genetically engineered poxviruses for recombinant gene expression, vaccination, and safety. *Proc. Natl. Acad. Sci. USA* 1996;93(21):11341-11348.

[261] Guo, PX; Goebel, S; Perkus, ME; Taylor, J; Norton, E; Allen, G; Languet, B; Desmettre, P; Paoletti, E. Coexpression by vaccinia virus recombinants of equine herpesvirus 1 glycoproteins gp13 and gp14 results in potentiated immunity. *J. Virol.* 1990;64(5):2399-2406.

[262] Huemer, HP; Strobl, B; Nowotny, N. Use of apathogenic vaccinia virus MVA expressing EHV-1 gC as basis of a combined recombinant MVA/DNA vaccination scheme. *Vaccine* 2000;18(14):1320-1326.

[263] Audonnet, JC; Mumford, JA; Jessett, DM; Pardo, MC; Taylor, J; Tartaglia, J; Minke, JM. Safety and efficacy of a canarypox-EHV recombinant vaccine in horses. In: U. Wernery JFW, J.A. Mumford and O-R. Kaaden., editor. Equine Infectious Diseases VIII: Proceedings of the 8th International Conference on Equine Infectious Diseases. Newmarket, UK: RandW Publications (Newmarket); 1998. p. 118-119.

[264] Wilson, WD; Rossdale, PD. Effect of age on the serological responses of thoroughbred foals to vaccination with an inactivated EHV-1/EHV-4 vaccine. In: U.Wernery JFW, J.A.Mumford and O-R.Kaaden., editor. Equine Infectious Diseases VIII: *Proceedings of the 8th International Conference on Equine Infectious Diseases*. Newmarket, UK: RandW Publications (Newmarket); 1999. p. 428.

[265] Lopez, AM; Hines, MT; Palmer, GH; Knowles, DP; Alperin, DC; Hines, SA. Analysis of anamnestic immune responses in adult horses and priming in neonates induced by a DNA vaccine expressing the vapA gene of Rhodococcus equi. *Vaccine* 2003;21(25-26):3815-3825.

[266] Trapp, S; von Einem, J; Hofmann, H; Kostler, J; Wild, J; Wagner, R; Beer, M; Osterrieder, N. Potential of equine herpesvirus 1 as a vector for immunization. *J. Virol.* 2005;79(9):5445-5454.

[267] Rosas, CT; Konig, P; Beer, M; Dubovi, EJ; Tischer, BK; Osterrieder, N. Evaluation of the vaccine potential of an equine herpesvirus type 1 vector expressing bovine viral diarrhea virus structural proteins. *J. Gen. Virol.* 2007;88(Pt 3):748-757.

[268] Rosas, CT; Tischer, BK; Perkins, GA; Wagner, B; Goodman, LB; Osterrieder, N. Live-attenuated recombinant equine herpesvirus type 1 (EHV-1) induces a neutralizing antibody response against West Nile virus (WNV). *Virus Res.* 2007;125(1):69-78.

[269] Belak, S; Palfi, V; Tuboly, S; Bartha, L. Passive immunization of foals to prevent respiratory disease caused by equine herpesvirus type 2. *Zentralbl Veterinarmed B* 1980;27(9-10):826-30.

[270] Morein, B; Merza, M. Vaccination against herpesviruses, Fiction or Reality? *Scandinavian Journal of Infectious Diseases* 1991;Supplement 78:110-118.

[271] Morein, B; Lövgren, K; Rönnberg, B; Sjolander, A; Villacrés-Erikson, M. Immunostimulating complexes. Clinical potential in vaccine development. *Clin. Immunother* 1995;3:461-475.

[272] Rollinson, EA; White, G. Relative activities of acyclovir and BW759 against Aujeszky's disease and equine rhinopneumonitis viruses. *Antimicrob Agents Chemother* 1983;24(2):221-6.

[273] Smith, KO; Galloway, KS; Hodges, SL; Ogilvie, KK; Radatus, BK; Kalter, SS; Heberling, RL. Sensitivity of equine herpesviruses 1 and 3 in vitro to a new nucleoside analogue, 9-[[2-hydroxy-1-(hydroxymethyl) ethoxy] methyl] guanine. *Am. J. Vet. Res.* 1983;44(6):1032-5.

[274] Wilkins, P. Acyclovir in the treatment of EHV-1 myeloencephalopathy. In: 22nd Annual Meeting of the American College of Veterinary Internal Medicine; 2004; Minneapolis, USA; 2004. p. 170-172.

[275] Garre, B; van der Meulen, K; Nugent, J; Neyts, J; Croubels, S; De Backer, P; Nauwynck, H. In vitro susceptibility of six isolates of equine herpesvirus 1 to acyclovir, ganciclovir, cidofovir, adefovir, PMEDAP and foscarnet. *Vet. Microbiol.* 2007;122(1-2):43-51.

[276] Garre, B; Shebany, K; Gryspeerdt, A; Baert, K; van der Meulen, K; Nauwynck, H; Deprez, P; De Backer, P; Croubels, S. Pharmacokinetics of acyclovir after intravenous infusion of acyclovir and after oral administration of acyclovir and its prodrug valacyclovir in healthy adult horses. *Antimicrob Agents Chem.other* 2007;51(12):4308-14.

[277] Maes, A; Garre, B; Desmet, N; van der Meulen, K; Nauwynck, H; De Backer, P; Croubels, S. Determination of acyclovir in horse plasma and body fluids by high-performance liquid chromatography combined with fluorescence detection and heated electrospray ionization tandem mass spectrometry. *Biomed. Chromatogr* 2008.

[278] Maxwell, LK; Bentz, BG; Bourne, DW; Erkert, RS. Pharmacokinetics of valacyclovir in the adult horse. *J. Vet. Pharmacol. Ther.* 2008;31(4):312-20.

[279] Murray, MJ; del Piero, F; Jeffrey, SC; Davis, MS; Furr, MO; Dubovi, EJ; Mayo, JA. Neonatal equine herpesvirus type 1 infection on a thoroughbred breeding farm. *J. Vet. Intern. Med.* 1998;12(1):36-41.

[280] Friday, PA; Scarratt, WK; Elvinger, F; Timoney, PJ; Bonda, A. Ataxia and paresis with equine herpesvirus type 1 infection in a herd of riding school horses. *J. Vet. Intern. Med.* 2000;14(2):197-201.

[281] Grayson-Jockey Club. Two-pronged attack on equine herpesvirus. *Grayson-Jockey Club Research Today* 2007;24(4):1.

In: Herpesviridae Viral Structure, Life Cycle and Infections ISBN 978-1-60692-947-6
Editor: Toma R. Gluckman

Chapter 3

Herpesvirus and Musculoskeletal Diseases

Roberto Álvarez-Lafuente[1] and Benjamín Fernández-Gutiérrez[2*]

[1] Service of Neurology, Hospital Clínico San Carlos, Lagos s/n, 28040 Madrid, Spain

[2] Service of Rheumatology, Hospital Clínico San Carlos, Lagos s/n, 28040 Madrid, Spain

Abstract

The purpose of this article is to review the results and conclusions of our group in previous studies of herpesvirus infections in three different musculoskeletal diseases: rheumatoid arthritis, giant cell arteritis and osteoarthritis. The presence of Epstein-Barr virus (EBV) and human herpesvirus 6 (HHV-6) genomes in blood, synovial fluid, and serum samples of patients with rheumatoid arthritis in a higher proportion than in healthy donors; the presence of HHV-6 and Varicella-zoster virus (VZV) in temporal artery biopsies of patients with giant cell arteritis; and the higher viral DNA prevalence of VZV in mesenchymal stem cells of osteoarthritis patients than in healthy controls, all these results take together suggested a possible involvement of the herpesviruses in the pathogeny of these diseases. Furthermore, recent insights have added new value information that should be analyzed to better understand those previous results; in the last years, a huge number of articles have been published on this topic, and different possible mechanisms have been suggested to explain the role of the herpesviruses in the musculoskeletal diseases; a review of these new hypothesis we will also be performed.

Keywords: Cytomegalovirus, Epstein-Barr virus, human herpesvirus 6, Varicella-zoster virus, quantitative PCR, rheumatoid arthritis, giant cell arteritis, osteoarthritis, mesenchymal stem cells.

---

* Corresponding Author: Benjamín Fernández-Gutiérrez
Servicio de Reumatología. Hospital Clínico San Carlos, Profesor Martín Lagos s/n, 28040 Madrid. Spain
Telephone: 34-91-330 36 15. Fax: 34-91-330 34 14; E-mail address: bfernandez.hcsc@salud.madrid.org.

Introduction. Herpesviruses and Musculoskeletal Diseases

Herpesviruses have been involved in the etiopathogeny of some musculoskeletal diseases. Although it is assumed that a genetic background is needed, and some genetic factors have been associated with most of the musculoskeletal diseases, the genetic is insufficient to explain, among others, the variation in geographic prevalence and the temporal fluctuation in the incidence of these diseases. Different environmental factors, like viruses and bacterias, have been investigated in the last years, but herpesviruses are the main focus of attention as we can infer from the reports that we can find in the literature. Some characteristics of these viruses have made to them the most likely candidates (1): they are ubiquitous, since musculoskeletal diseases are common throughout the world; they persist within the body, since these diseases are chronic and manifest as recurrent flares; they show direct or indirect tropism for the joints, given the predominantly articular lesions; and they are capable of altering host immune responses. The purpose of this article is to review the results and conclusions of our group in previous studies of herpesvirus infections in rheumatoid arthritis (RA), giant cell arteritis (GCA) and osteoarthritis (OA); a review of the recent reports on this topic will also be performed.

Herpesviruses and Rheumatoid Arthritis

RA is the most common chronic inflammatory joint disease (1), and one of the most common immune-mediated diseases (2), in which non-suppurative inflammation of the synovium is frequently associated with a variety of extra-articular manifestations (3); although the pathogenesis of RA is still poorly understood, involvement of both cellular and humoral autoimmune mechanisms has been clearly demonstrated (2). The multifactorial pathophysiology of RA involves both genetic and environmental influences (4). Genetic factors are important in disease susceptibility; accumulating knowledge on the genetic underpinnings of RA have confirmed a role for several Class II HLAs, i.e., HLA-DRB1*01, DRB1*04, and corresponding subtypes that contain the shared epitope. Familial clustering of RA has been documented, and concordance for RA has been found in 15% to 30% of monozygotic twin pairs. Nevertheless, genetic factors fail to completely explain the occurrence of RA, and environmental exposures are probably crucial as well. A viral trigger of RA in the genetically predisposed has been hypothesized for many years (5-13). A virus could act as an adjuvant in the development of autoimmunity, non-specifically stimulating innate immune responses, including mast cells, dendritic cells, Toll-like receptors and complement receptors (14).

Thus, in a previous report of our group (15), with the aim to assess the relevance of viral infection in RA, we studied the prevalence and viral load of the human herpesviruses, cytomegalovirus (CMV), Epstein-Barr virus (EBV) and human herpesvirus 6 (HHV-6) in serum and peripheral blood mononuclear cells (PBMCs) of RA patients. A total of 133 PBMCs samples (61 of RA patients and 72 of normal donors) and 136 serum samples (59 from RA patients and 77 from healthy donors), were analyzed by quantitative real-time polymerase chain reaction for the DNA prevalence and viral load of HHV-6, EBV and CMV. The results were as follows (Tables 1-3): i) in PBMCs samples, we found statistically significant differences for EBV in DNA prevalence (55.7% in RA patients vs. 33% in control group, p=0.009) and viral load (0 – 592.29 copies/μg of DNA for RA patients, vs. 0 – 40.4 copies/μg of DNA for controls, p=0.001). ii) In serum samples, we found a statistically significant difference for HHV-6 DNA prevalence (10.2% in RA patients vs. 0% in controls, p=0.006) and viral load (0 – 529.10 copies/μg of DNA for RA patients, vs. 0 copies/μg of DNA for controls, p=0.007). Therefore, we concluded that all these results suggested that herpesviruses might play a role in RA; however, other alternatives could not be completely ruled out: i) defects in cellular immunity in RA patients may result in a relatively high virus load; ii) RA patients could be more prone to infection/reactivation. Nevertheless, all these data raised the question of the usefulness of monitoring the DNA viral load in RA patients.

Table 1. DNA prevalence of HHV-6, EBV and CMV in RA patients and controls

	PBMCs			SERUM		
RA	**HHV-6**	EBV	CMV	**HHV-6**	**EBV**	**CMV**
Positives/n	20/61	34/61	15/61	6/59	0/59	1/59
DNA prevalence	32.8%	55.7%	24.6%	10.2%	0%	1,7%
CONTROLS						
Positives/n	21/72	24/72	15/72	0/77	0/77	0/77
DNA prevalence	29.2%	33.3%	20.8%	0%	0%	0%
p	0.65	0.009	0.6	0.006	1	0.4

Data were analyzed by the Chi-Square test for PBMCs samples and by the Fisher exact test for serum samples.
PBMCs= peripheral blood mononuclear cells.

Table 2. HHV-6, EBV and CMV viral load in RA patients and controls

	PBMCs			SERUM		
RA	HHV-6	EBV	CMV	**HHV-6**	**EBV**	**CMV**
Range	0 - 92.3	0 - 592.3	0 - 240.9	0 - 529.1	0	0 - 45.9
Median	0	0	0	0	0	0
CONTROLS						
Range	0 - 13.8	0 - 40.4	0 - 22.7	0	0	0
Median	0	0	0	0	0	0
p	0.451	0.001	0.337	0.007	1	0.277

Viral load are in copies/μg DNA. Data were analyzed by the Mann-Whitney U test.
PBMCs = peripheral blood mononuclear cells.

Table 3. DNA prevalence of HHV-6, EBV and CMV in RA patients under 57 years and controls

	PBMCs			SERUM		
RA < 57 years	HHV-6	EBV	CMV	**HHV-6**	**EBV**	**CMV**
Positives/n	6/19	13/19	5/19	3/19	0/19	0/19
DNA prevalence	31.6%	68.4%	26.3%	15.8%	0%	0%
CONTROLS						
Positives/n	21/72	24/72	15/72	0/77	0/77	0/77
DNA prevalence	29.2%	33.3%	20.8%	0%	0%	0%
p	0.83	0.006	0.6	0.0005	1	1

Data were analyzed by the Chi-Square test for PBMCs samples and by the Fisher exact test for serum samples.

PBMCs= peripheral blood mononuclear cells

Following publication of this report, other studies have been published on this topic in the last three years that added new information to the possible involvement of these viruses in RA. Thus, Mirkinson et al. (16) showed the case of a 3-year-old patient with biopsy-proven HHV-6 encephalitis that developed a clinical condition consistent with systemic-onset juvenile idiopathic arthritis (SoJIA) and responsive to synthetic interleukin-1 (IL-1) receptor therapy. This suggested both a temporal relationship between HHV-6 infection and the development of SoJIA and the likely involvement of IL-1 in his disease. The authors concluded that his case suggests that future prospective studies in new-onset SoJIA should include an evaluation for HHV-6 infection.

However, the strongest evidences relating environmental factors with RA have been found for EBV. Thus, in a recent report, Lünemann JD et al. (17) determined both EBV-specific T cell and B cell responses and cell-associated EBV DNA copies in patients with RA and demographically matched healthy virus carriers. Patients with RA showed increased and broadened IgG responses to lytic and latent EBV-encoded Ags and 7-fold higher levels of EBV copy numbers in circulating blood cells. Additionally, patients with RA exhibited substantial expansions of CD8(+) T cells specific for pooled EBV Ags expressed during both B cell transformation and productive viral replication and the frequency of CD8(+) T cells specific for these Ags correlated with cellular EBV copy numbers. In contrast, CD4(+) T cell responses to EBV and T cell responses to human CMV Ags were unchanged, altogether arguing against a defective control of latent EBV infection in RA. The authors conclude that these data show that the regulation of EBV infection is perturbed in RA and suggest that increased EBV-specific effector T cell and Ab responses are driven by an elevated EBV load in RA.

In another recent report, Pratesi et al. (2) synthesized multiple peptides derived from EBV-encoded Epstein-Barr nuclear antigen 1 (EBNA-1) substituting the arginines with citrulline, to test the hypothesis that deimination of viral sequences containing Arg–Gly repeats could generate epitopes recognized by anti–citrullinated protein antibodies (ACPAs) that are present in rheumatoid arthritis (RA) sera. Anti–cyclic citrullinated peptide antibodies were purified by affinity chromatography and tested on a panel of in vitro deiminated proteins. Their ability to bind in vivo deiminated proteins was evaluated by immunoprecipitation, using EBV-infected cell lines. Antibodies specific for a peptide corresponding to the EBNA-135–58 sequence containing citrulline instead of arginine (viral citrullinated peptide [VCP]) were detected in 50% of RA sera and in <5% of normal and disease control sera. In addition, affinity purified anti-VCP antibodies from RA sera reacted with filaggrin-derived citrullinated peptides, with deiminated fibrinogen, and with deiminated recombinant EBNA-1. Moreover, anti-VCP antibodies immunoprecipitated, from the lysate of calcium ionophore–stimulated lymphoblastoid cell lines, an 80-kd band that was reactive with a monoclonal anti–EBNA-1 antibody and with anti–modified citrulline antibodies. The authors conclude that these data indicate that anti-ACPAs react with a viral deiminated protein and suggest that EBV infection may play a role in the induction of these RA-specific antibodies. The same group published another report on this topic with the same conclusions (18).

Regarding clinical evidence of antiviral prodrugs for RA, Agarwal et al. (19) recently reported an interesting case of new therapy of patients with RA, in which acyclovir, an antiviral drug that slows the growth and spread of the herpes virus, induced the remission of active RA as well as acute disseminated VZV infection. After 2 weeks of acyclovir treatment, the patient noticed a marked improvement in his joint symptoms. For the next 24 months (at least until author's last follow-up), the RA remained in remission without the need for any disease-modifying drug. The authors suggested that clinical remission of RA is an expression of suppressed autoimmune process after the infection with VZV. However, they think that it could be infer that acyclovir inactivated an inflamed EBV infected synovial cells because EBV is in the same group of herpes virus (20).

Whether the observed abnormalities in EBV-directed immune responses and EBV viral loads are a cause or a consequence of RA remains a mystery. Through its potential for molecular mimicry, by polyclonal activation of B cells, or via some other mechanism, EBV or an EBV-specific immune response could be a trigger for the development of RA in genetically predisposed patients. Alternatively, an innate or acquired immune defect in those with or at risk for RA could handicap the host's ability to suppress this chronic viral infection. This suggests that in those patients with RA, T cell control of latent EBV infection is defective (21).

Therefore, the links between RA and the EBV are numerous and complex. Some of them probably occur also with other diseases and may be related to RA-induced dysimmunity; the EBV is a ubiquitous virus that can modify host responses and adapt to its environment (1). The role for the EBV, and more specifically the EBV burden, in RA is under close scrutiny; future studies will determine whether the EBV burden should be monitored over time in RA patients.

In conclusion, the EBV is a strong candidate that may act at several levels of the pathophysiology of RA; however, many unanswered questions remain regarding potential direct and indirect roles for the EBV and other human herpesviruses like HHV-6 in RA.

Herpesviruses and Giant Cell Arteritis

GCA or temporal arteritis is a relatively common systemic vasculitis affecting medium and large arteries, especially the extracranial branches of the carotid arteries (22), and it has the histological appearance of a granulomatous inflammatory process. When present in cranial arteries, this inflammatory process may cause ischaemia of a variety of structures including the optic disc, with subsequent rapid onset of blindness (23). While the alterations in cellular architecture of affected vessels have been well described (24), the aetiological basis of these alterations has not yet been identified. Giant cell arteritis represents a highly complex immune response that is driven by interferon-γ producing T lymphocytes, macrophages in the vascular wall, and maladaptive arterial response to tissue injury (25-26). The incidence of GCA is 15–25 per 100,000 in at-risk populations (27). Susceptible persons are usually older than 50 years, and incidence rates increase with advancing age (28). The cause of GCA is unknown. Some familial accumulation and the association with certain HLA-DR haplotypes seem to indicate a genetic predisposition. Variations in the incidence of GCA have been reported in different parts of the world, suggesting that environmental or genetic factors may be involved (29-30). However, the nature of the ''trigger'' (or triggers) of this inflammatory response have not yet been identified. As with many autoimmune diseases, infectious agents have been suspected as possible initiators of the inflammatory process in GCA (31). Flu-like symptoms are often seen at the onset of the disease and are followed by an acute phase response, and molecular studies on GCA have suggested a possible link between infection and GCA. Furthermore, the sudden onset and segmental distribution that characterize GCA are reminiscent of recurrent herpetic lesions. In addition, some factors postulated to contribute to reactivation of latent herpesvirus, eg, sunlight (32) and hormonal disturbances, are possible triggering factors for GCA. The temporal arteries receive a portion of their innervation from the trigeminal ganglia, (33) which are a major repository of latent herpesviruses (34). Therefore, the reactivation of latent herpesviruses might contribute to the pathogenesis of GCA involving the temporal arteries (35).

To analyze the hypothesis that an environmental factor might play a role in the pathogenesis of GCA, our group evaluated the prevalence and viral load of Parvovirus B19 (B19), Varicella zoster virus (VZV) and HHV-6 in temporal artery biopsy (TAB) specimens of GCA patients (36). We investigated 113 TAB specimens from 113 patients suspected of having GCA: 57 with biopsy-proven GCA as GCA group, and 56 with controls. We extracted DNA from biopsies and quantitative real-time polymerase chain reaction (PCR) assay was performed to establish the prevalence and viral load of B19, VZV and HHV-6. Amplification of human β-globin gene was used as internal positive control. The results were as follows (Tables 4-6): B19 was detected in 54.4% with a median viral load of 45.2 [0 – 180.2] copies/μg of DNA in GCA group vs. 37.5% and 0 [0 – 66.7] copies/μg of DNA in control group, p= 0.07 for DNA prevalence and p= 0.007 for viral load. Among B19 positive samples, 21 biopsy-proven GCA patients (67.8%) had more than 10^2 B19 copies/μg of DNA vs. 5 (23.8%) controls; there is a statistically significant association between histologic evidence of GCA and a high viral load of B19 DNA in TAB tissue, p = 0.001. However, no statistical significant difference was found for VZV (p= 0.94 for DNA prevalence; p=0.76 for viral load) and HHV-6 (p= 0.89 for DNA prevalence; p=0.64 for viral load) when compared

GCA and control groups. These findings suggested that B19 seems to play a role in the etiopathology of GCA, particularly in those patients with high viral load, but no evidence was found for VZV and HHV-6.

Table 4. DNA prevalence of B19, VZV and HHV-6 in TAB specimens of GCA patients and in control group

	GCA (n = 57)	CG* (n = 56)	p
B19	31 (54.4%)	21 (37.5%)	0.07
HHV-6	20 (35.1%)	19 (33.9%)	0.89
VZV	18 (31.6%)	18 (32.1%)	0.94

* CG: control group

Table 5. B19, VZV and HHV-6 viral load in GCA patients and control group

VIRAL LOAD*	GCA	CG**	p
B19	45.2 [0 – 180.2]	0 [0 – 66.7]	0.007
HHV-6	0 [0 – 47.8]	0 [0 – 37.7]	0.64
VZV	0 [0 – 25.8]	0 [0 – 26.4]	0.76

*Viral loads are expressed in genomes /µg of DNA as a median with their percentiles 25 and 75 in brackets.

** CG: control group

Table 6. B19, VZV and HHV-6 viral load ranges in positive GCA patients and controls

Viral load range*	B19		HHV-6		VZV	
	GCA	CG**	GCA	CG	GCA	GC
10^1 - 10^2	10 (32.2%)	16 (76.2%)	15 (75%)	16 (84.2%)	14 (77.8%)	18 (100%)
10^2 - 10^3	19 (61.3%)	5 (23.8%)	5 (25%)	3 (15.8%)	4 (22.2%)	0 (0%)
> 10^3	2 (6.5%)	0 (0%)	0 (0%)	0 (0%)	0 (0%)	0 (0%)

*Viral loads are expressed in genomes /µg of DNA

** CG: control group

Powers et al. (35) published a report the same year (2005) about the GCA affecting the cranial arteries; this is a disease of unknown cause that causes blindness, stroke, and other morbidity. Its sudden onset and segmental distribution are suggestive of diseases that involve viral reactivation, and cranial arteries are known to be innervated by ganglia that harbor herpes simplex virus (HSV). They used a high-sensitivity polymerase chain reaction assay to test for HSV DNA in specimens from 39 consecutive temporal artery biopsies performed for suspected GCA. HSV DNA was detected in 21 (88%) of 24 histologically positive and 8 (53%) of 15 histologically negative specimens (P = .027; Fisher exact test). Analysis of 10 renal artery samples from age-matched control subjects using the same assay showed no detectable HSV DNA. The authors conclude that detectable HSV DNA is correlated with histologically confirmed GCA in this patient population.

However, in other two articles published in the last two years, the authors have not found any result supporting the possible involvement of herpesvirus in the etiology of the GCA. The manuscript of Cankovic et al. (37), a study that analyzed GCA biopsy specimens using real-time quantitative polymerase chain reaction for the detection of HSV1, cytomegalovirus, and Epstein–Barr virus DNAs, failed to confirm an association between HSV1 and GCA, revealing no viral genome in 35 biopsy specimens of histologically positive temporal arteries. Cooper et al. (38) used PCR to detect the presence of Chlamydia pneumoniae, parvovirus B19 and all the human herpes viruses except HHV-8 in temporal artery biopsy specimens; samples from 37 temporal artery biopsies with histological evidence of arteritis and 66 samples from histologically negative temporal artery biopsies, all from different patients, were negative for C. pneumoniae, HSV, VZV, EBV, and HHV7 DNA. From the 37 histologically positive specimens two were positive for HHV6, two for CMV and two for parvovirus B19 DNA. Parvovirus B19 DNA was also detected in five histologically negative biopsies, one positive for HCMV DNA and a further one was positive for HHV6 DNA. Therefore, there was no statistically significant difference to the presence of virus DNA in the two types of specimens (P=0.538). The authors concluded that this study does not support a role for C. pneumoniae, parvovirus B19 or human herpes viruses in the pathogenesis of temporal arteritis.

Therefore, molecular studies support the concept that GCA is an antigen-driven process associated with chronic inflammation and mediated by CD4+ T cells (39); but, because of the predilection of GCA for affecting elderly individuals, the reactivation of a latent infection has been hypothesized as a disease trigger (40). In this regard, herpesviruses, for example the VZV, are known to produce latent infections and can also lead to T-cell-mediated inflammation. Furthermore, some herpesviruses, for example HSV, induce a pathologic finding that is a hallmark of GCA: giant cell formation (41). Finally, VZV, CMV, and HHV-6 have a vascular tropism and they may induce endothelial damage (42-43). To date, however, studies of herpesviruses in GCA have not yielded consistent results.

Herpesviruses, Mesenchymal Stem Cells and Osteoarthritis

Osteoarthritis (OA) is a disease of the entire joint that is ultimately associated with articular cartilage loss and progressive joint degeneration (44). The etiology of OA varies among individuals, with possible roles for systemic factors, such as genetics and obesity, as well as for local biomechanical factors, such as muscle weakness, joint laxity, and traumatic injury. Joint deterioration occurs over extended periods of time, and the diverse molecular mechanisms that mediate pathogenic events of early, mid, and late disease are not yet fully understood. In OA, the synovium, bone, and cartilage are each well established as sites that can be involved in the pathophysiological mechanisms that can lead to progressive joint degeneration (45). Recent investigations on the mesenchymal stem cell (MSC) offer a new perspective for bone and cartilage tissue regeneration. MSCs have the capacity to differentiate into a variety of connective tissue cells including bone, cartilage, tendon, muscle, and adipose tissue (46). These cells are easily isolated from bone marrow and can be expanded in culture through many generations, while retaining their capacity to differentiate when exposed to appropriate signals. However, it has been described that patients submitted to autologous stem cells transplants could suffer from viral infection because of reactivation (47-48), and that, allogeneic stem cell transplantation could be complicated by herpesvirus reactivation (49).

In a recent report of our group (50), we investigated whether there is a possible viral transmission using mesenchymal stem cells (MSCs) in autologous or allogeneic transplantation in the context of OA patients. With this purpose, we analyzed the presence of B19, VZV, and HHV-6 was studied in MSCs from bone marrow (BM) of patients with OA and healthy donors. MSCs were prepared from BM aspirates obtained from 18 patients undergoing joint replacement as a result of OA and from 10 healthy donors. DNA was extracted from primary MSCs culture established from these cells and quantitative real time polymerase chain reaction was performed to analyse the prevalence and viral load of B19, VZV and HHV-6. We found a total viral DNA prevalence of 16.7% (3/18) among OA patients: 1/18 was positive for B19, 2/18 for VZV, and 0/18 for HHV-6. In the control group, we found a total viral DNA prevalence of 20% (2/10); the two positives belonged to B19. We did not find any statistical significant difference (Table 7). This first approach to the viral prevalence in MSCs of BM in OA patients seem showed a low risk of viral transmission or reactivation in a possible MSCs transplantation. However, additional studies by other laboratories would be needed to confirm these results.

In the last year, another report has developed other interesting aspects of the possible infection of the MSCs by the herpesviruses. Smirnov et al. (51) have demonstrated that MSCs in BM are permissive to productive CMV infection, and that CMV alters the function of MSCs: (i) by changing the repertoire of cell surface molecules in BM-MSCs, CMV modifies the pattern of interaction between BM-MSCs and hematopoietic cells; (ii) CMV infection of BM-MSCs undergoing adipogenic or osteogenic differentiation impaired the process of differentiation. In conclusion, their experiments demonstrate that BM-derived MSCs are permissive to productive CMV infection, and that CMV can significantly alter the function of MSCs. They propose the following scenario. After reactivation of CMV from its latency in hematopoietic progenitor cells in BM, MSCs, residing in close vicinity, may represent the first easily accessible target for successful replication and dissemination of the virus. Therefore, frequently occurring CMV reactivations may result in the depletion of uncommitted MSCs from BM and/or may lead to the substantial loss of MSC potential for renewal and ability to differentiate into specialized cells and tissues. This may have severe consequences. For example, CMV-caused depletion and inability of MSCs to support osteoblast regeneration may contribute to the development of osteoporosis in elderly people. Similarly, CMV mediated deterioration of MSCs may result in impaired regeneration of cartilage tissues and, therefore, contribute to the pathogenesis of arthritis. The infection could also alter cytokine milieu in BM. These changes may affect hematopoiesis and change the properties and functions of immune progenitor cells.

Table 7. Prevalences and viral loads of B19, VZV, and HHV-6 in MSCs of OA patients and controls

	OA patients		Controls		%OA vs. %Controls	
	Pos */n (%)	V.L.**	Pos./n (%)	V.L.	p	O.R. *** (CI 95%)
TOTAL	3 / 18 (16.7%)	29.7	2 / 10 (20%)	13.4	0.825	0.8 (0.1-8.8)
B19	1 / 18 (5.6%)	61.2	2 / 10 (20%)	13.4	0.236	0.2 (0.1-4.2)
VZV	2 / 18 (11.2%)	14.4	0 / 10 (0%)	-	0.274	- -
HHV-6	0 / 18 (0%)	-	0 / 10 (0%)	-	-	- -

* Pos = positive samples; ** V.L. = viral load, in copies / μg of DNA; ***O.R. = Odds ratio

Therefore, frequent virus reactivations in BM cells and subsequent productive herpesviruses infection of MSCs may be an underlying cause of various pathological conditions; thus, the presence of viral particles of these ubiquitous viruses should be monitored in order to prevent a possible reactivation.

Conclusion

In conclusion, there are not definitive evidences relating human herpesviruses with the pathogenesis of the musculoskeletal diseases. However, in the last years, there is an increasing body of evidence obtained through different molecular biology studies. Furthermore, while the heterogeneity is easily assumed for the genetic predisposition in these diseases, most of the results related to the environmental susceptibility are refuted because viruses are only found in a subset of patients, although statistical significant differences with controls are shown in different studies. Perhaps, it could be possible that more than one virus could be involved in the pathogenesis of some of this diseases through several common mechanisms that have been previously suggested. In this scenario, human herpesviruses could play an important role since most of them share some general characteristics that have made to them the most likely candidates to perturb the immune system.

References

[1] Toussirot E, Roudier J. Pathophysiological links between rheumatoid arthritis and the Epstein-Barr virus: An update. *Joint Bone Spine,* 74 (2007) 418-426.

[2] Pratesi F, Tommasi C, Anzilotti C, Chimenti D, Migliorini P. Deiminated Epstein-Barr Virus Nuclear Antigen 1 Is a Target of Anti–Citrullinated Protein Antibodies in Rheumatoid Arthritis. *Arthr Rheum*. 2006; 54: 733-741.

[3] Kumar V, Cotran RS, Robbins SL. In: Basic pathology. 7th ed. Philadelphia: W.B. Saunders; 2003. p. 103–64.

[4] Albani S, Carson DA, Roudier J. Genetic and environmental factors in the immune pathogenesis of rheumatoid arthritis. *Rheum Dis Clin North Am.* 1992;18:729-39.

[5] Albert LJ, Inman RD: Molecular mimicry and autoimmunity. *N Engl J Med.* 1999, 341:2068-2074.

[6] Bonneville M, Scotet E, Peyrat MA, Saulquin X, Houssaint E: Epstein-Barr virus and rheumatoid arthritis. *Rev Rhum Engl Ed.* 1998, 65:365-368.

[7] Alspaugh MA, Jensen FC, Rabin H, Tan EM: Lymphocytes transformed by Epstein-Barr virus. Induction of nuclear antigen reactive with antibody in rheumatoid arthritis. *J Exp Med.* 1978, 147:1018-1027.

[8] Cooke SP, Rigby SP, Griffiths DJ, Venables PJ: Viral studies in rheumatic disease. *Ann Med Interne* (Paris) 1998, 149:30-33.

[9] Dostal C, Newkirk MM, Duffy KN, Paleckova A, Bosak V, Cerna M, Zd'arsky E, Zvarova J: Herpes viruses in multicase families with rheumatoid arthritis and systemic lupus erythematosus. *Ann N Y Acad Sci.* 1997, 815:334-337.

[10] Inman RD: Infectious etiology of rheumatoid arthritis. *Rheum Dis Clin North Am.* 1991, 17:859-870.

[11] Carty SM, Snowden N, Silman AJ: Should infection still be considered as the most likely triggering factor for rheumatoid arthritis? *J Rheumatol.* 2003, 30:425-429.

[12] Griffiths DJ: Rheumatoid arthritis: a viral aetiology? *Hosp Med.* 2000, 61:378-379.

[13] Masuko-Hongo K, Kato T, Nishioka K: Virus-associated arthritis. *Best Pract Res Clin Rheumatol.* 2003, 17:309-318.

[14] Fairweather D, Frisancho-Kiss S, Rose NR: Viruses as adjuvants for autoimmunity: evidence from Coxsackievirus-induced myocarditis. *Rev Med Virol.* 2005, 15:17-27.

[15] Alvarez-Lafuente R, Fernandez-Gutierrez B, de Miguel S, Jover JA, Rollin R, Loza E, Clemente D, Lamas JR. Potential relationship between herpes viruses and rheumatoid arthritis. Analysis with quantitative real-time polymerase chain reaction. *Ann Rheum Dis*. 2005 ;64:1357-1359.

[16] Mirkinson LJ, Nagle D, Kadom N, Jones OY. Anakinra therapy in a child with systemic-onset juvenile rheumatoid arthritis after human herpesvirus 6 encephalitis. *J Clin Rheumatol.* 2006; 12: 83-6.
[17] Lünemann JD, Frey O, Eidner T, Baier M, Roberts S, Sashihara J, Volkmer R, Cohen JI, Hein G, Kamradt T, Münz C. Increased frequency of EBV-specific effector memory CD8+ T cells correlates with higher viral load in rheumatoid arthritis. *J Immunol.* 2008;181:991-1000.
[18] Anzilotti C, Merlini G, Pratesi F, Tommasi C, Chimenti D, Migliorini P. Antibodies to viral citrullinated peptide in rheumatoid arthritis. *J Rheumatol.* 2006;33:647-51.
[19] Agarwal V, Singh R, Chauhan S. Remission of rheumatoid arthritis after acute disseminated varicella-zoster infection. *Clin Rheumatol.* 2006;21:1–2.
[20] Sawada S, Takei M, Inomata H, Nozaki T, Shiraiwa H. What is after cytokine-blocking therapy, a novel therapeutic target—Synovial Epstein-Barr virus for rheumatoid arthritis. *Autoimmun Rev.* 2007;6:126-30.
[21] Costenbader KH, Karlson EW. Epstein–Barr virus and rheumatoid arthritis: is there a link? *Arthritis Res Ther.* 2006; 8: 204.
[22] Weyand CM. The pathogenesis of giant cell arteritis. *J Rheumatol.* 2000;27:517–22.
[23] Goodman BW Jr. 1979. Temporal arteritis. *Am J Med.* 67:839–852.
[24] Weyand CM, Goronzy JJ. 2000. Pathogenic principles in giant cell arteritis. *Int J Cardiol.* 75:S9–S15.
[25] Weyand CM, Goronzy JJ. Giant cell arteritis as an antigen-driven disease. *Rheum Dis Clin North Am.* 1995;21:1027– 39.
[26] Weyand CM, Goronzy JJ. Arterial wall injury in giant cell arteritis. *Arthritis Rheum.* 1999;42:844–53.
[27] Lawrence RC, Helmick CG, Arnett FC, et al. Estimates of the prevalence of arthritis and selected musculoskeletal disorders in the United States. *Arthritis Rheum.* 1998;41:778– 99.
[28] Machado EB, Michet CJ, Ballard DJ, et al. Trends in incidence and clinical presentation of temporal arteritis in Olmsted County, Minnesota, 1950–1985. *Arthritis Rheum.* 1988;31:745– 9.
[29] Weyand CM, Hunder NN, Hicok KC, Hunder GG, Goronzy JJ. HLADRB1 alleles in polymyalgia rheumatica, giant cell arteritis, and rheumatoid arteritis. *Arthritis Rheum.* 1994;37:514–20.
[30] Dababneh A, Gonzalez-Gay MA, Garcia-Porruaet C, et al. Giant cell arteritis and polymyalgia rheumatica can be differentiated by distinct patterns of HLA class II association. *J Rheumatol.* 1998;25:2140– 5.
[31] Russo MG, Waxman J, Abdoh AA, Serebro LH. Correlation between infection and the onset of the giant cell (temporal) arteritis syndrome A trigger mechanism? *Arthritis Rheum.* 1995;38:374–80.
[32] O'Brien JP, Regan W. Actinically degenerate elastic tissue: the prime antigen in the giant cell (temporal) arteritis syndrome? New data from the posterior ciliary arteries. *Clin Exp Rheumatol.* 1998;16:39-48.
[33] Uddman R, Edvinsson L, Hara H. Axonal tracing of autonomic nerve fibers to the superficial temporal artery in the rat. Cell Tissue Res. 1989;256:559-565.

[34] Liesegang TJ. The biology of herpes simplex and Varicella zoster virus infections. *Int Ophthalmol Clin*. 1993;33:81-93.
[35] Powers JF, Bedri S, Hussein S, Salomon RN, Tischler AS. High prevalence of herpes simplex virus DNA in temporal arteritis biopsy specimens. *Am J Clin Pathol.* 2005;123:261– 4.
[36] Álvarez-Lafuente R, Fernández-Gutiérrez B, Jover JA, Judez E, Loza E, Clemente D, Garcia-Asenjo JA, Lamas JR. Human Parvovirus B19, Varicella zoster virus and Herpesvirus 6 in temporal artery biopsies of giant cell arteritis patients. Analysis with quantitative real-time polymerase chain reaction. *Ann Rheum Dis.* 2005 ;64:780-2.
[37] Cankovic M, Zarbo RJ. Failure to detect human herpes simplex virus, cytomegalovirus and Epstein-Barr virus viral genomes in giant cell arteritis biopsy specimens by real-time quantitative polymerase chain reaction. *Cardiovasc Pathol.* 2006; 15:280–286.
[38] Cooper RJ, D'Arcy S, Kirby M, Al-Buhtori M, Rahman MJ, Proctor L, Bonshek RE. Infection and Temporal Arteritis: A PCR-Based Study to Detect Pathogens in Temporal Artery Biopsy Specimens. *J Med Virol.* 2008; 80: 501-505.
[39] Weyand CM. Vasculitis: a dialogue between the artery and the immune system. In: Hoffman GS, Weyand CM, editors. Inflammatory diseases of blood vessels. New York: Marcel Dekker; 2002. pp. 1–12.
[40] Rodriguez-Pla A, Stone JH. Vasculitis and systemic infections. *Curr Op Rheumatol.* 2006, 18: 39–47.
[41] Teitelbaum CS, Streeten BW, Dawson CR. Histopathology of herpes simplex virus keratouveitis. *Curr Eye Res.* 1987; 6:189–194.
[42] Ross R. The pathogenesis of atherosclerosis: a perspective for the 1990s. *Nature,* 1993; 362:801–809.
[43] Weyand CM. Vasculitis: a dialogue between the artery and the immune system. In: Hoffman GS, Weyand CM, editors. Inflammatory diseases of blood vessels. New York: Marcel Dekker; 2002. pp. 1–12.
[44] Jones EA, Crawford A, English A, Henshaw K, Mundy J, Corscadden D, Chapman T, Emery P, Hatton P, McGonagle D. Synovial Fluid Mesenchymal Stem Cells in Health and Early Osteoarthritis. *Arthritis Rheum*. 2008; 58: 1731-40.
[45] Abramson S, Krasnokutsky S. Biomarkers in Osteoarthritis. *Bull NYU Hosp Jt Dis.* 2006; 64: 77-81.
[46] Caplan AI. Mesenchymal stem cells: cell-based reconstructive therapy in orthopedics. *Tissue Eng*. 2005;11:1198-211.
[47] Behzad-Behbahani A, Pouransari R, Tabei SZ, Rahiminejad MS, Robati M, Yaghobi R, *et al*. Risk of viral transmission via bone marrow progenitor cells versus umbilical cord blood hematopoietic stem cells in bone marrow transplantation. *Transplant Proc*. 2005;37:3211-2.
[48] Dini G, Castagnola E, Comoli P, van Tol MJ, Vossen JM. Infections after stem cell transplantation in children: state of the art and recommendations. *Bone Marrow Transplant*, 2001; Suppl 1:S18-21.
[49] Imbert-Marcille BM, Tang XW, Lepelletier D, Besse B, Moreau P, Billaudel S, *et al.* Human herpesvirus 6 infection after autologous or allogeneic stem cell transplantation:

a single-center prospective longitudinal study of 92 patients. *Clin Infect Dis.* 2000;31:881-6.

[50] Rollin R, Álvarez-Lafuente R, Marco F, Jover JA, Hernandez-García C, Rodríguez-Navas C, López-Durán L, Fernández-Gutiérrez B. Human Parvovirus B19, Varicela Zoster virus, and Humanherpesvirus-6 in mesenchymal stem cells of patients with osteoarthritis: analysis with quantitative real time polymerase chain reaction. *Osteoarthr Cartilage,* 2007; 15: 475-478.

[51] Smirnov SV, Harbacheuski R, Lewis-Antes A, Zhu H, Rameshwar P, Kotenko SV. Bone-marrow-derived mesenchymal stem cells as a target for cytomegalovirus infection: Implications for hematopoiesis, self-renewal and differentiation potential. *Virology,* 2007; 360: 6-16.

In: Herpesviridae Viral Structure, Life Cycle and Infections ISBN 978-1-60692-947-6
Editor: Toma R. Gluckman

Chapter 4

Herpesvirus MicroRNAs in Infection and Cancer

Andrea J. O'Hara and Dirk P. Dittmer
University of North Carolina at Chapel Hill, Chapel Hill, North Carolina, USA

Abstract

MicroRNAs (miRNAs) are a class of small non-coding functional RNAs that mediate post-transcriptional regulation of target mRNAs in a sequence-specific manner. They affect a wide variety of cellular processes, ranging from cellular differentiation, proliferation, apoptosis, metabolism, and infection to cancer. Over the past few years, miRNAs have been shown to be encoded in a number of herpesvirus genomes. These DNA viruses utilize the highly conserved host machinery to produce their own virally encoded miRNAs. These viral-encoded miRNAs are important regulators in both viral life cycle and virus-host interaction, specifically viral oncogenesis.

Introduction

MiRNAs are generally transcribed by RNA polymerase II (Figure 1) [Lee, 2004]. The capped, polyadenylated RNA transcript is known as the primary miRNA (pri-miRNA), which may contain one or several miRNAs [Cai, 2004]. Within the pri-miRNA transcript, the miRNA forms a ~80 bp hairpin stem-loop structure, known as the pre-miRNA [Cullen, 2004]. The pre-miRNA hairpin stem-loop structure is recognized and cleaved from the pri-miRNA transcript by Drosha and DGCR8 [Lee, 2003; Denli, 2004; Gregory, 2004; Tomari, 2005]. The pre-miRNA is then exported from the nucleus into the cytoplasm by Exportin 5 and its cofactor Ran [Yi, 2003; Lund, 2004; Zeng, 2004]. The remainder of the pri-miRNA transcript remains in the nucleus and is degraded [Cai, 2005]. The pre-miRNA is then bound by the RNAse III enzyme Dicer, which cleaves the terminal loop of the pre-miRNA yielding the 21-23 bp miRNA duplex product [Bartel, 2004; Cullen, 2004; Chendrimada, 2005; Elbashir, 2001a; Elbashir, 2001b; Hutvagner, 2001]. Dicer subsequently facilitates the assembly of one of the miRNA strands into the RNA-induced silencing complex (RISC) [Chendrimada, 2005; Hammond, 2000; Maniataki, 2005; Tomari, 2004]. The unincorporated strand of the mature miRNA is released and degraded. The RISC complex containing the miRNA strand is now ready to function on its target mRNA.

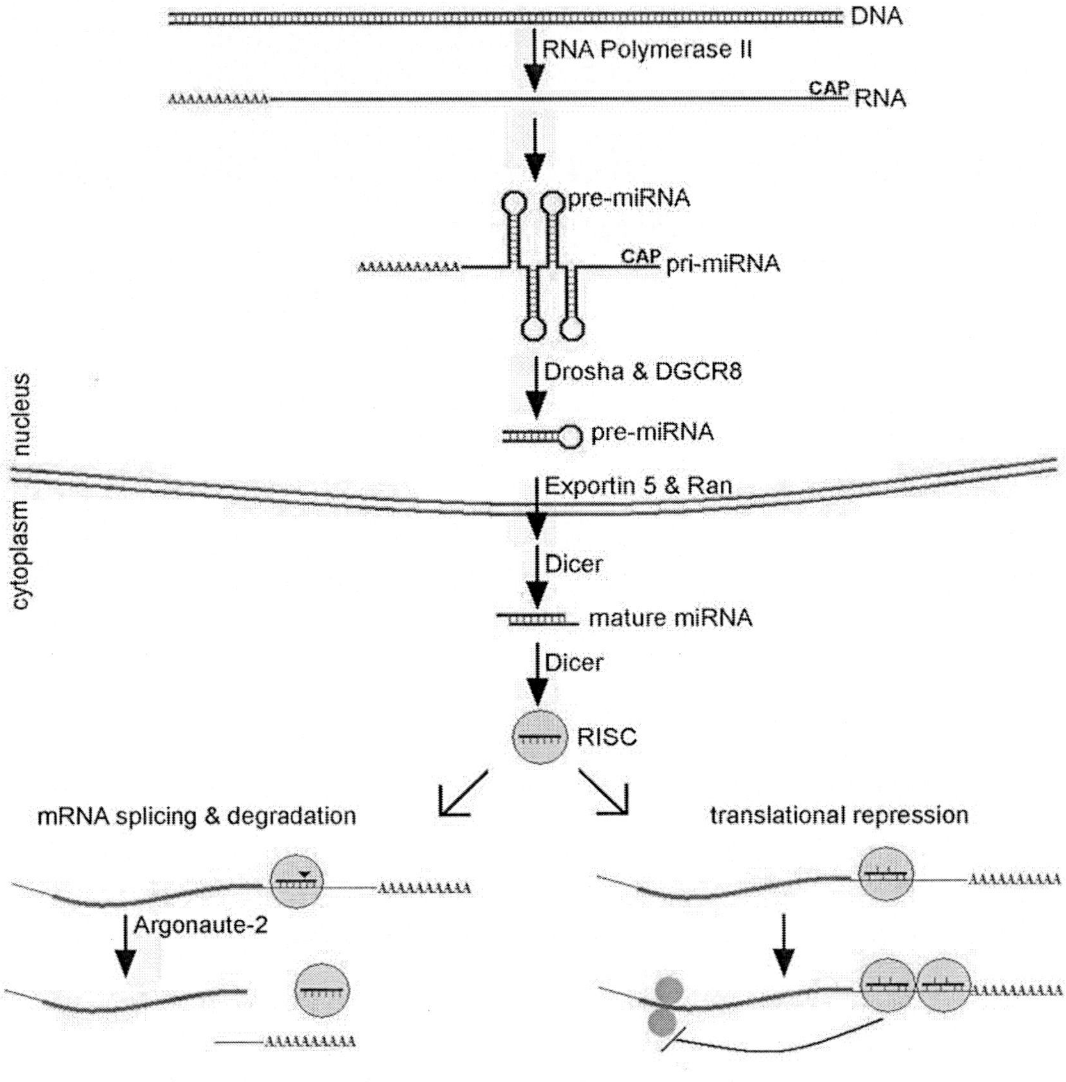

Figure 1. MiRNA Processing and Action.

The miRNA within the RISC complex directs RISC to a complementary mRNA species [Schwarz, 2002; Brown, 2005]. The 5' 2-8 residues of the miRNA, or "seed sequence", engages in Watson-Crick base pairing with its target mRNA [Lewis, 2005]. If a perfect match is encountered, Argonaute-2 within the RISC complex can function to cleave the mRNA, which will then be degraded [Liu, 2004; Meister, 2004; Liu, 2005; Zeng, 2003; Yekta, 2004; Hutvagner, 2002; Bagga, 2005]. More commonly, imperfect binding will occur, which results in translational repression of the target mRNA [Olsen, 1999; Zeng, 2002; Doench, 2004]. This typically requires several RISC complexes bound to the target mRNA [Doench, 2004].

MiRNAs require limited homology beyond the seed sequence to act on a target mRNA, which reduces the need for conservation. Therefore, an expected lack of miRNA sequence homology in viruses is present, attributable in part to a higher rate of mutation and the potentially faster evolution of viruses, as compared to eukaryotes. For instance, I human gamma herpesvirus Epstein-Barr Virus (EBV), a lymphocryptovirus, and Kaposi sarcoma-associated herpesvirus (KSHV), a rhadinovirus, are separated by 60-80 million years. In this case, the lack of conservation of miRNAs between genomes is not surprising. Genomes that are not as far divided, such as EBV and rhesus lymphocryptovirus (rLCV), within the lymphocryptovirus subfamily, contain several similar miRNAs, suggesting some level of conservation and therefore a possible selective advantage [Cai, 2006a]. Conversely, KSHV and rhesus rhadinovirus (RRV), within the rhadinovirus subfamily, do not contain sequence homologous miRNAs, though in both cases the viral miRNA clusters are positional homologs.

Currently, miRNAs have been confirmed in 12 herpesviruses: herpes simplex virus-1 and -2, human, mouse and chimpanzee cytomegalovirus, Epstein-Barr virus, rhesus lymphocryptovirus, mouse gammaherpesvirus-68, Kaposi's sarcoma-associated herpesvirus, rhesus rhadinovirus and Marek's disease virus-1 and -2. Table 1 gives a summary of each herpesvirus, including the number of viral miRNAs, names of viral miRNAs and references of the papers originally describing the discovery of the miRNAs.

Herpes Simplex Virus – 1 (HSV-1, HHV-1)

HSV-1 is an alpha herpesvirus. Like most alpha herpesviruses, it has a relatively short reproductive cycle, spreads rapidly in culture and establishes latent infections primarily in sensory ganglia. HSV-1, which typically causes oro-facial infection, can eventually establish latency in trigeminal ganglia in humans. Interestingly, growing numbers of genital herpes (over 50% of primary episodes) have been attributed to HSV-1 [Xu, 2002]. As is commonly true with latent infection, viral reactivation and reoccurrence of infection can occur. Though the disease is generally mild in most individuals, HSV infection can cause life-threatening illness, namely Herpes simplex encephalitis.

The HSV genome is over 150 kbp in length and encodes nearly 80 gene products. Computational analysis predicted several HSV-1 viral miRNAs [Pfeffer, 2005]. Northern blot analysis and cloning eventually identified a single miRNA gene [Cui, 2006]. Time course analysis indicated HSV1-miR-H1 expression kinetics resembled that of a late gene product, detectable starting 4 hours post infection and remaining high after 8 hours post infection [Cui, 2006]. Subsequent cDNA sequencing recovered an additional 7 mature miRNAs from 5 additional miRNA gene loci [Umbach, 2008]. These viral miRNAs were transcribed in both infected cell culture models and in the trigeminal ganglia of latently infected mice. Four of the viral miRNAs derive from the second exon of the spliced ~6.3kb latency associated

Table 1. Herpesvirus miRNAs

Virus (Host)	miRNA Gene	Acession Number	Mature miRNA	Sequence	Reference
HSV-1 (Human)	HSV1-miR-H1	MI0004730	HSV1-miR-H1	uggaaggacgggaaguggaag	7
	HSV1-miR-H2	MI0008937	HSV1-miR-H2-5p	ucgcacgcgcccggcacagacu	18
			HSV1-miR-H2-3p	ccugagccagggacgagugcgacu	18
	HSV1-miR-H3	MI0008938	HSV1-miR-H3	cugggacugugcgguuggga	18
	HSV1-miR-H4	MI0008939	HSV1-miR-H4-5p	gguagaguuugacaggcaagca	18
			HSV1-miR-H4-3p	cuugccugucuaacucgcuagu	18
	HSV1-miR-H5	MI0008940	HSV1-miR-H5	gucagagauccaaacccuccgg	18
	HSV1-miR-H6	MI0008941	HSV1-miR-H6	cacuucccguccuuccauccc	18
HSV-2 (Human)	HSV2-miR-I		HSV2-miR-I	uagugcuugccugucuaacuc	17
HCMV (Human)	HCMV-miR-UL22A	MI0001678	HCMV-miR-UL22A	uaacuagccuucccgugaga	9,12,14
			HCMV-miR-UL22A*	ucaccagaaugcuaguuuguag	9,12,14
	HCMV-miR-UL36	MI0001679	HCMV-miR-UL36	ucguugaagacaccuggaaaga	10,12,14
			HCMV-miR-UL36*	uuuccagguguuuucaacgugc	10,12,14
	HCMV-miR-UL70	MI0003688	HCMV-miR-UL70-5p	ugcgucucggccucguccaga	10
			HCMV-miR-UL70-3p	ggggaugggcuggcgcgcgg	10
	HCMV-miR-UL112	MI0001680	HCMV-miR-UL112	aagugacggugagauccaggcu	12,14
	HCMV-miR-US4	MI0003687	HCMV-miR-US4	cgacauggacgugcagggggau	10
	HCMV-miR-US5-1	MI0001682	HCMV-miR-US5-1	ugacaagccugacgagagcgu	10,12,14
	HCMV-miR-US5-2	MI0001683	HCMV-miR-US5-2	uuaugauaggugugacgauguc	10,12,14
	HCMV-miR-US25-1	MI0001684	HCMV-miR-US25-1	aaccgcucaguggcucggacc	9,12,14
			HCMV-miR-US25-1*	uccgaacgcuaggucgguucuc	9,12,14

Virus (Host)	miRNA Gene	Acession Number	Mature miRNA	Sequence	Reference
	HCMV-miR-US25-2	MI0001685	HCMV-miR-US25-2-5p	agcggucuguucagguggauga	12,14
			HCMV-miR-US25-2-3p	auccacuuggagagcucccgcgg	12,14
	HCMV-miR-US33	MI0001686	HCMV-miR-US33-5p	gauugugcccggaccgugggcg	12,14
			HCMV-miR-US33-3p	ucacgguccgagcacaucca	12,14
mCMV (Mouse)	mCMV-miR-M23-1	MI0006252	mCMV-miR-M23-1-5p	cucgguacggacggggaaccgu	1,8
			mCMV-miR-M23-1-3p	cuccugcgucggcccgaggcc	1,8
	mCMV-miR-M23-2	MI0006253	mCMV-miR-M23-2	augggggccucggucaagcgg	1,8
			mCMV-miR-M23-2*	ugaacguguccccuaucggugg	1,8
	mCMV-miR-M44-1	MI0006254	mCMV-miR-M44-1	uaucuuuuuccagagccgcggu	8
	mCMV-miR-M55-1	MI0006255	mCMV-miR-M55-1	uggugaucggcgugcuagccgu	8
	mCMV-miR-M87-1	MI0006258	mCMV-miR-M87-1	aggcagccgucggcagcggcagc	8
	mCMV-miR-M95-1	MI0006260	mCMV-miR-M95-1-5p	ggucgugggcuugugucgcuug	1,8
			mCMV-miR-M95-1-3p	agcgacgucggaccgcgacggc	1,8
	mCMV-miR-m01-1	MI0006246	mCMV-miR-M1-1	agaggagaauaacgucgaacgg	8
	mCMV-miR-m01-2	MI0006247	mCMV-miR-M1-2	gaagagaaucggguuggaacggu	1,8
			mCMV-miR-M1-2*	cguucgacacgguuuccuucga	1,8
	mCMV-miR-m01-3	MI0006248	mCMV-miR-M1-3	cggugaagcgacuguugccucga	1,8
			mCMV-miR-M1-3*	cgaggaacgcucgcuucacggc	1,8
	mCMV-miR-m01-4	MI0006249	mCMV-miR-M1-4	uccuaugcuaacacgugcgcgug	1,8
			mCMV-miR-M1-4*	cgccgcgugguagcauuagaac	1,8
	mCMV-miR-m21-1	MI0006250	mCMV-miR-M21-1	auaggggacacguucaagccg	1,8
	mCMV-miR-m22-1	MI0006251	mCMV-miR-M22-1	uuccccguccguaccgaggcca	1,8
	mCMV-miR-m59-1	MI0006256	mCMV-miR-M59-1	uuagcagugccucgaccgucag	8
	mCMV-miR-m59-2	MI0006257	mCMV-miR-M59-2	cccgaagagcccucacagagcc	8
	mCMV-miR-m88-1	MI0006259	mCMV-miR-M88-1	cagaagucgaugucggggucu	1,8
			mCMV-miR-M88-1*	augaccgacccccugacaucgg	1,8

Table 1. Continued

Virus (Host)	miRNA Gene	Acession Number	Mature miRNA	Sequence	Reference
	mCMV-miR-m107-1	MI0006261	mCMV-miR-M107-1-5p	cggucacucgucucgagucacc	1,8
			mCMV-miR-M107-1-3p	ugcucgcgucgagugaccgcuc	1,8
	mCMV-miR-m108-1	MI0006262	mCMV-miR-M108-1	uuucugacgguggcucgugucg	1,8
			mCMV-miR-M108-1*	ucacgagcaaccgcccgaaaug	1,8
	mCMV-miR-m108-2	MI0006263	mCMV-miR-M108-2-5p.2	ucacucgucgcgagcggucac	1,8
			mCMV-miR-M108-2-5p.1	gcggucacucgacgcgagcaccg	1,8
EBV (Human)	EBV-miR-BART1	MI0001067	EBV-miR-BART1-3p	uagcaccgcuauccacuauguc	5,12,13
			EBV-miR-BART1-5p	ucuuaguggaagugacgugcugug	5,12,13
	EBV-miR-BART2	MI0001068	EBV-miR-BART2-5p	uauuuucugcauucgcccuugc	12,13
			EBV-miR-BART2-3p	aaggagcgauuuggagaaaauaaa	12,13
	EBV-miR-BART3	MI0003725	EBV-miR-BART3	cgcaccacuagucaccaggugu	5,11,12
			EBV-miR-BART3*	accuaguguuaguguugugcu	5,11,12
	EBV-miR-BART4	MI0003726	EBV-miR-BART4	gaccugaugcugcuggugugcu	5,11,12
	EBV-miR-BART6	MI0003728	EBV-miR-BART6-3p	cggggaucggacuagccuuaga	5,11,12
			EBV-miR-BART6-5p	uaagguugguccaauccauagg	5,11,12
	EBV-miR-BART7	MI0003729	EBV-miR-BART7	caucauaguccaguguccaggg	5,11,12
			EBV-miR-BART7*	ccuggaccuugacuaugaaaca	5,11,12
	EBV-miR-BART8	MI0003730	EBV-miR-BART8	uacgguuuccuagauuguacag	5,11,12
			EBV-miR-BART8*	gucacaaucuauggggucguaga	5,11,12
	EBV-miR-BART9	MI0003731	EBV-miR-BART9	uaacacuucaugggucccguagu	5,11,12
			EBV-miR-BART9*	uacuggacccugaauuggaaac	5,11,12
	EBV-miR-BART10	MI0003732	EBV-miR-BART10	uacauaaccauggaguuggcugu	5,11,12
			EBV-miR-BART10*	gccaccucuuugguucuguaca	5,11,12

Virus (Host)	miRNA Gene	Acession Number	Mature miRNA	Sequence	Reference
	EBV-miR-BART11	MI0003733	EBV-miR-BART11-5p	ucagacaguuuggugcgcuaguug	5,11,12
			EBV-miR-BART11-3p	acgcacaccaggcugacugcc	5,11,12
	EBV-miR-BART12	MI0003734	EBV-miR-BART12	uccugugguguuugguguggguu	5,11,12
	EBV-miR-BART13	MI0003735	EBV-miR-BART13*	aaccggcucguggcucguacag	5,11,12
			EBV-miR-BART13	uguaacuugccagggacggcuga	5,11,12
	EBV-miR-BART14	MI0003736	EBV-miR-BART14	uaaaugcugcaguaguagggau	5,11,12
			EBV-miR-BART14*	uacccuacgcugccgauuuaca	5,11,12
	EBV-miR-BART15	MI0004988	EBV-miR-BART15	gucagugguuuuguuuccuuga	11,12
	EBV-miR-BART16	MI0004989	EBV-miR-BART16	uuagauagagugggugugugcucu	11,12
	EBV-miR-BART17	MI0004990	EBV-miR-BART17-5p	uaagaggacgcaggcauacaag	11,12
			EBV-miR-BART17-3p	uguaugccugguguccccuuagu	11,12
	EBV-miR-BART18	MI0004991	EBV-miR-BART18-3p	uaucggaaguuugggcuucguc	11,12
			EBV-miR-BART18-5p	ucaaguucgcacuuccuauaca	11,12
	EBV-miR-BART19	MI0004992	EBV-miR-BART19-5p	acauuccccgcaaacaugacaug	11,12
			EBV-miR-BART19-3p	uuuuguuugcuugggaaugcu	11,12
	EBV-miR-BART20	MI0004993	EBV-miR-BART20-5p	uagcaggcaugucuucauucc	11,12
			EBV-miR-BART20-3p	caugaaggcacagccuguuacc	11,12
	EBV-miR-BHRF1-1	MI0001064	EBV-miR-BHRF1-1	uaaccugaucagccccggaguu	12,13
	EBV-miR-BHRF1-2	MI0001065	EBV-miR-BHRF1-2*	aaauucuguugcagcagauagc	12,13
			EBV-miR-BHRF1-2	uaucuuuugcggcagaaauuga	12,13
	EBV-miR-BHRF1-3	MI0001066	EBV-miR-BHRF1-3	uaacgggaaguguguaagcaca	
rLCV (Simian)	rLCV-miR-rL1-1	MI0003737	rLCV-miR-rL1-1	uaaccugaucagccccggggguu	5
	rLCV-miR-rL1-10	MI0003746	rLCV-miR-rL1-10	uagugcgccggugaccugauag	5
	rLCV-miR-rL1-11	MI0003747	rLCV-miR-rL1-11	ugacacucgauaggauacgggg	5
	rLCV-miR-rL1-12	MI0003748	rLCV-miR-rL1-12-5p	agaccagaccaugcacaguggg	5
			rLCV-miR-rL1-12-3p	aacggugcauggacuggcuaga	5

Table 1. Continued

Virus (Host)	miRNA Gene	Acession Number	Mature miRNA	Sequence	Reference
	rLCV-miR-rL1-13	MI0003749	rLCV-miR-rL1-13	gaucauagccaguguccaggga	5
	rLCV-miR-rL1-14	MI0003750	rLCV-miR-rL1-14-5p	ucggacggucuggugcgcuugau	5
			rLCV-miR-rL1-14-3p	ucgcacaucaggcugaacgac	5
	rLCV-miR-rL1-15	MI0003751	rLCV-miR-rL1-15	uccuguagaguauggguggguuu	5
	rLCV-miR-rL1-16	MI0003752	rLCV-miR-rL1-16-5p	agcaggcaugucuucauucc	5
			rLCV-miR-rL1-16-3p	caugaaacacauggccuguucc	5
	rLCV-miR-rL1-2	MI0003738	rLCV-miR-rL1-2	uaucuuuugcgggggaauuucca	5
	rLCV-miR-rL1-3	MI0003739	rLCV-miR-rL1-3	cgcaccucgccgucucuacugcu	5
	rLCV-miR-rL1-4	MI0003740	rLCV-miR-rL1-4-3p	caccacacgauccacuaggucu	5
			rLCV-miR-rL1-4-5p	accuaguaauugugcgguguu	5
	rLCV-miR-rL1-5	MI0003741	rLCV-miR-rL1-5-3p	cgcaccacuuuucacuaggugu	5
			rLCV-miR-rL1-5-5p	aaccuagugccggugaugugcu	5
	rLCV-miR-rL1-6	MI0003742	rLCV-miR-rL1-6-5p	uuuaguggaagugacgugcugug	5,12
			rLCV-miR-rL1-6	uagcaccgcuauccacuauguc	5,12
	rLCV-miR-rL1-7	MI0003743	rLCV-miR-rL1-7	cgagguaaacaucggcuuacug	5
	rLCV-miR-rL1-8	MI0003744	rLCV-miR-rL1-8	uaaggugaauauagcugcccauug	5,12
	rLCV-miR-rL1-9	MI0003745	rLCV-miR-rL1-9	ucgaugcaugguccccccuuagu	5
MHV-68 (Mouse)	MGHV-miR-M1-1	MI0001669	MGHV-miR-M1-1	uagaaauggccguacuuccuuu	12,15
	MGHV-miR-M1-2	MI0001670	MGHV-miR-M1-2	cagacccccucucccccucuuu	12,15
	MGHV-miR-M1-3	MI0001671	MGHV-miR-M1-3	gaggugagcaggaguugcgcuu	12,15
	MGHV-miR-M1-4	MI0001672	MGHV-miR-M1-4	ucgaggagcacguguuauucua	12,15
	MGHV-miR-M1-5	MI0001673	MGHV-miR-M1-5	agaguugagaucgggucgucuc	12,15
	MGHV-miR-M1-6	MI0001674	MGHV-miR-M1-6	ugaaacugugugagguggguuuu	12,15

Virus (Host)	miRNA Gene	Acession Number	Mature miRNA	Sequence	Reference
	MGHV-miR-M1-7	MI0001675	MGHV-miR-M1-7-5p	aaagguggaggugcgguaaccu	12,15
			MGHV-miR-M1-7-3p	gauaucgcgcccaccuuuauu	12,15
	MGHV-miR-M1-8	MI0001676	MGHV-miR-M1-8	agcacucacugggggguuugguc	12,15
	MGHV-miR-M1-9	MI0001677	MGHV-miR-M1-9	ucacauuugccuggaccuuuuu	12,15
KSHV	KSHV-miR-K12-2	MI0002476	KSHV-miR-K12-2	aacuguaguccgggucgaucug	4,6
(Human)	KSHV-miR-K12-1	MI0002475	KSHV-miR-K12-1	auuacaggaaacuggguguaagc	4,6,12,14,15
	KSHV-miR-K12-11	MI0002474	KSHV-miR-K12-11	uuaaugcuuagccuguguccga	6,12,14,15
	KSHV-miR-K12-12	MI0004987	KSHV-miR-K12-4-3p	uagaauacugaggccuagcuga	11
			KSHV-miR-K12-12	accaggccaccauuccucuccg	11
	KSHV-miR-K12-3	MI0002483	KSHV-miR-K12-3	ucacauucugaggacggcagcga	4,6,12,14,15
			KSHV-miR-K12-3*	ucgcggucacagaaugugaca	4,6,12,14,15
	KSHV-miR-K12-4	MI0002482	KSHV-miR-K12-4-5p	agcuaaaccgcaguacucuagg	4,6,12,14,15
	KSHV-miR-K12-5	MI0002481	KSHV-miR-K12-5	uaggaugccuggaacuugccgg	4,6,12,14,15
	KSHV-miR-K12-6	MI0002480	KSHV-miR-K12-6-3p	ugaugguuuucgggcuguugag	4,6,12,14,15
			KSHV-miR-K12-6-5p	ccagcagcaccuaauccaucgg	4,6,12,14,15
	KSHV-miR-K12-8	MI0002478	KSHV-miR-K12-8	uaggcgcgacugagagagcacg	4,6,12,14,15
	KSHV-miR-K12-9	MI0002477	KSHV-miR-K12-9	cuggguauacgcagcugcguaa	4,6,12,14,15
			KSHV-miR-K12-9*	acccagcugcguaaaccccgcu	4,6,12,14,15
RRV	RRV-miR-rR1-1	MI0005718	RRV-miR-rR1-1	cgaucgcaccuuuggccggccgg	16
(Simian)			RRV-miR-rR1-1*	ggccaccgaggaugcgguc	16
	RRV-miR-rR1-2	MI0005719	RRV-miR-rR1-2	auacggcgcugcacgguugga	16
	RRV-miR-rR1-3	MI0005720	RRV-miR-rR1-3	cccgaugagcaguuagucc	16
	RRV-miR-rR1-4	MI0005721	RRV-miR-rR1-4*	cucguuaaccgcccucccgaga	16
			RRV-miR-rR1-4	uggggagggcggucagcgcgcg	16
	RRV-miR-rR1-5	MI0005722	RRV-miR-rR1-5	ccggaacccaaagacacgugcccg	16

Table 1. Continued

Virus (Host)	miRNA Gene	Acession Number	Mature miRNA	Sequence	Reference
	RRV-miR-rR1-6	MI0005723	RRV-miR-rR1-6*	cgauguacgcccuuucgcagu	16
			RRV-miR-rR1-6	cgcggaaaggugugcacaucgua	16
	RRV-miR-rR1-7	MI0005724	RRV-miR-rR1-7-5p	uggagagcaguuaacgugcguuc	16
			RRV-miR-rR1-7-3p	cgcacgucgauugcucucuag	16
MDV-1 (Chicken)	MDV1-miR-M31	MI0008337	MDV1-miR-M31	ugcuacagucgugagcagaucaa	3
	MDV1-miR-M1	MI0005093	MDV1-miR-M1*	ugcugcgcaugaaagagcga	2,3,20
			MDV1-miR-M1	ugcuuguucacugugcggca	2,3,20
	MDV1-miR-M10	MI0006988	MDV1-miR-M10-5p	gcguugucucguagagguccag	3,20
			MDV1-miR-M10-3p	ucgaaaucucuacgagauaaca	3,20
	MDV1-miR-M11	MI0006989	MDV1-miR-M11-3p	ugaguuacauggucaggggauu	20
			MDV1-miR-M11-5p	uuuuccuuaccguguagcuuaga	20
	MDV1-miR-M12	MI0006990	MDV1-miR-M12	ugcauaauacggaggguucu	2,3,20
	MDV1-miR-M13	MI0006991	MDV1-miR-M13	gcauggaaacguccugggaaa	20
			MDV1-miR-M2	guuguauucugcccgguaguccg	2,3,20
	MDV1-miR-M3	MI0005095	MDV1-miR-M3	augaaaaugugaaaccucucccgc	2,3,20
	MDV1-miR-M4	MI0005096	MDV1-miR-M4	uuaaugcuguaucggaacccuuc	2,3,20
			MDV1-miR-M4*	aagguucugacagcaugacc	2,3,20
	MDV1-miR-M5	MI0005097	MDV1-miR-M5*	aaccguaugcgaucacauugac	2,3,20
			MDV1-miR-M5	uguguaucguggucgucuacugu	2,3,20
	MDV1-miR-M6	MI0005098	MDV1-miR-M6-5p	ucuguuguuccguaguguucuc	2,3,20
			MDV1-miR-M6-3p	gagaucccugcgaaaugacagu	2,3,20
	MDV1-miR-M7	MI0005099	MDV1-miR-M7	uguuaucucggggagaucccgau	2,3,20
			MDV1-miR-M7*	ucgagaucucuacgagauuacag	2,3,20

Virus (Host)	miRNA Gene	Acession Number	Mature miRNA	Sequence	Reference
	MDV1-miR-M8	MI0005100	MDV1-miR-M8-5p	uauuguucugugguugguuucg	2,3,20
			MDV1-miR-M8-3p	gugaccucuacggaacaauagu	2,3,20
	MDV1-miR-M9	MI0006987	MDV1-miR-M9*	aaacuccgagggcaggaaaaag	20
			MDV1-miR-M9	uuuucuccuuccccccggaguu	20
MDV-2 (Chicken)	MDV2-miR-M14	MI0005882	MDV2-miR-M14-3p	ucaggaaguuccgugcccgaa	19
			MDV2-miR-M14-5p	gugugguacggugcacccugaga	19
	MDV2-miR-M15	MI0005883	MDV2-miR-M15*	uggaagggaaaggcaaaccgga	19
			MDV2-miR-M15	uggugugguuuuucccuuccaucgca	19
	MDV2-miR-M16	MI0005884	MDV2-miR-M16	cauccagucuguuuuggcaucuga	19
	MDV2-miR-M17	MI0005885	MDV2-miR-M17*	aguccuucccggguccccuaga	19
			MDV2-miR-M17	uaggacaaccgggacggacagg	19
	MDV2-miR-M18	MI0005886	MDV2-miR-M18-3p	caaugccugcggagagaaaga	19
			MDV2-miR-M18-5p	uguuuucucucaggcuggcauugc	19
	MDV2-miR-M19	MI0005887	MDV2-miR-M19	caugccccccuccgaggguagc	19
	MDV2-miR-M20	MI0005888	MDV2-miR-M20*	uccuuagcgugggugccugaga	19
			MDV2-miR-M20	ucaaguacugcgcgcaaggaccg	19
	MDV2-miR-M21	MI0005889	MDV2-miR-M21*	ucccuccuucgcggggugcuuga	19
			MDV2-miR-M21	gagcaccacgccgauggacggaga	19
	MDV2-miR-M22	MI0005890	MDV2-miR-M22*	uaguggcuugcuuguaggcugu	19
			MDV2-miR-M22	ucuuacacgcacgucacucugguc	19
	MDV2-miR-M23	MI0005891	MDV2-miR-M23	augguccgugguacgguguccu	19
	MDV2-miR-M24	MI0005892	MDV2-miR-M24	uuagaugccgucagggaaagau	19
	MDV2-miR-M25	MI0005893	MDV2-miR-M25-3p	caugcacuacuccgggggguaggac	19
			MDV2-miR-M25-5p	ccuccuucggacgagugcuugccg	19
	MDV2-miR-M26	MI0005894	MDV2-miR-M26	uccuuugugcugugugugaga	19

Table 1. Continued

Virus (Host)	miRNA Gene	Acession Number	Mature miRNA	Sequence	Reference
	MDV2-miR-M27	MI0005895	MDV2-miR-M27-3p	gcgucgagcaccgugcuggaggaa	19
			MDV2-miR-M27-5p	cuucguccgguguucgaggcgu	19
	MDV2-miR-M28	MI0005896	MDV2-miR-M28*	cgaggguaggcgcagaggaaaucg	19
			MDV2-miR-M28	uuuucucgacgccuacccucggcg	19
	MDV2-miR-M29	MI0005897	MDV2-miR-M29	ucuucacguaccucucuauggcu	19
	MDV2-miR-M30	MI0005898	MDV2-miR-M30	caacacucccucggacgcagca	19

[1] Buck, A.H., et al., Discrete clusters of virus-encoded micrornas are associated with complementary strands of the genome and the 7.2-kilobase stable intron in murine cytomegalovirus. *J Virol*, 2007. 81(24): p. 13761-70.

[2] Burnside, J., et al., Marek's disease virus encodes MicroRNAs that map to meq and the latency-associated transcript. *J Virol*, 2006. 80(17): p. 8778-86.

[3] Burnside, J. and R.W. Morgan, Genomics and Marek's disease virus. *Cytogenet Genome Res*, 2007. 117(1-4): p. 376-87.

[4] Cai, X., et al., Kaposi's sarcoma-associated herpesvirus expresses an array of viral microRNAs in latently infected cells. *Proc Natl Acad Sci U S A*, 2005. 102(15): p. 5570-5.

[5] Cai, X., et al., Epstein-Barr virus microRNAs are evolutionarily conserved and differentially expressed. *PLoS Pathog*, 2006a. 2(3): p. e23.

[6] Cai, X. and B.R. Cullen, Transcriptional origin of Kaposi's sarcoma-associated herpesvirus microRNAs. *J Virol*, 2006b. 80(5): p. 2234-42.

[7] Cui, C., et al., Prediction and identification of herpes simplex virus 1-encoded microRNAs. *J Virol*, 2006. 80(11): p. 5499-508.

[8] Dolken, L., et al., Mouse cytomegalovirus microRNAs dominate the cellular small RNA profile during lytic infection and show features of posttranscriptional regulation. *J Virol*, 2007. 81(24): p. 13771-82.

[9] Dunn, W., et al., Human cytomegalovirus expresses novel microRNAs during productive viral infection. *Cell Microbiol*, 2005. 7(11): p. 1684-95.

[10] Grey, F., et al., Identification and characterization of human cytomegalovirus-encoded microRNAs. *J Virol*, 2005. 79(18): p. 12095-9.

[11] Grundhoff, A., C.S. Sullivan, and D. Ganem, A combined computational and microarray-based approach identifies novel microRNAs encoded by human gamma-herpesviruses. *Rna*, 2006. 12(5): p. 733-50.

[12] Landgraf, P., et al., A mammalian microRNA expression atlas based on small RNA library sequencing. *Cell*, 2007. 129(7): p. 1401-14.

[13] Pfeffer, S., et al., Identification of microRNAs of the herpesvirus family. *Nat Methods*, 2005. 2(4): p. 269-76.

[14] Pfeffer, S., et al., Identification of virus-encoded microRNAs. *Science*, 2004. 304(5671): p. 734-6.

[15] Samols, M.A., et al., Cloning and identification of a microRNA cluster within the latency-associated region of Kaposi's sarcoma-associated herpesvirus. *J Virol*, 2005. 79(14): p. 9301-5.

[16] Schafer, A., et al., Cloning and analysis of microRNAs encoded by the primate gamma-herpesvirus rhesus monkey rhadinovirus. Virology, 2007. 364(1): p. 21-7.

[17] Tang, S., et al., An acutely and latently expressed herpes simplex virus 2 viral microRNA inhibits expression of ICP34.5, a viral neurovirulence factor. *Proc Natl Acad Sci U S A*, 2008. 105(31): p. 10931-6.

[18] Umbach, J.L., et al., MicroRNAs expressed by herpes simplex virus 1 during latent infection regulate viral mRNAs. *Nature*, 2008. 454(7205): p. 780-3.

[19] Yao, Y., et al., Marek's disease virus type 2 (MDV-2)-encoded microRNAs show no sequence conservation with those encoded by MDV-1. *J Virol*, 2007. 81(13): p. 7164-70.

[20] Yao, Y., et al., MicroRNA profile of Marek's disease virus-transformed T-cell line MSB-1: predominance of virus-encoded microRNAs. *J Virol*, 2008. 82(8): p. 4007-15.

[21] The Wellcome Trust Sanger Institute. miRBase. http://microrna.sanger.ac.uk/.

transcript (LAT) locus of the HSV-1 genome, with LAT able to fold into the expected precursor stem-loop structure for each miRNA. Folding of the resulting pri-miRNA into a structure containing multiple hairpins may offer added stability, which may explain the high level of stability of the LAT transcript. The LAT transcript is the only viral gene product expressed at abundant levels during latency [Stevens, 1987], suggesting viral miRNA expression is highly important in maintaining HSV-1 latency.

HSV1-miR-H2, -H3, -H4, and -H6 all have predicted viral targets. HSV1-miR-H2 is antisense to the immediate-early infected cell protein 0 (ICP0) transcript. Co-transfection experiments indicated that ICP0 protein levels were reduced upon HSV1-miR-H2 expression. This is due to a translational repression and not mRNA degradation, despite perfect target homology [Umbach, 2008]. ICP0 is not essential for viral replication but promotes lytic infection [Hagglund, 2004]. ICP0 null mutant viruses are defective for progression through a productive lytic life cycle [Stow, 1986]. The effect of decreased ICP0 protein, an immediate early HSV-1 transcriptional activator, is a push towards latency of the virus. Thus, HSV1-miR-H2 expression may promote or maintain viral latency. HSV1-miR-H3 and -H4 were found to be complementary to ICP34.5 though it was not directly examined as a target. Finally, HSV1-miR-H6 is predicted to target ICP4, an immediate early protein. ICP4 is required for maximal levels of all early and late gene expression [Clements, 1977; Knipe, 1978; Preston, 1979; Watson, 1980]. It is involved in both specific and nonspecific DNA binding and interacts with transcription factors [Kristie, 1986; Michael, 1988]. ICP4 mutants are unable to express early, and therefore late, lytic genes without exposure to sodium butyrate [Poon, 2006]. Thus, ICP4 is required for lytic replication and its down regulation would result in a shift towards latency. Finally, loss of the LAT transcript, which would include loss of all HSV-1 viral miRNAs, results in a loss of cell protection and increased levels of apoptosis [Inman, 2001]. It is therefore likely that all these viral miRNAs may be working in part to start or maintain viral latency. Consequently, a viral miRNA deletion virus would preferentially enter the lytic rather than the latent phase of the viral life cycle.

Herpes Simplex Virus – 2 (HSV-2, HHV-2)

HSV-2 is also an alpha herpesvirus. HSV-2 infection typically causes genital herpes and can establish latency in dorsal root ganglia in humans. Neonatal HSV infection, acquired intrapartum, is highly symptomatic and often lethal. As with HSV-1, HSV-2 recurrent infection can be either symptomatic or asymptomatic [Roizman, 2001]. In general, HSV-2 infection recurs more frequently than HSV-1 infection [Benedetti, 1994; Lafferty, 1987].

The HSV-2 genome is 154 kb and encodes nearly 80 gene products. Extensive conservation between HSV-1 and HSV-2 genomes exists, with average sequence identity of approximately 83% [Dolan, 1998]. Computational analysis had previously indicated putative miRNA genes in the LAT region of the HSV-2 genome [Pfeffer, 2005]. Sequencing of small RNAs eventually revealed one such miRNA, HSV2-miR-I [Tang, 2008]. This sequence was conserved among multiple HSV-2 strains. HSV2-miR-I is located in LAT exon 2 and is antisense to ICP34.5, a key viral neurovirulence factor. HSV2-miR-I is detectable in infected cell culture, in active and latently infected guinea pig dorsal root ganglia and in human latently infected sacral dorsal root ganglia. Because HSV2-miR-I is located antisense to ICP34.5, ICP34.5 was considered a likely target of HSV2-miR-I. Further experiments revealed that HSV2-miR-I does in fact regulate ICP34.5 protein expression by RISC-mediated mRNA degradation. ICP34.5 is a late gene involved in active virus replication. Specifically, ICP34.5 is involved in a pathway to which final effect is to shut off PKR activation and induction of interferon (IFN) [Williams, 2001]. This pathway is normally activated in HSV infection due the presence of double-stranded RNA produced during active infection. A loss of ICP34.5 expression would result in an increase in IFN, which is generally not a desirable effect for the virus. However, during latency, these ds-RNAs are not produced. Therefore, down regulation of ICP34.5 would result in the establishment and maintenance of viral latency.

Marek's Disease Virus – 1 (MDV-1)

MDV-1, an alpha herpesvirus, infects epithelial cells, T lymphocytes and B lymphocytes in chickens. However, fully productive infection occurs only in feather follicle epithelium. MDV-1 causes Marek's disease, a lymphoid cell infiltration or lymphomatuous tumor in the peripheral nerves and gonads [Witter, 1997].

The MDV-1 genome is nearly 178 kbp long and encodes 87 genes. MDV-1 has 14 miRNA genes encoding 23 mature miRNAs in two clusters [Burnside, 2006; Yao, 2008; Burnside, 2007]. The first cluster consists of MDV1-miR-M1 to -M5, -M9, -M11, -M12, and -M31, which flank the meq oncogene. The meq gene is the strongest candidate for an oncogene in MDV-1; its expression is important for transformation of lymphoblastoid cells [Xie, 1996], Rat-2 cells [Liu, 1998], Df-1 cells [Himly, 1998; Levy, 2005] and the formation of MDV oncogenesis [Lupiani, 2004]. Because MDV1-miRs-M1 to -M5 are oriented around the meq locus, with MDV1-miR-M2 through -M5 in the same orientation, it is possible that these miRNAs are contributing to meq–induced oncogenesis. MDV1-miR-M6 to -M8, -M10 and -M13 are clustered in a large intron of the latency-associated transcript MSR. Additonally, because both the meq locus and latency-associated transcript are expressed during latency, these miRNAs may also function to establish or maintain latency.

Deep sequencing analysis of multiple MDV-1 strains indicated high levels of sequence homology. Analysis of miRNA expression indicated MDV-1 miRNAs were differentially expressed between different strains, with MDV1-miR-M6 to -M8 showing no change in expression, while MDV1-miR-M2, -M4, -M5, and -M12 were expressed on varying levels in tumors depending on infection strain. Genomic clustering of the miRNAs would suggest common pri-miRNA transcripts. However, differential expression indicates a level of regulation beyond transcription, most like via miRNA processing. MDV1-miR-m4 had the highest level of miRNA expression in MDV-1, accounting for nearly 72% of all MDV-1 miRNAs. Many targets were suggested for the MDV-1 miRNAs, but none has yet been confirmed. Nonetheless, given the extremely high expression of MDV1-miR-m4, it is likely to play an important role in MDV-1 pathogenesis.

Marek's Disease Virus – 2 (MDV-2)

MDV-1 and MDV-2 diverged about 26 million years ago. Like MDV-1, MDV-2 is also an alpha herpesvirus, with the genome about 164 kbp long, encoding 76 genes. While genes within the UL and US regions of the two viruses are highly conserved, many open reading frames are unique to MDV-1. Moreover, while MDV-1 causes T-cell lymphomas in chickens, MDV-2 is non-oncogenic.

With the discovery of MDV-1 miRNAs, the search began for MDV-2 miRNAs. 17 miRNA MDV-2 genes were found, which encode 27 mature miRNAs [Yao, 2007]. These 17 miRNA genes are clustered in two regions of the genome, with 16 clustered in the same orientation in a 4.2 kb TR_L/IR_L region. Four putative ORFs exist in this cluster and eight miRNA genes were located in the coding regions of these genes. The clustering of these miRNAs in one region with the same orientation suggests a common precursor mRNA transcript. The only miRNA not in this cluster, MDV2-miR-M17, is located in the IR_s/RT_s region, oriented opposite ICP4. This suggests ICP4 as a possible MDV2-miR-M17 target, though this has not yet been confirmed. No other targets are known for the remaining MDV-2 miRNAs.

Human Cytomegalovirus (HCMV, HHV-5)

The beta herpesvirus HCMV is associated with congenital diseases and post-transplant complications [Pass, 2001]. It is the only herpesvirus that exhibits natural transplacental transmission. CMV infection in the US among individuals over 6 years of age is above 58% [Staras, 2006]. Following initial infection, infectious virus is found in virtually all bodily fluids for months to years post infection [Mocarski, 2001]. Like most beta herpesviruses, HCMV has a long reproductive cycle and exhibits slow viral spread in culture. Cytomegalia, or enlarged infected cells, are a hallmark of this herpesvirus family. HCMV specifically infects human fibroblast, endothelial, epithelial and astrocyte cells. Unlike some other herpesviruses, it is not significantly associated with any cancers. At 230 kb with over 150 unique ORFs, HCMV has the largest genome of all herpesviruses.

While viral miRNAs are typically clustered in the latency region of the genome, 16 HCMV miRNAs are located in 10 positions across the genome [Pfeffer, 2005; Grey, 2005; Dunn, 2005]. These miRNA genes are clustered (6 genes) and unclustered (4 genes) and transcribed from strands opposite to described ORFs, in intergenic regions or within introns [Pfeffer, 2005; Grey, 2005; Dunn, 2005]. These miRNAs were also highly expressed during the lytic stage of the viral life cycle.

Multiple experiments determined several targets of the viral miRNAs. HCMV-miR-UL112-1 targets the viral immediate early gene-72 (IE72) product, an immediate early trans-activator. Repression of IE72 results in attenuation of acute replication and therefore a switch to latency [Grey, 2008; Grey, 2007]. When HCVM-miR-UL112-1 is expressed, a decrease in protein expression is observed, indicating mRNA cleavage and degradation mediated by the miRNA. HCMV-miR-UL112-1 specifically binds cellular major histocompatibility complex class I-related chain B (MICB), which upsets binding with natural killer cell activating receptor NKG2D, resulting in evasion from natural killer cell attack [Stern-Ginossar, 2007]. This is an example of a viral miRNA directly down-regulating a host immune defense gene, providing a means of evading host immune response. Finally, HCMV-miR-UL112-1 also suppresses protein levels of viral gene IE1 by transcriptional repression [Murphy, 2008]. IE1 is required to execute the virus transcriptional program, the regulation of which would influence the choice between latency and lytic replication. Though IE1 is not required for viral replication at high multiplicities of infection (MOI), at MOI below 1 PFU/cell IE1 mutant viruses show replication attenuation. At MOI below 0.1 PFU/cell there is a complete failure to replicate [Gawn, 2002]. Overall, HCMV-miR-UL112-1 is involved in host immune evasion and down regulation of lytic proteins, resulting in the establishment of viral latency. To date, no targets have been confirmed for the other HCMV miRNAs. Chimpanzee cytomegalovirus (CCMV) is highly related with many conserved miRNAs, however few experiments have been done with this virus so very little is confirmed.

Mouse Cytomegalovirus (MCMV)

Given the findings of viral miRNAs in HCMV, further research was done to determine the presence of viral miRNAs in its murine homolog, MCMV. Like HCMV, MCMV is a beta herpesvirus. However, HCMV and MCMV share no detectable DNA sequence homology. MCMV has a large tissue tropism and grows to high titer in the salivary glands, liver and spleen of immunocompromised mice.

The MCMV genome is about 230 kbp long and contains over 165 genes. Computational analysis revealed the presence of multiple miRNA genes. Cloning of small miRNA pools and northern blotting confirmed the presence of 18 miRNA genes encoding for 28 mature miRNAs [Buck, 2007; Dolken, 2007]. As in HCMV, the MCMV miRNAs are spread out throughout the genome, some in clusters, on both DNA strands. Furthermore, the miRNA genes are intergenic, intronic and occasionally within or opposite an ORF. Kinetic experiments indicate that the viral miRNAs are expressed during the lytic portion of the viral life cycle, consistent with immediate-early and early expression [Buck, 2007; Dolken, 2007]. At late infection time points, MCMV miRNAs become highly abundant, surpassing expression levels of highly abundant cellular miRNAs, suggesting a level of competition between the two types of miRNAs [Dolken, 2007]. No conservation of sequence or location was observed between MCMV and HCMV, suggesting the miRNAs may function on host targets as opposed to viral ones.

Epstein-Barr Virus (EBV, HHV-4)

Like many gamma herpesviruses, EBV replicates in lymphoblastoid cells but can infect other cell types. EBV primarily infects human B cells but can infect T cells and epithelial cells as well. A gamma herpesvirus and a lymphocryptovirus, its genome is about 170 kbp in length and contains approximately 82 genes. Following B cell infection, the virus goes latent and typically forms a nuclear DNA episome, which can later be reactivated. EBV DNA can also integrate into chromosomal DNA. EBV infection is generally benign but can cause B- and T-cell lymphomas, as well as EBV-associated gastric carcinoma [Kieff, 2001; Kim do, 2007]. EBV infection is widespread in the human population, with over 90% of adults positive for antibodies to the viral capsid [Henle, 1969].

The first reported cloning and detection of small RNAs was found in a Burkitt's Lymphoma cell line latently infected with EBV [Pfeffer, 2004]. 4% of the recovered cDNAs were viral sequences. The 23 miRNA genes found in EBV are distributed into two distinct clusters. One cluster contains 3 miRNA genes, EBV-miR-BHRF1-1, -2 and -3, which encode for 4 mature miRNAs, and is located proximal to the BHRF1 open-reading frame [Pfeffer, 2004; Cai, 2006a; Grundhoff, 2006]. The other cluster contains 20 miRNA genes encoding 35 mature miRNAs. 2 miRNAs, EBV-miR-BART-1 and -2, are located with the BART gene, while an additional set of 13 EBV BART miRNAs map to a ~12 kb intronic region within the BART gene [Pfeffer, 2004; Cai, 2006a; Grundhoff, 2006]. These miRNA clusters are differentially expressed with the 3 member BHRF-1 cluster expressed exclusively in stage III latency, while all of the 20 member BART cluster are predominantly expressed during stage II latency. However, an induction of the miRNA expression is seen during lytic reactivation [Cai, 2006a].

The transcriptional origin of the miRNA clusters was determined. The expression of the 13 miRNA genes located within the intronic region of the BART gene directly coincides with BART expression, indicating the BART mRNA as the pri-miRNA transcript for these miRNAs [Cai, 2006a] and the P1 promoter [de Jesus, 2003; Sadler, 1995; Chen, 2005]. Several stable intermediates containing BART miRNAs are detectable, indicating splice variants and preferential processing to mature miRNAs [Edwards, 2008]. The BHRF1 miRNAs have differential splicing according to latency stage, in association with BHRF1 mRNA. This includes expression of a 1.3 kb transcript of miR-BHRF-1, BHRF1 open reading frame and EBV-miR-BHRF-2 during latency III, and expression of a 1.4 kb transcript of BHRF1 mRNA, EBV-miR-BHRF-2 and EBV-miR-BHRF-3 during induction of EBV replication in latency I [Xing, 2007].

Several EBV miRNA targets are known. The BART cluster 1 miRNAs are reported to target the expression of viral LMP1 protein [Lo, 2007]. The BART cluster 1 regulates LMP1 translation, as mRNA levels are not consistent with protein levels. LMP1 is required for transformation of primary B-lymphocytes to long-term lymphoblastoid cell lines (LCL) [Dirmeier, 2003; Dirmeier, 2005; Kaye, 1999; Kaye, 1995; Kaye, 1993; Kilger, 1998]. LMP1 also activates NF-KB, the inactivation of which results in rapid apoptosis [Cahir-McFarland, 2002; Cahir-McFarland, 2000; Cahir-McFarland]. However, elevated expression of LMP1 can result in growth inhibition [Eliopoulos, 1996]. MiRNA regulation indicates the importance of tightly controlled LMP1 expression for EBV pathogenesis. One known target of the EBV-miR-BART2 is the viral mRNA BALF5, which encodes EBV DNA polymerase [Pfeffer, 2004; Barth, 2008]. This target mRNA is transcribed from the opposite strand as EBV-miR-BART-2 and is cleaved in the area of homology, reducing the full-length 5.0 kb mRNA to 3.7 kb [Furnari, 1993]. The purpose of this function is not entirely understood, but could be involved in the establishment of latency or inhibition of lytic EBV replication. EBV-miR-BART5 is targets the cellular mRNA "p53 Up-regulated Modulator of Apoptosis", or PUMA [Choy, 2008]. Reduction of EBV-miR-BART5 or induction of PUMA can trigger apoptosis in EBV infected cells. Thus, EBV-miR-BART5 expression reduces PUMA levels, which aids in cell survival. EBV-miR-BHRF1-3 is known to target CXCL-11, an IFN-inducible T-cell attracting chemokine [Xia, 2008]. CXCL-11 has potent anti-tumor activity in laboratory animals, thus its down-regulation promotes EBV-related transformation [Hensbergen, 2005]. All together, the EBV miRNAs function to establish and maintain latency and eventually oncogenesis.

Rhesus Lymphocryptovirus (rLCV, Rh-LCV)

RLCV and EBV are primate lymphocryptoviruses that have diverged in sequence in parallel to the evolution of their primate host species. RLCV and EBV evolutionarily diverged between 13 and 23 million years ago [Gerner, 2004]. The rLCV genome is 171 kb and contains nearly 80 genes. Sequence analysis indicates a 65% shared homology between EBV and rLCV, with the structural proteins being most highly conserved and latent proteins being less conserved [Rivailler, 2002].

cDNA cloning of latently infected rhesus B cells identified 16 miRNA genes in two distinct clusters, expressing a total of 22 mature miRNAs [Cai, 2006a]. One miRNA, rLCV-miR-rL1-1 is located adjacent to the rLCV BHRF1 gene. The other 14 miRNA genes, expressing the remaining 20 mature miRNAs, are located adjacent to the rLCV BART locus. Eight of the mature miRNAs, derived from six miRNA genes, are conserved to EBV, especially in the seed sequence region of the mature miRNA [Cai, 2006a]. Additionally, the genomic order and orientation of the conserved miRNAs is also maintained.

To determine the level of conservation of the viral miRNAs, sequence homology of different regions of the miRNA gene were compared between EBV and rLCV [Cai, 2006a]. While the mature miRNA sequence and base of the hairpin stem-loop are important in the processing and function of the miRNA gene, the sequence of the terminal loop is relatively irrelevant, as long as an open structure is maintained. Comparison of each of these regions in the conserved miRNAs revealed the mature miRNA and base sequence were 89% and 84% conserved, respectively, compared to 68% of the terminal loop [Cai, 2006a]. As the overall genome sequence homology is 65% conserved, this indicates conservation is specific to the functional portions of the miRNA gene [Rivailler, 2002]. The extensive level of conservation between EBV and rLCV miRNAs, despite significant sequence divergence in other viral latent genes, indicates the targets for these miRNAs are also probably conserved. Currently no rLCV miRNA targets have been confirmed.

Mouse Gammaherpesvirus – 68 (MHV-68)

MHV-68 is evolutionarily related to the human gamma herpesviruses EBV and KSHV [Speck, 1999]. Its genome is approximately 119 kbp long and encodes 81 genes. MHV-68 infection in mice causes acute productive infection in the lungs and splenic lymphoproliferation due to viral latency in splenic B cells [Weck, 1996; Usherwood, 1996b; Usherwood, 1996a; Sunil-Chandra, 1992b; Sunil-Chandra, 1992a].

Along with computational predictions, nine MHV-68 miRNAs were cloned from latently infected mouse B lymphoma S11 cells [Pfeffer, 2005]. All nine of the viral miRNAs map to a 6 kbp region near ORF M1, immediately downstream of predicted viral tRNA genes. Sequence analysis identified 5 additional miRNA genes, though expression of these genes has not been confirmed. Like EBV and KSHV, the viral miRNAs are expressed during latency. However, unlike most miRNAs, the MHV-68 miRNAs are transcribed by RNA pol-III [Pfeffer, 2005]. Each of these transcripts contains a tRNA and one to two pre-miRNAs, as confirmed by northern blot analysis. RNA pol-III promoters are generally unregulated in any cell type. This explains previous reports of viral tRNA-like sequences expressed in the germinal centers of mice latently infected by MHV68 [Bowden, 1997]. These tRNA-like molecules are most likely nonfunctional remnants from the expressed promoter region of the miRNA genes and not true tRNAs. Aside from different transcription, the structure of MHV-68 pre-miRNAs is also unusual, with a short hairpin structure [Pfeffer, 2005]. This may indicate that the processing and export is distinct from other herpesvirus and cellular miRNA maturation. Loss of the miRNA region was shown to result in defects in the establishment of splenic latency though not peritoneal cells, indicating viral miRNAs function to establish latency though miRNA targets may be tissue specific [Clambey, 2002].

Kaposi's Sarcoma-Associated Herpesvirus (KSHV, HHV-8)

KSHV is a human gamma herpesvirus that primarily infects B-cell and endothelial cells. It is the etiological agent of Kaposi's Sarcoma, a highly vascular endothelial tumor found in immunocompromised patients. KSHV is also associated with pleural effusion lymphoma (PEL), a highly aggressive body cavity-based lymphoma, and multicentric Castleman's disease [Chang, 1994]. Its genome is approximately 137 kbp in length and encodes 83 genes. Upon entry of the linear viral DNA into the nucleus, the DNA is rapidly circularized to form a nuclear episome. Once episomal, the viral DNA can attach to the cellular DNA via viral scaffolding protein LANA. In vitro models suggest that cells typically switch to a latent life cycle 24-48 hours post infection, with approximately 1-3% of cells undergoing spontaneous lytic reactivation [Ganem, 2001].

To date, 12 miRNA genes encoding 14 mature miRNAs have been identified from latently infected PEL cell lines [Cai, 2005; Pfeffer, 2005; Samols, 2005; Grundhoff, 2006]. All 12 miRNAs encoded by KSHV are expressed in latently infected cells [Cai, 2006b; Samols, 2005]. These are all found within the latency region of the genome, with 10 of the 12 miRNAs located in an intergenic region between latency gene K12 (kaposin) and orf71 (v-flip) [Cai, 2005; Pfeffer, 2005; Samols, 2005; Grundhoff, 2006]. MiRNA expression occurs via promoters located 5' to orf72 and orf73 and requires read-through of a leaky poly-(A) site at orf71. This results in several different mRNA products that encode viral miRNAs [Cai, 2006b; Pearce, 2005]. KSHV-miR-K12-2 is located in the 3' UTR of the K12 gene while KSHV miRNA miR-K10 is located in the middle of the viral K12 open reading frame. Both miRNAs can use the upstream promoters that produce the alternatively spliced K12 mRNA. As a result, K12 translation and miR-k10 production are mutually exclusive [Pfeffer, 2005;

Cai, 2005; Samols, 2005]. K12 products kaposin A, B and C have important functions in cell growth and cytokine production [McCormick, 2005; Kliche, 2001]. Because over-expression of these products can be deleterious to the cell, KSHV-miR-K12-10 and KSHV-miR-K12-12 production may be tightly regulated to ensure that sufficient levels of both miRNAs, as well as kaposin mRNAs, are maintained.

Sequence analysis of the viral miRNA genes indicates a high level of conservation in both mature miRNA sequence and terminal loop sequence in KS, MCD and PEL [Marshall, 2007; O'Hara and Chugh, unpublished]. This suggests a tight level of selection on the KSHV miRNAs, presumably due to the importance of mRNA targeting in all KSHV malignancies. To date, few KSHV miRNA targets have been found. Expression profiling from the ectopic expression of the viral miRNA cluster in 293 cells indicated several possible miRNA targets. QRT-PCR and northern blotting confirmed that thrombospondin 1 (THBS1) protein is the target of several KSHV miRNAs: KSHV-miR-K12-1, KSHV-miR-K12-3-3p, KSHV-miR-K12-6-3p and KSHV-miR-K12-11 [Samols, 2007]. THBS1 is a matricellular glycoprotein that regulates proliferation and angiogenesis by activating latent TGF-B through direct binding [Bornstein, 2001; Lawler, 2002; Schultz-Cherry, 1995; de Fraipont, 2001]. Further analysis of KSHV miRNAs has indicated seed sequence homology of KSHV-miR-K12-11 with cellular miR-155 [Skalsky, 2007; Gottwein, 2007]. Indeed, expression of cellular miR-155 is low when KSHV-miR-K12-11 is expressed. This indicates both miRNAs probably regulate a common set of targets, and given miR-155's known role in B-cell transformation, KSHV-miR-K12-11 is probably contributing to B-cell tumorigenesis in KSHV infection [Clurman, 1989; Costinean, 2006; Eis, 2005].

Rhesus Monkey Rhadinovirus (RRV)

RRV is a simian rhadinovirus closely related to KSHV that infects B-cells and endothelial cells of immunocompromised rhesus macaques. Its genome is about 133 kbp in length and encodes 89 genes. Given the high level of similarity between KSHV and RRV, several studies were carried out to determine if viral miRNAs were also present in RRV. Upon latent infection of RRV in rhesus monkey vascular endothelial cell cultures (MVECs), cDNA cloning revealed the presence of 11 mature viral miRNAs [Schafer, 2007]. Computer analysis identified 7 viral miRNA genes, 6 of which were readily folded into the characteristic hairpin stem-loop structure of pre-miRNAs. The presence of all 11 mature miRNAs was confirmed by primer extension analysis, including the miRNA that computational analysis could not structurally confirm. Importantly, all 7 miRNA genes are clustered in a conserved intergenic region. In KSHV, the viral miRNAs are located between K12/kaposin and orf71 (vFLIP) [Cai, 2005; Pfeffer, 2005; Samols, 2005; Grundhoff, 2006]. RRV lacks a kaposin gene and therefore all the viral miRNAs are located between orf69 and orf71.

As in KSHV, all RRV viral miRNAs are located in the same orientation. In KSHV, this allows for miRNA expression through promoters located 5' to orf72 and orf73 and requires read-through of a leaky poly-(A) site at orf71 [Cai, 2006b; Pearce, 2005]. Lytic and latent promoters have been identified 5' of orf73 in RRV and a consensus poly-(A) site is present in orf71, suggesting a similar mechanism of processing may occur [DeWire, 2005]. Unlike KSHV, viral miRNA expression increases dramatically during lytic reactivation of RRV [Schafer, 2007]. This is likely due to a strong lytic promoter located immediately 5' of the orf73 gene which is lacking in KSHV [DeWire, 2005]. Though none of the 11 mature RRV miRNAs bore any sequence homology to the KSHV miRNAs, genomic location and orientation suggest that these miRNAs are generally conserved between genomes. Differences in sequence are likely due to sequence divergence between the two genomes. Despite differences in sequence, it is possible that RRV viral miRNAs may have similar targets and functions as the KSHV viral miRNAs.

Conclusion

There are several popular theories for why viruses encode miRNAs. Given that miRNAs act on the mRNA level and not the protein level, any effects the miRNA may have will take hours or even days to develop. This suggests that viruses most likely encode miRNAs to establish long-term or latent infections. As targeting experiments have shown, a number of viral miRNAs target viral mRNAs, with the result being establishment or maintenance of latency. In HSV-1, HSV1-miR-H2 targets ICP0, a protein required for progression through the lytic life cycle [Umbach, 2008]. HSV1-miR-H6 targets ICP4, also required for lytic progression [Umbach, 2008]. HCMV-miR-UL112-1 targets IE72, the repression of which results in attenuation of acute replication [Grey, 2007; Grey, 2008]. Expression of any of these viral miRNAs results in reduced expression of a viral mRNA required for lytic replication. All of these are examples of viral miRNAs regulating viral mRNAs in an attempt to establish and maintain viral latency.

Alternatively, viral miRNAs may function to overwhelm host miRNA machinery, out-competing or diverting the host from its normal cellular functions. In KSHV miRNA cloning experiments, the viral miRNAs made up one fourth of all cloned miRNAs in the latently infected BCBL cell line [Pfeffer, 2005]. Given constraints on viral genome size, the small size of the miRNA gene (<200 bp) is certainly appealing [Cullen, 2004]. This is especially true when a miRNA gene can regulate hundreds of target mRNAs [Lim, 2005].

Because many herpesviruses are known to cause cancer, miRNA involvement in oncogenesis is probable. Viral miRNAs may be acting as potential oncogenes or may be facilitating oncogenesis in target tissues. As oncogenes, viral miRNAs could have direct effects on the induction of oncogenesis. On the other hand, miRNAs may act indirectly to modulate oncogenesis driven by other viral or cellular factors. Evidence of this is already found in cellular miRNAs. The expression of the miR-17-92 cluster significantly accelerated lymphogenesis in mice with the c-myc oncogene driven by the immunoglobulin heavy-chain enhancer Eμ [He, 2005]. These tumors were also able to evade apoptosis. Among viral miRNAs, EBV-miR-BART5 targets PUMA, decreasing levels of this pro-apoptotic factor, resulting in increased cell survival [Choy, 2008]. And in MDV-1, a number of miRNAs cluster around the meq oncogene [Burnside, 2006; Burnside, 2007; Yao, 2008]. With viral miRNAs clustered around the meq locus, in the same orientation, these miRNAs may be aiding in meq oncogenesis.

Another possibility is that viral miRNAs facilitate oncogenesis by aiding in the evasion of innate and adaptive immune responses. This is especially likely considering the need to evade immune responses in order to establish latency, a requirement for oncogenesis in herpesviruses. In MHV, a variant of the virus that was unable to avoid inflammation, a common immune response, was rapidly cleared by the immune system and was found to lack a region of the genome that encompassed all 9 MHV68 miRNAs [Macrae, 2001]. In HCMV, HCMV-miR-UL112-1 targets MICB, resulting in evasion from nature killer cell attack as a means of evading the host immune response [Stern-Ginossar, 2007]. This is an example of a viral miRNA targeting a cellular mRNA, resulting in evasion of host immune response. Evasion of host immune response can promote oncogenesis.

Given the number of miRNAs encoded by each virus and the number of targets each miRNA may act upon, the viral miRNAs may work on each and every one of these functions. None of these possible functions are mutually exclusive. Evidence to this idea is seen in HCMV. HCMV-miR-UL112-1 has been shown to target viral and cellular mRNAs. The resulting effect of viral targeting includes attenuation of acute viral replication resulting in a viral switch to latency. Meanwhile, cellular targeting results in down regulation of MICB, resulting in host immune evasion. The miRNA is able to target all of these mRNAs simultaneously, despite the wide range of effects. MiRNAs allow a highly specific way of simultaneously regulating a wide variety of virus and host cell functions and are therefore important regulators in viral life cycle, virus-host interaction and viral oncogenesis.

References

Bagga, S., Bracht, J., Hunter, S., et al. (2005). Regulation by let-7 and lin-4 miRNAs results in target mRNA degradation. *Cell, 122*, 553-563.

Bartel, D.P. (2004). MicroRNAs: genomics, biogenesis, mechanism, and function. *Cell, 116*, 281-297.

Barth, S., Pfuhl, T., Mamiani, A., et al. (2008). Epstein-Barr virus-encoded microRNA miR-BART2 down-regulates the viral DNA polymerase BALF5. *Nucleic Acids Res, 36*, 666-675.

Benedetti, J., Corey, L. and Ashley, R. (1994). Recurrence rates in genital herpes after symptomatic first-episode infection. *Ann Intern Med, 121*, 847-854.

Bornstein, P. (2001). Thrombospondins as matricellular modulators of cell function. *J Clin Invest, 107*, 929-934.

Bowden, R.J., Simas, J.P., Davis, A.J., et al. (1997). Murine gammaherpesvirus 68 encodes tRNA-like sequences which are expressed during latency. *J Gen Virol, 78 (Pt 7)*, 1675-1687.

Brown, K.M., Chu, C.Y. and Rana, T.M. (2005). Target accessibility dictates the potency of human RISC. *Nat Struct Mol Biol, 12*, 469-470.

Buck, A.H., Santoyo-Lopez, J., Robertson, K.A., et al. (2007). Discrete clusters of virus-encoded micrornas are associated with complementary strands of the genome and the 7.2-kilobase stable intron in murine cytomegalovirus. *J Virol, 81*, 13761-13770.

Burnside, J., Bernberg, E., Anderson, A., et al. (2006). Marek's disease virus encodes MicroRNAs that map to meq and the latency-associated transcript. *J Virol, 80*, 8778-8786.

Burnside, J. and Morgan, R.W. (2007). Genomics and Marek's disease virus. *Cytogenet Genome Res, 117*, 376-387.

Cahir-McFarland, E.D., Davidson, D.M., Schauer, S.L., et al. (2000). NF-kappa B inhibition causes spontaneous apoptosis in Epstein-Barr virus-transformed lymphoblastoid cells. *Proc Natl Acad Sci U S A, 97*, 6055-6060.

Cahir-McFarland, E. and Kieff, E. (2002). NF-kappaB inhibition in EBV-transformed lymphoblastoid cell lines. *Recent Results Cancer Res, 159*, 44-48.

Cahir-McFarland, E.D., Carter, K., Rosenwald, A., et al. (2004). Role of NF-kappa B in cell survival and transcription of latent membrane protein 1-expressing or Epstein-Barr virus latency III-infected cells. *J Virol, 78*, 4108-4119.

Cai, X., Hagedorn, C.H. and Cullen, B.R. (2004). Human microRNAs are processed from capped, polyadenylated transcripts that can also function as mRNAs. *Rna, 10*, 1957-1966.

Cai, X., Lu, S., Zhang, Z., et al. (2005). Kaposi's sarcoma-associated herpesvirus expresses an array of viral microRNAs in latently infected cells. *Proc Natl Acad Sci U S A, 102*, 5570-5575.

Cai, X., Schafer, A., Lu, S., et al. (2006a). Epstein-Barr virus microRNAs are evolutionarily conserved and differentially expressed. *PLoS Pathog, 2*, e23.

Cai, X. and Cullen, B.R. (2006b). Transcriptional origin of Kaposi's sarcoma-associated herpesvirus microRNAs. *J Virol, 80*, 2234-2242.

Chang, Y., Cesarman, E., Pessin, M.S., et al. (1994). Identification of herpesvirus-like DNA sequences in AIDS-associated Kaposi's sarcoma. *Science, 266*, 1865-1869.

Chen, H., Huang, J., Wu, F.Y., et al. (2005). Regulation of expression of the Epstein-Barr virus BamHI-A rightward transcripts. *J Virol, 79*, 1724-1733.

Chendrimada, T.P., Gregory, R.I., Kumaraswamy, E., et al. (2005). TRBP recruits the Dicer complex to Ago2 for microRNA processing and gene silencing. *Nature, 436*, 740-744.

Choy, E.Y., Siu, K.L., Kok, K.H., et al. (2008). An Epstein-Barr virus-encoded microRNA targets PUMA to promote host cell survival. *J Exp Med, 205*, 2551-2560.

Clambey, E.T., Virgin, H.W.t. and Speck, S.H. (2002). Characterization of a spontaneous 9.5-kilobase-deletion mutant of murine gammaherpesvirus 68 reveals tissue-specific genetic requirements for latency. *J Virol, 76*, 6532-6544.

Clements, J.B., Watson, R.J. and Wilkie, N.M. (1977). Temporal regulation of herpes simplex virus type 1 transcription: location of transcripts on the viral genome. *Cell, 12*, 275-285.

Clurman, B.E. and Hayward, W.S. (1989). Multiple proto-oncogene activations in avian leukosis virus-induced lymphomas: evidence for stage-specific events. *Mol Cell Biol, 9*, 2657-2664.

Costinean, S., Zanesi, N., Pekarsky, Y., et al. (2006). Pre-B cell proliferation and lymphoblastic leukemia/high-grade lymphoma in E(mu)-miR155 transgenic mice. *Proc Natl Acad Sci U S A, 103*, 7024-7029.

Cui, C., Griffiths, A., Li, G., et al. (2006). Prediction and identification of herpes simplex virus 1-encoded microRNAs. *J Virol, 80*, 5499-5508.

Cullen, B.R. (2004). Transcription and processing of human microRNA precursors. *Mol Cell, 16*, 861-865.

de Fraipont, F., Nicholson, A.C., Feige, J.J., et al. (2001). Thrombospondins and tumor angiogenesis. *Trends Mol Med, 7*, 401-407.

de Jesus, O., Smith, P.R., Spender, L.C., et al. (2003). Updated Epstein-Barr virus (EBV) DNA sequence and analysis of a promoter for the BART (CST, BARF0) RNAs of EBV. *J Gen Virol, 84*, 1443-1450.

Denli, A.M., Tops, B.B., Plasterk, R.H., et al. (2004). Processing of primary microRNAs by the Microprocessor complex. *Nature, 432*, 231-235.

DeWire, S.M. and Damania, B. (2005). The latency-associated nuclear antigen of rhesus monkey rhadinovirus inhibits viral replication through repression of Orf50/Rta transcriptional activation. *J Virol, 79*, 3127-3138.

Dirmeier, U., Neuhierl, B., Kilger, E., et al. (2003). Latent membrane protein 1 is critical for efficient growth transformation of human B cells by epstein-barr virus. *Cancer Res, 63*, 2982-2989.

Dirmeier, U., Hoffmann, R., Kilger, E., et al. (2005). Latent membrane protein 1 of Epstein-Barr virus coordinately regulates proliferation with control of apoptosis. *Oncogene, 24*, 1711-1717.

Doench, J.G. and Sharp, P.A. (2004). Specificity of microRNA target selection in translational repression. *Genes Dev, 18*, 504-511.

Dolan, A., Jamieson, F.E., Cunningham, C., et al. (1998). The genome sequence of herpes simplex virus type 2. *J Virol, 72*, 2010-2021.

Dolken, L., Perot, J., Cognat, V., et al. (2007). Mouse cytomegalovirus microRNAs dominate the cellular small RNA profile during lytic infection and show features of posttranscriptional regulation. *J Virol, 81*, 13771-13782.

Dunn, W., Trang, P., Zhong, Q., et al. (2005). Human cytomegalovirus expresses novel microRNAs during productive viral infection. *Cell Microbiol, 7*, 1684-1695.

Edwards, R.H., Marquitz, A.R. and Raab-Traub, N. (2008). Epstein-Barr virus BART microRNAs are produced from a large intron prior to splicing. *J Virol, 82*, 9094-9106.

Eis, P.S., Tam, W., Sun, L., et al. (2005). Accumulation of miR-155 and BIC RNA in human B cell lymphomas. *Proc Natl Acad Sci U S A, 102*, 3627-3632.

Elbashir, S.M., Harborth, J., Lendeckel, W., et al. (2001a). Duplexes of 21-nucleotide RNAs mediate RNA interference in cultured mammalian cells. *Nature, 411*, 494-498.

Elbashir, S.M., Lendeckel, W. and Tuschl, T. (2001b). RNA interference is mediated by 21- and 22-nucleotide RNAs. *Genes Dev, 15*, 188-200.

Eliopoulos, A.G., Dawson, C.W., Mosialos, G., et al. (1996). CD40-induced growth inhibition in epithelial cells is mimicked by Epstein-Barr Virus-encoded LMP1: involvement of TRAF3 as a common mediator. *Oncogene, 13*, 2243-2254.

Furnari, F.B., Adams, M.D. and Pagano, J.S. (1993). Unconventional processing of the 3' termini of the Epstein-Barr virus DNA polymerase mRNA. *Proc Natl Acad Sci U S A, 90*, 378-382.

Ganem, D. (2001). Kaposi's Sarcoma-associated Herpesvirus. In P.M. Howley, D.E.G., R.A. Lamb, M.A. Martin, B. roizman, S.E, Straus, and D.M. Knipe (Eds.), *Fields Virology (*4, 2848-2888). Philadelphia: Lippincott Williams & Wilkins.

Gawn, J.M. and Greaves, R.F. (2002). Absence of IE1 p72 protein function during low-multiplicity infection by human cytomegalovirus results in a broad block to viral delayed-early gene expression. *J Virol, 76*, 4441-4455.

Gerner, C.S., Dolan, A. and McGeoch, D.J. (2004). Phylogenetic relationships in the Lymphocryptovirus genus of the Gammaherpesvirinae. *Virus Res, 99*, 187-192.

Gottwein, E., Mukherjee, N., Sachse, C., et al. (2007). A viral microRNA functions as an orthologue of cellular miR-155. *Nature, 450*, 1096-1099.

Gregory, R.I., Yan, K.P., Amuthan, G., et al. (2004). The Microprocessor complex mediates the genesis of microRNAs. *Nature, 432*, 235-240.

Grey, F., Antoniewicz, A., Allen, E., et al. (2005). Identification and characterization of human cytomegalovirus-encoded microRNAs. *J Virol, 79*, 12095-12099.

Grey, F., Meyers, H., White, E.A., et al. (2007). A human cytomegalovirus-encoded microRNA regulates expression of multiple viral genes involved in replication. *PLoS Pathog, 3*, e163.

Grey, F. and Nelson, J. (2008). Identification and function of human cytomegalovirus microRNAs. *J Clin Virol, 41*, 186-191.

Grundhoff, A., Sullivan, C.S. and Ganem, D. (2006). A combined computational and microarray-based approach identifies novel microRNAs encoded by human gamma-herpesviruses. *Rna, 12*, 733-750.

Hagglund, R. and Roizman, B. (2004). Role of ICP0 in the strategy of conquest of the host cell by herpes simplex virus 1. *J Virol, 78*, 2169-2178.

Hammond, S.M., Bernstein, E., Beach, D., et al. (2000). An RNA-directed nuclease mediates post-transcriptional gene silencing in Drosophila cells. *Nature, 404*, 293-296.

He, L., Thomson, J.M., Hemann, M.T., et al. (2005). A microRNA polycistron as a potential human oncogene. *Nature, 435*, 828-833.

Henle, G., Henle, W., Clifford, P., et al. (1969). Antibodies to Epstein-Barr virus in Burkitt's lymphoma and control groups. *J Natl Cancer Inst, 43*, 1147-1157.

Hensbergen, P.J., Wijnands, P.G., Schreurs, M.W., et al. (2005). The CXCR3 targeting chemokine CXCL11 has potent antitumor activity in vivo involving attraction of CD8+ T lymphocytes but not inhibition of angiogenesis. *J Immunother, 28*, 343-351.

Himly, M., Foster, D.N., Bottoli, I., et al. (1998). The DF-1 chicken fibroblast cell line: transformation induced by diverse oncogenes and cell death resulting from infection by avian leukosis viruses. *Virology, 248*, 295-304.

Hutvagner, G., McLachlan, J., Pasquinelli, A.E., et al. (2001). A cellular function for the RNA-interference enzyme Dicer in the maturation of the let-7 small temporal RNA. *Science, 293*, 834-838.

Hutvagner, G. and Zamore, P.D. (2002). A microRNA in a multiple-turnover RNAi enzyme complex. *Science, 297*, 2056-2060.

Inman, M., Perng, G.C., Henderson, G., et al. (2001). Region of herpes simplex virus type 1 latency-associated transcript sufficient for wild-type spontaneous reactivation promotes cell survival in tissue culture. *J Virol, 75*, 3636-3646.

Kaye, K.M., Izumi, K.M. and Kieff, E. (1993). Epstein-Barr virus latent membrane protein 1 is essential for B-lymphocyte growth transformation. *Proc Natl Acad Sci U S A, 90*, 9150-9154.

Kaye, K.M., Izumi, K.M., Mosialos, G., et al. (1995). The Epstein-Barr virus LMP1 cytoplasmic carboxy terminus is essential for B-lymphocyte transformation; fibroblast cocultivation complements a critical function within the terminal 155 residues. *J Virol, 69*, 675-683.

Kaye, K.M., Izumi, K.M., Li, H., et al. (1999). An Epstein-Barr virus that expresses only the first 231 LMP1 amino acids efficiently initiates primary B-lymphocyte growth transformation. *J Virol, 73*, 10525-10530.

Kieff, E., and A.B. Rickinson. (2001). Epstein-Barr virus and its replication. In P.M. Howley, D.E.G., R.A. Lamb, M.A. Martin, B. roizman, S.E, Straus, and D.M. Knipe (Eds.), *Fields Virology (*4, 2511-2573). Philadelphia: Lippincott Williams & Wilkins.

Kilger, E., Kieser, A., Baumann, M., et al. (1998). Epstein-Barr virus-mediated B-cell proliferation is dependent upon latent membrane protein 1, which simulates an activated CD40 receptor. *Embo J, 17*, 1700-1709.

Kim do, N., Chae, H.S., Oh, S.T., et al. (2007). Expression of viral microRNAs in Epstein-Barr virus-associated gastric carcinoma. *J Virol, 81*, 1033-1036.

Kliche, S., Nagel, W., Kremmer, E., et al. (2001). Signaling by human herpesvirus 8 kaposin A through direct membrane recruitment of cytohesin-1. *Mol Cell, 7*, 833-843.

Knipe, D.M., Ruyechan, W.T., Roizman, B., et al. (1978). Molecular genetics of herpes simplex virus: demonstration of regions of obligatory and nonobligatory identity within diploid regions of the genome by sequence replacement and insertion. *Proc Natl Acad Sci U S A, 75*, 3896-3900.

Kristie, T.M. and Roizman, B. (1986). DNA-binding site of major regulatory protein alpha 4 specifically associated with promoter-regulatory domains of alpha genes of herpes simplex virus type 1. *Proc Natl Acad Sci U S A, 83*, 4700-4704.

Lafferty, W.E., Coombs, R.W., Benedetti, J., et al. (1987). Recurrences after oral and genital herpes simplex virus infection. Influence of site of infection and viral type. *N Engl J Med, 316*, 1444-1449.

Landgraf, P., Rusu, M., Sheridan, R., et al. (2007). A mammalian microRNA expression atlas based on small RNA library sequencing. *Cell, 129*, 1401-1414.

Lawler, J. (2002). Thrombospondin-1 as an endogenous inhibitor of angiogenesis and tumor growth. *J Cell Mol Med, 6*, 1-12.

Lee, Y., Ahn, C., Han, J., et al. (2003). The nuclear RNase III Drosha initiates microRNA processing. *Nature, 425*, 415-419.

Lee, Y., Kim, M., Han, J., et al. (2004). MicroRNA genes are transcribed by RNA polymerase II. *Embo J, 23*, 4051-4060.

Levy, A.M., Gilad, O., Xia, L., et al. (2005). Marek's disease virus Meq transforms chicken cells via the v-Jun transcriptional cascade: a converging transforming pathway for avian oncoviruses. *Proc Natl Acad Sci U S A, 102*, 14831-14836.

Lewis, B.P., Burge, C.B. and Bartel, D.P. (2005). Conserved seed pairing, often flanked by adenosines, indicates that thousands of human genes are microRNA targets. *Cell, 120*, 15-20.

Lim, L.P., Lau, N.C., Garrett-Engele, P., et al. (2005). Microarray analysis shows that some microRNAs downregulate large numbers of target mRNAs. *Nature, 433*, 769-773.

Liu, J.L., Ye, Y., Lee, L.F., et al. (1998). Transforming potential of the herpesvirus oncoprotein MEQ: morphological transformation, serum-independent growth, and inhibition of apoptosis. *J Virol, 72*, 388-395.

Liu, J., Carmell, M.A., Rivas, F.V., et al. (2004). Argonaute2 is the catalytic engine of mammalian RNAi. *Science, 305*, 1437-1441.

Liu, J., Valencia-Sanchez, M.A., Hannon, G.J., et al. (2005). MicroRNA-dependent localization of targeted mRNAs to mammalian P-bodies. *Nat Cell Biol, 7*, 719-723.

Lo, A.K., To, K.F., Lo, K.W., et al. (2007). Modulation of LMP1 protein expression by EBV-encoded microRNAs. *Proc Natl Acad Sci U S A, 104*, 16164-16169.

Lund, E., Guttinger, S., Calado, A., et al. (2004). Nuclear export of microRNA precursors. *Science, 303*, 95-98.

Lupiani, B., Lee, L.F., Cui, X., et al. (2004). Marek's disease virus-encoded Meq gene is involved in transformation of lymphocytes but is dispensable for replication. *Proc Natl Acad Sci U S A, 101*, 11815-11820.

Macrae, A.I., Dutia, B.M., Milligan, S., et al. (2001). Analysis of a novel strain of murine gammaherpesvirus reveals a genomic locus important for acute pathogenesis. *J Virol, 75*, 5315-5327.

Maniataki, E. and Mourelatos, Z. (2005). A human, ATP-independent, RISC assembly machine fueled by pre-miRNA. *Genes Dev, 19*, 2979-2990.

Marshall, V., Parks, T., Bagni, R., et al. (2007). Conservation of virally encoded microRNAs in Kaposi sarcoma--associated herpesvirus in primary effusion lymphoma cell lines and in patients with Kaposi sarcoma or multicentric Castleman disease. *J Infect Dis, 195*, 645-659.

McCormick, C. and Ganem, D. (2005). The kaposin B protein of KSHV activates the p38/MK2 pathway and stabilizes cytokine mRNAs. *Science, 307*, 739-741.

Meister, G., Landthaler, M., Patkaniowska, A., et al. (2004). Human Argonaute2 mediates RNA cleavage targeted by miRNAs and siRNAs. *Mol Cell, 15*, 185-197.

Michael, N., Spector, D., Mavromara-Nazos, P., et al. (1988). The DNA-binding properties of the major regulatory protein alpha 4 of herpes simplex viruses. *Science, 239*, 1531-1534.

Mocarski, E.S., Shenk, T. and Pass, R.F. (2001). Cytomegaloviruses. In P.M. Howley, D.E.G., R.A. Lamb, M.A. Martin, B. roizman, S.E, Straus, and D.M. Knipe (Eds.), *Fields Virology (*4, 2703-2773). Philadelphia: Lippincott Williams & Wilkins.

Murphy, E., Vanicek, J., Robins, H., et al. (2008). Suppression of immediate-early viral gene expression by herpesvirus-coded microRNAs: implications for latency. *Proc Natl Acad Sci U S A, 105*, 5453-5458.

Olsen, P.H. and Ambros, V. (1999). The lin-4 regulatory RNA controls developmental timing in Caenorhabditis elegans by blocking LIN-14 protein synthesis after the initiation of translation. *Dev Biol, 216*, 671-680.

Pass, R.F. (2001). Cytomegalovirus. In P.M. Howley, D.E.G., R.A. Lamb, M.A. Martin, B. roizman, S.E, Straus, and D.M. Knipe (Eds.), *Fields Virology* 2675-2706). Philadelphia: Lippincott Williams & Wilkins.

Pearce, M., Matsumura, S. and Wilson, A.C. (2005). Transcripts encoding K12, v-FLIP, v-cyclin, and the microRNA cluster of Kaposi's sarcoma-associated herpesvirus originate from a common promoter. *J Virol, 79*, 14457-14464.

Pfeffer, S., Zavolan, M., Grasser, F.A., et al. (2004). Identification of virus-encoded microRNAs. *Science, 304*, 734-736.

Pfeffer, S., Sewer, A., Lagos-Quintana, M., et al. (2005). Identification of microRNAs of the herpesvirus family. *Nat Methods, 2*, 269-276.

Poon, A.P., Gu, H. and Roizman, B. (2006). ICP0 and the US3 protein kinase of herpes simplex virus 1 independently block histone deacetylation to enable gene expression. *Proc Natl Acad Sci U S A, 103*, 9993-9998.

Preston, C.M. (1979). Control of herpes simplex virus type 1 mRNA synthesis in cells infected with wild-type virus or the temperature-sensitive mutant tsK. *J Virol, 29*, 275-284.

Rivailler, P., Jiang, H., Cho, Y.G., et al. (2002). Complete nucleotide sequence of the rhesus lymphocryptovirus: genetic validation for an Epstein-Barr virus animal model. *J Virol, 76*, 421-426.

Roizman, B., Knipe, D. and Whitley, R. (2001). Herpes Simplex Viruses. In P.M. Howley, D.E.G., R.A. Lamb, M.A. Martin, B. roizman, S.E, Straus, and D.M. Knipe (Eds.), *Fields Virology (*4, 2503-2602). Philadelphia: Lippincott Williams & Wilkins.

Sadler, R.H. and Raab-Traub, N. (1995). The Epstein-Barr virus 3.5-kilobase latent membrane protein 1 mRNA initiates from a TATA-Less promoter within the first terminal repeat. *J Virol, 69*, 4577-4581.

Samols, M.A., Hu, J., Skalsky, R.L., et al. (2005). Cloning and identification of a microRNA cluster within the latency-associated region of Kaposi's sarcoma-associated herpesvirus. *J Virol, 79*, 9301-9305.

Samols, M.A., Skalsky, R.L., Maldonado, A.M., et al. (2007). Identification of cellular genes targeted by KSHV-encoded microRNAs. *PLoS Pathog, 3*, e65.

Schafer, A., Cai, X., Bilello, J.P., et al. (2007). Cloning and analysis of microRNAs encoded by the primate gamma-herpesvirus rhesus monkey rhadinovirus. *Virology, 364*, 21-27.

Schultz-Cherry, S., Chen, H., Mosher, D.F., et al. (1995). Regulation of transforming growth factor-beta activation by discrete sequences of thrombospondin 1. *J Biol Chem, 270*, 7304-7310.

Schwarz, D.S., Hutvagner, G., Haley, B., et al. (2002). Evidence that siRNAs function as guides, not primers, in the Drosophila and human RNAi pathways. *Mol Cell, 10*, 537-548.

Skalsky, R.L., Samols, M.A., Plaisance, K.B., et al. (2007). Kaposi's sarcoma-associated herpesvirus encodes an ortholog of miR-155. *J Virol, 81*, 12836-12845.

Speck, S.H. and Virgin, H.W. (1999). Host and viral genetics of chronic infection: a mouse model of gamma-herpesvirus pathogenesis. *Curr Opin Microbiol, 2*, 403-409.

Staras, S.A., Dollard, S.C., Radford, K.W., et al. (2006). Seroprevalence of cytomegalovirus infection in the United States, 1988-1994. *Clin Infect Dis, 43*, 1143-1151.

Stern-Ginossar, N., Elefant, N., Zimmermann, A., et al. (2007). Host immune system gene targeting by a viral miRNA. *Science, 317*, 376-381.

Stevens, J.G., Wagner, E.K., Devi-Rao, G.B., et al. (1987). RNA complementary to a herpesvirus alpha gene mRNA is prominent in latently infected neurons. *Science, 235*, 1056-1059.

Stow, N.D. and Stow, E.C. (1986). Isolation and characterization of a herpes simplex virus type 1 mutant containing a deletion within the gene encoding the immediate early polypeptide Vmw110. *J Gen Virol, 67 (Pt 12)*, 2571-2585.

Sunil-Chandra, N.P., Efstathiou, S., Arno, J., et al. (1992a). Virological and pathological features of mice infected with murine gamma-herpesvirus 68. *J Gen Virol, 73 (Pt 9)*, 2347-2356.

Sunil-Chandra, N.P., Efstathiou, S. and Nash, A.A. (1992b). Murine gammaherpesvirus 68 establishes a latent infection in mouse B lymphocytes in vivo. *J Gen Virol, 73 (Pt 12)*, 3275-3279.

Tang, S., Bertke, A.S., Patel, A., et al. (2008). An acutely and latently expressed herpes simplex virus 2 viral microRNA inhibits expression of ICP34.5, a viral neurovirulence factor. *Proc Natl Acad Sci U S A, 105*, 10931-10936.

Tomari, Y., Matranga, C., Haley, B., et al. (2004). A protein sensor for siRNA asymmetry. *Science, 306*, 1377-1380.

Tomari, Y. and Zamore, P.D. (2005). MicroRNA biogenesis: drosha can't cut it without a partner. *Curr Biol, 15*, R61-R64.

Umbach, J.L., Kramer, M.F., Jurak, I., et al. (2008). MicroRNAs expressed by herpes simplex virus 1 during latent infection regulate viral mRNAs. *Nature, 454*, 780-783.

Usherwood, E.J., Ross, A.J., Allen, D.J., et al. (1996a). Murine gammaherpesvirus-induced splenomegaly: a critical role for CD4 T cells. *J Gen Virol, 77 (Pt 4)*, 627-630.

Usherwood, E.J., Stewart, J.P., Robertson, K., et al. (1996b). Absence of splenic latency in murine gammaherpesvirus 68-infected B cell-deficient mice. *J Gen Virol, 77 (Pt 11)*, 2819-2825.

Watson, R.J. and Clements, J.B. (1980). A herpes simplex virus type 1 function continuously required for early and late virus RNA synthesis. *Nature, 285*, 329-330.

Weck, K.E., Barkon, M.L., Yoo, L.I., et al. (1996). Mature B cells are required for acute splenic infection, but not for establishment of latency, by murine gammaherpesvirus 68. *J Virol, 70*, 6775-6780.

The Wellcome Trust Sanger Institute. miRBase. http://microrna.sanger.ac.uk/.

Williams, B.R. (2001). Signal integration via PKR. *Sci STKE, 2001*, RE2.

Witter, R.L. (1997). Increased virulence of Marek's disease virus field isolates. *Avian Dis, 41*, 149-163.

Xia, T., O'Hara, A., Araujo, I., et al. (2008). EBV microRNAs in primary lymphomas and targeting of CXCL-11 by ebv-mir-BHRF1-3. *Cancer Res, 68*, 1436-1442.

Xie, Q., Anderson, A.S. and Morgan, R.W. (1996). Marek's disease virus (MDV) ICP4, pp38, and meq genes are involved in the maintenance of transformation of MDCC-MSB1 MDV-transformed lymphoblastoid cells. *J Virol, 70*, 1125-1131.

Xing, L. and Kieff, E. (2007). Epstein-Barr virus BHRF1 micro- and stable RNAs during latency III and after induction of replication. *J Virol, 81*, 9967-9975.

Xu, F., Schillinger, J.A., Sternberg, M.R., et al. (2002). Seroprevalence and coinfection with herpes simplex virus type 1 and type 2 in the United States, 1988-1994. *J Infect Dis, 185*, 1019-1024.

Yao, Y., Zhao, Y., Xu, H., et al. (2007). Marek's disease virus type 2 (MDV-2)-encoded microRNAs show no sequence conservation with those encoded by MDV-1. *J Virol, 81*, 7164-7170.

Yao, Y., Zhao, Y., Xu, H., et al. (2008). MicroRNA profile of Marek's disease virus-transformed T-cell line MSB-1: predominance of virus-encoded microRNAs. *J Virol, 82*, 4007-4015.

Yekta, S., Shih, I.H. and Bartel, D.P. (2004). MicroRNA-directed cleavage of HOXB8 mRNA. *Science, 304*, 594-596.

Yi, R., Qin, Y., Macara, I.G., et al. (2003). Exportin-5 mediates the nuclear export of pre-microRNAs and short hairpin RNAs. *Genes Dev, 17*, 3011-3016.

Zeng, Y., Wagner, E.J. and Cullen, B.R. (2002). Both natural and designed micro RNAs can inhibit the expression of cognate mRNAs when expressed in human cells. *Mol Cell, 9*, 1327-1333.

Zeng, Y., Yi, R. and Cullen, B.R. (2003). MicroRNAs and small interfering RNAs can inhibit mRNA expression by similar mechanisms. *Proc Natl Acad Sci U S A, 100*, 9779-9784.

Zeng, Y. and Cullen, B.R. (2004). Structural requirements for pre-microRNA binding and nuclear export by Exportin 5. *Nucleic Acids Res, 32*, 4776-4785.

In: Herpesviridae Viral Structure, Life Cycle and Infections ISBN 978-1-60692-947-6
Editor: Toma R. Gluckman

Chapter 5

Asymptomatic Alphaherpesvirus Reactivation

***Randall J. Cohrs*[1], *David M. Koelle*[2], *Matthew C. Schuette*[3], *Satish Mehta*[4], *Duane Pierson*[5], *Donald H. Gilden*[1,6] *and James M. Hill*[7]**

[1]Department of Neurology, University of Colorado School of Medicine, Denver, Colorado, USA

[2]Vaccine and Infectious Diseases Institute, Fred Hutchinson Cancer Research Institute, Seattle, Washington, USA

[3]Department of Mathematics, William Jewell College, Liberty, Missouri

[4]Enterprise Advisory Services, Inc., Houston, Texas, USA

[5]Space Life Sciences, NASA, Lyndon B. Johnson Space Center, Houston, Texas, USA

[6]Department of Microbiology, University of Colorado School of Medicine, Denver, Colorado, USA

[7]Departments of Ophthalmology (LSU Eye Center), Pharmacology, Microbiology, and the Neuroscience Center, Louisiana State University Health Sciences Center, New Orleans, Louisiana, USA

Abstract

Human alphaherpesviruses include types 1 and 2 herpes simplex virus (HSV) and varicella zoster virus (VZV). All human alphaherpesviruses are neurotropic. After primary infection, these viruses become latent in cranial nerve ganglia (HSV-1 and VZV), in dorsal root ganglia (VZV), in sacral ganglia (HSV-2 and VZV) and in autonomic ganglia (VZV). During latency, virus gene expression is restricted and no infectious virus is produced.

Primary HSV-1 infection usually occurs in childhood and results in few lesions in the head and neck, but primary infection can also be asymptomatic. The classical diseases of HSV-1 reactivations are fever blisters and ocular herpes. Recent reports demonstrating frequent shedding of shedding of HSV-1 DNA in the absence of disease, suggests that a small percentage of neurons reactivate to yield virus that is detected on ocular and oral surfaces.

Primary HSV-2 infection typically develops in sexually active individuals. Primary infections range from asymptomatic seroconversion to typical primary disease (i.e., genital herpes). HSV-2 shedding, both symptomatic and asymptomatic, are more frequent in the first couple of years after seroconversion. Asymptomatic virus shedding can be divided into two groups: unrecognized shedding, in which symptoms or lesions are present but go un-noticed or are misdiagnosed; and strict asymptomatic shedding, in which the subject has no symptoms and even a skilled clinician is unable to note any abnormality on physical exam. Therapies that reduce symptomatic recurrences may be less effective against strict asymptomatic shedding and transmission (Corey and Wald, 2008). Herein, data concerning the contribution of asymptomatic shedding to HSV transmission as well as the biology of HSV-2 shedding are reviewed.

Primary VZV infection typically results in childhood varicella (chickenpox). VZV reactivation, predominately in the elderly, most often results in zoster (shingles), but virus may spread to the spinal cord to cause myelitis or to blood vessels of the brain to cause vasculopathy. VZV reactivation often produces prolonged pain after zoster (post herpetic neuralgia). While the clinical features of VZV reactivation are well recognized, subclinical VZV reactivation and shedding has recently been reported in astronauts. Physical and physiological stressors associated with spaceflight (Taylor et al., 1992; White and Averner, 2001; Williams, 2003) appear to induce virus reactivation and subsequent shedding of VZV in saliva (Mehta et al., 2004; Cohrs et al., 2008). Herein, asymptomatic VZV reactivation during space flight, in ground-based space flight analogs, and in the general population will be reviewed as well as a mathematical model estimating the contribution of asymptomatic VZV reactivation to virus epidemiology presented.

1. Alphaherpesviruses

The Herpesviridae family includes over 115 members from multiple species. All are large, enveloped, double-stranded DNA-containing viruses which replicate in the nucleus of the infected cell and are characterized by life-long latency in their native host. Herpesviruses are further grouped into subfamilies (alphaherpesvirinae, betaherpesvirinae, and gammaherpesvirinea) based on shared biological characteristics including host range, length of replication cycle and site of latency. (Roizman and Morse, 1978). Alphaherpesviruses have a predilection for epithelial cells where productive infection occurs, and neurons where the virus becomes latent. In tissue culture, alphaherpesviruses have a short reproductive cycle (8 – 24 hrs) characterized by a rapidly spreading infection leading to cell lysis. The genomes of alphaherpesviruses contain unique long and unique short regions, each flanked by internal and terminal repeat sequences. Alphaherpesviruses are grouped at the genus level (Simplexvirus, Varicellovirus, Mardivirus, Iltovirus) based on DNA structure and host species. The genome of representative members from each alphaherpesvirus subfamily have been sequenced and range in size from 110 kilobase pairs (kbp) to 164 kbp with a potential coding capacity of 70-85 genes (Table 1).

Table 1. The Alphaherpesvirus

Accession Number	Name	Size (bp)[a]	ORFs[b]	Sub-Family	Host
NC001806	Human Herpesvirus Type 1	152261	77	Simplexvirus	Human
NC001798	Human Herpesvirus Type 2	154746	77	Simplexvirus	Human
NC006623	Cercopithecine Herpesvirus Type 2	150715	75	Simplexvirus	Baboon
NC005261	Cercopithecine Herpesvirus Type 1	156789	75	Simplexvirus	Monkey
NC001348	Human Herpesvirus Type 3	124884	73	Varicellovirus	Human
NC004812	Cercopithecine Herpesvirus Type 9	124784	74	Varicellovirus	Monkey
NC001491	Equid Herpesvirus Type 1	150224	80	Varicellovirus	Horse
NC001844	Equid Herpesvirus Type 4	145597	79	Varicellovirus	Horse
NC001847	Bovine Herpesvirus Type 1	135301	70	Varicellovirus	Cow
NC005264	Bovine Herpesvirus Type 5	137821	70	Varicellovirus	Cow
NC006560	Suid Herpesvirus Type 1	143461	70	Varicellovirus	Pig
NC002229	Gallid Herpesvirus Type 2	117874	85	Madvirus	Chicken
NC002577	Gallid Herpesvirus Type 3	164270	76	Madvirus	Chicken
NC002686	Meleagrio Herpesvirus Type 1	159160	79	Madvirus	Turkey
NC007653	Gallid Herpesvirus Type 1	148687	79	Iltovirus	Chicken
NC006151	Psittacid Herpesvirus Type 1	163025	77	Iltovirus	Parrot

a; bp, base pairs
b; open reading frames

The human alphaherpesviruses (HSV1 and 2 and VZV) are prevalent in the population worldwide. In immunocompetent individuals, primary infection of mucosal epithelial cells results in local virus replication. Primary HSV infection typically resolves without obvious local or systemic dissemination; however, in the case of VZV, virus is transferred to tonsillar T-cells which transmit virus to the skin, where varicella develops (Ku et al., 2005). During primary infection, the human alphaherpesivurses gain access to ganglionic neurons. Virus particles lacking the outer envelope travel to the nucleus via retrograde microtubular-assisted transport. The virus genome enters the nucleus where the viral DNA termini join covalently and the genome assumes an "endless" concatameric or circular form coated with histones. The specific posttranslational modifications present on the histones repress transcription of the majority of virus genes. In this latent state, the virus can reside unnoticed for the life of the host. However, when latent virus reactivates, disease is often more severe than that produced by primary infection.

HSV-1, HSV-2 and VZV share a similar basic genomic structure which consists of covalently joined long and short segments (Figure 1). The long DNA segment (~108 kbp, HSV; ~104 kbp, VZV) contains a long sequence of unique DNA (U_L) flanked by terminal (TR_L) and internal repeated (IR_L) DNA. Similarly, the short DNA segment (~27 kbp, HSV; ~20kbp, VZV) contains a short sequence of unique DNA (U_S) flanked by its attendant terminal (TR_S) and internal repeated (IR_S) DNA. The size and location of open reading frames (ORF) indicate a greater degree of genetic homology between HSV-1 and HSV-2 than between either HSV types or VZV. In addition, the ~9.2 kbp DNA repeats flanking HSV U_L are reduced to 88 bp in the VZV genome. All human alphaherpesviruses contain an origin of DNA replication (*ori*) located within IR_S and TR_S, and both HSV types contain an *ori* mapping near the center of U_L. Consequently both HSV long and short DNA segments invert to form four equimolar genomic isomers, whereas only the short VZV DNA segment undergoes major inversion resulting in two isomeric forms of the virus genome.

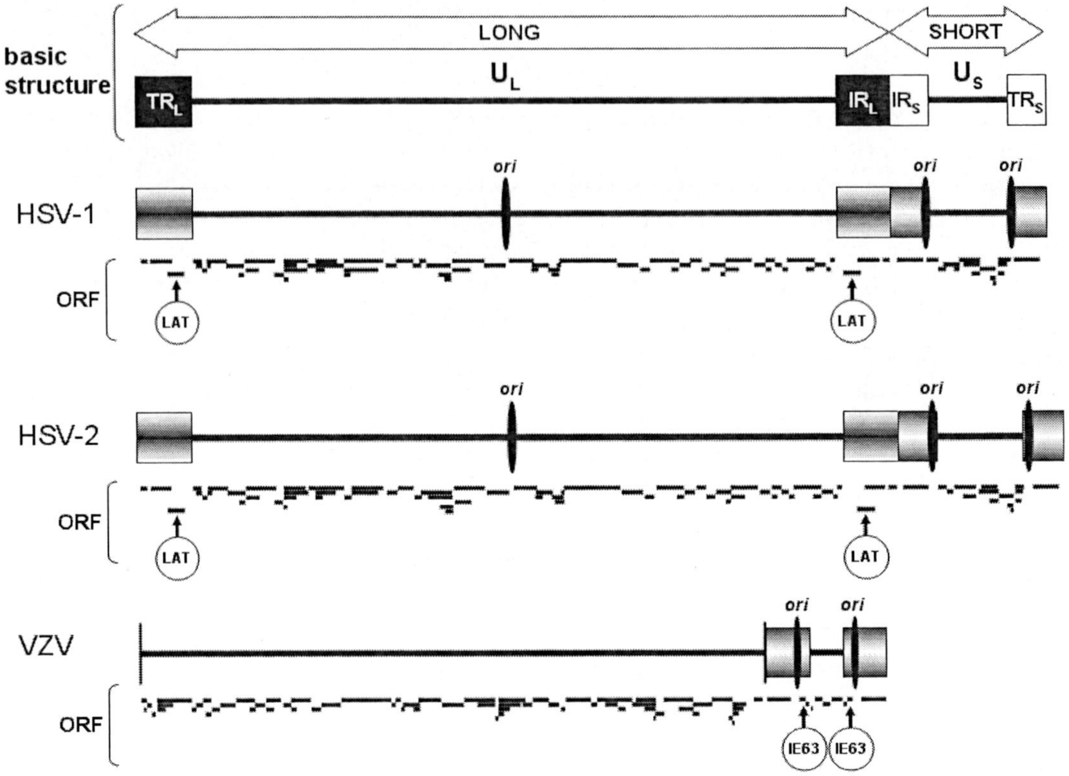

Figure 1. Anatomy of alphaherpesvirus genome. The basic alphaherpesviruse genomic structure consists of long and short covalently joined DNA segments. The long segment contains terminal (TR_L) and internal (IR_L) inverted repeated DNA. Similarly, the short segment contains terminal (TR_L) and internal (IR_L) inverted repeated DNA. The gemonic structure of HSV-1, HSV-2 and VZV are diagramed showing the relative location of the predicted open reading frames (ORFs) and origin of DNA replication (*ori*). Both HSV-1 and HSV-2 transcribe a latency associated transcript (LAT) which is located within the TRL and IRL. However, the homologous region of DNA is not present in VZV and the virus transcript most reliably associated with latent infection encodes the immediate-early protein 63 (IE63).

Clues to the mechanisms by which human alphaherpesviruses reactivate require a full understanding of the physical state of virus nucleic acid and virus gene expression in latently infected cells. Both latent HSV-1 and VZV DNA are latent in ganglionic neurons, and sometimes both viruses are found in the same cell (Theil et al., 2003). The major latency associated transcript (LAT; Figure 1) detected in HSV-1 latently infected neurons is a small (~2 kb) stable intron spliced from a larger (8.5 kb) primary (Wagner et al., 1988). The primary LAT transcript maps within HSV-1 TR_L/IR_L. Since this region is not present in the VZV genome, it is probable that VZV has evolved a different mechanism to maintain latency. Analysis of multiple, latently infected human ganglia reveals that VZV latency is characterized by transcription of at least 5 viral genes, of which the immediate early gene 63 (IE63; Figure 1) is the most prevalent and abundant (Cohrs and Gilden, 2007). The mechanism by which both HSV-1 LAT and VZV IE63 maintain latency is under intense investigation, and may involve inhibition of apoptosis (Branco and Fraser, 2005; Hood et al., 2006).

2. Human Herpesvirus Type 1 (HSV-1)

Herpes simplex virus type 1 is a significant, and prevalent, human pathogen that can cause herpes labialis, ocular keratitis, facial lesions, herpetic whitlow, stomatitis, and, rarely, encephalitis. This section will focus primarily on the most common aspects of ocular and oral facial HSV-1 infections. Herpes labialis (fever blister) is much more frequent than ocular herpes, with an estimated 32% to 45% of the population of the United States experiencing at least one specific herpetic lesion incident (Miller and Danaher, 2008; Hobbs et al., 2008; Spruance et al., 1977, 1984). The incidence of herpetic ocular disease, a major cause of blindness in industrialized nations, is estimated to be between 5.9 and 20 per 100,000 per year (Kaye and Choudhary, 2006; Liesegang, 2001). In the United States, approximately 500,000 individuals per year experience herpetic eye disease (Leisegang, 2001). Hence, the estimate of ocular herpetic disease occurrences is 2% to 4% (Kaye and Choudhary, 2006).

Asymptomatic HSV-1 Shedding

HSV-1 infections were described as early as 2500 BC (Roizman and Whitley, 2001), but the first isolation of infectious HSV-1 from the oral cavity was in 1953 (Buddingh et al., 1953). This clinical study was done at the LSU School of Medicine in New Orleans, where saliva of 553 healthy volunteers (185 children <15 yrs and 368 adults >15 yrs) from the Charity Hospital of Louisiana were analyzed for infectious HSV-1. The results showed that infectious HSV-1 was detected at a rate 3 times greater in saliva from adults than children (Table 2). Although the experiments were conducted more than 55 years ago, comparison of data collected in 1953 with more recent studies demonstrates a general correlation between HSV-1 detection in saliva with virus isolation, and also attests to the efficiency of virus detection in 1953.

The first report of detection of infectious HSV-1 in tears appeared in 1967 (Kaufman et al., 1967) (Table 3). Thirty-six percent (4/11) of eye swabs from healthy individuals were positive for infectious HSV-1. While the anatomical site from which infectious HSV-1 originated remained unknown, four years later, Stevens and Cook (Stevens and Cook, 1971) detected HSV-1 latency in the peripheral nervous system by assessing the appearance of infectious HSV-1 following *ex vivo* incubation of the neural tissue. This led to the conclusion that HSV-1 detection in tear fluid most likely represented a consequence of neuronal reaction. Two new studies on HSV-1 DNA in tears and saliva (Kaufman et al, 2005) and studies on HSV-1 DNA in a large number (174) of human TG (Hill et al, 2008) support the early studies of Stevens and Cook (1971) and Kaufman et al (1967) related to the site of HSV-1 latency and the frequency of HSV-1 shedding in tears and saliva.

Table 2. Asymptomatic shedding of infectious HSV-1 detected by cell culture from oral samples of healthy subjects

Author(s), Year	N	Individuals: total positive/ total subjects	Shedding frequency: total positive samples/total samples	Sample frequency: number of samples/subject
Spruance, 1984	8	8/8 (100%)	47/637 (7.4%)	105
Douglas & Couch, 1970	10	8/10 (80%)	11/494 (2.2%)	~49
Okinaga, 2000	10	4/10 (40%)	4/870 (0.5%)	87
Kaufman, 1967	35	6/35 (17.1%)	6/700 (0.9%)	20
Tateishi et al, 1994	1000	27/1000 (2.7%)	27/1000 (2.7%)	one
Buddingh et al, 1953	368*	30/368 (8.2%)	30/368 (8.2%)	one
Buddingh et al, 1953	185**	5/185 (2.4%)	5/185 (2.7%)	one
Lindgren et al, 1968	418	8/418 (1.9%)	8/2204(0.4%)	5-6
Hatherley et al., 1980	384	37/384 (9.6%)	47/1536 (3.1%)	5
Kameyama et al, 1988	110	5/110 (4.5%)	70/7805 (0.9%)	61
Totals	**2528**	**134/2528 (5.3%)**	**249/15799(1.6%)**	

*adults
**children

Table 3. Asymptomatic shedding of infectious HSV-1 detected by cell culture from eye swabs (tears) of healthy subjects

Author(s), Year	N	Individuals: total positives/total subjects	Shedding frequency: total positive swabs/ total swabs	Swab frequency: number of swabs/subjects
Kaufman et al. 1967	35	11/35 (31%)	11/1400 (0.8%)	20*
Okinaga 2000	10	1/10 (10%)	1/1742 (0.06%)	~17
Khodadoost et al. 2004	10	1/10 (10%)	1/10 (10%)	one
Asbell et al. 1995	23	1/23 (5%)	1/23 (5%)	one
Kaye et al. 1990	24	0/24 (0/0)	0/752 (0%)	~ 31
Totals	**102**	**14/102 (14%)**	**14/3927 (0.4%)**	

N = Total number of subjects
*Each day both eyes of each subject was swabbed

Polymerase chain reaction (PCR) is an extremely sensitive technique used to identify and quantitate HSV DNA in fluids from humans. In addition, animal models have been developed which confirm and extend key biological findings obtained in clinical studies. Before summarizing the data on detection of asymptomatic shedding of HSV-1, a brief review of two clinical diseases, herpes keratitis (ocular disease) and herpes labialis (cold sores, fever blisters) is necessary. Ophthalmologists, dentists, dermatologists, infectious disease specialists, and general practitioners usually encounter three types of patients that seek diagnosis and treatment for potential HSV-1 infections. The first and the largest of these groups is accurately diagnosed, begin antiviral therapy, and have successful reduction of the herpetic lesions followed by rapid healing. The second group does not have an immediate or prompt successful response, but with an increase in the dose and/or frequency of the antiviral therapy, the lesions are reduced and success is achieved. A final group appears to have an infection that is resistant to intense, multiple antiviral therapies. While this is usually not serious in immunocompetent patients with herpetic skin lesions, resistant herpetic ocular infections are a cause for concern. Patients with ocular herpes can experience repeated herpetic corneal and stromal lesions and ultimately, irreversible stromal damage. If the lesion appears in the central axis of the cornea, a transplant to restore vision may be required.

At least two possibilities could account for the failure of antiherpetic therapy: the genetics of the virus and the genetics of the host. With regard to viral genetics, animal models of HSV-1 latency and reactivation have identified HSV-1 strains which reactivate with different frequencies (Hill et al., 1978). Greater than 95% of clinical HSV-1 strains appear to reactivate with low or moderate frequency, and only a small percentage (<5.0%) reactivate with high frequency (Hill et al, 1987; Toma et al, 2008).

With regard to host genetics, in a mouse model of HSV-1 latency and reactivation, recent studies indicate that the ApoE e4 allele is a known risk factor for the development of ocular herpes (Hill et al., 2007; Bhattacharjee et al., 2008). In humans, the ApoE e4 is a risk factor for herpes labialis (Lin et al., 1995). Finally, the worst case scenario may be an individual who is homozygous for the e4 allele of ApoE who harbors the latent high phenotypic reactivator of HSV-1 (Burgos et al., 2003, 2005, 2006, and 2007). This individual would be expected to have frequent reactivation episodes and shed high copy numbers of HSV-1 (Hill et al., 2007).

Rates and Patterns of HSV-1 Asymptomatic Shedding

A review of existing PCR studies assessing HSV-1 DNA in the tears of asymptomatic, healthy volunteers show most studies have a low frequency (1 to 2 times per subject) of tear sampling (Table 4). Five of the 10 studies reported no detection of HSV-1 DNA. The largest study collected tears twice a day for 30 days from 50 subjects and analyzed approximately 2700 tear samples for HSV-1 DNA by PCR (Kaufman et al, 2005). In this study, viral DNA was detected at least once in 47 of 50 (94%) subjects. Interestingly, four seronegative subjects also shed HSV-1 DNA at least once during the 30 days of tear collection.

What is the possible explanation for seronegative subjects shedding HSV-1 DNA? First, and most likely, is that the sensitivity of the PCR is at least 1,000 times greater than the serology assay for HSV. Another possibility, considered unlikely, is that a subject had a recent HSV-1 inoculation and had not yet seroconverted. In most cases, we rule this hypothesis out due to the timing of shedding and the episodic shedding of the HSV-1 DNA.

Table 4. Asymptomatic shedding of HSV-1 detected by PCR from eye swabs (tears) of healthy subjects

Author(s), Year	N	Individuals: total positive/total subjects	Shedding frequency: total positive swabs/total swabs taken	Swab frequency: number of swabs/subject
Kaufman et al., 2005	50	47/50 (94%)	941/2708 (34.7%)	60
Abiko et al., 2002	22	5/22 (22.7%)	5/132 (3.7%)	Six
Robert et al., 2002	93	1/93 (1%)	1/186 (0.5%)	Two
Hidalgo et al., 1998	17	1/17 (5.9%)	1/17 (5.9%)	One
Kudo et al., 1996	25	1/25 (4%)	1/54 (1.8%)	One
Linder et al., 2005	10	0/10 (0%)	0/10 (0%)	One
Khodadoost et al., 2004	10	0/10 (0%)	0/10 (0%)	One
Fukuda et al., 2003	50	0/50 (0%)	0/50 (0%)	One
Koizumi et al., 1999	19	0/19 (0%)	0/38 (0%)	Two
Yamamoto et al., 1994	20	0/20 (0%)	0/20 (0%)	One
Totals	**316**	**55/316 (17%)**	**949/3225 (29%)**	

Table 5 summarizes studies assessing the presence of infectious HSV-1 from tears of asymptomatic, healthy volunteers. In most studies, infectious HSV-1 was not detected or detected in only one tear sample. However, when both eyes were swabbed once a day on each weekday for 5 consecutive weeks, 36% (4/11) of the samples contained infectious HSV-1. These studies used cell culture to detect infectious HSV-1. This procedure is known to be considerably less sensitive than PCR. Thus, one cannot directly compare PCR- and cell culture-based data.

Table 5. Asymptomatic shedding of infectious HSV-1 detected by cell culture from eye swabs (tears) of healthy subjects

Author(s), Year	N	Individuals: total positives/total subjects	Shedding frequency: total positive swabs/ total swabs	Swab frequency: number of swabs/subjects
Kaufman et al. 1967	35	11/35 (31%)	11/1400 (0.8%)	20*
Okinaga 2000	10	1/10 (10%)	1/1742 (0.06%)	~17
Khodadoost et al. 2004	10	1/10 (10%)	1/10 (10%)	one
Asbell et al. 1995	23	1/23 (5%)	1/23 (5%)	one
Kaye et al. 1990	24	0/24 (0/0)	0/752 (0%)	~ 31
Totals	**102**	**14/102 (14%)**	**14/3927 (0.4%)**	

N = Total number of subjects

*Each day both eyes of each subject was swabbed

A detailed review of 22 reports on HSV-1 shedding in the oral cavity reported that at least 70% of the U.S. population shed HSV-1 DNA at least once a month, that the rate of oral HSV-1 shedding is highly variable among individuals, and that even HSV-1 seronegative individuals can shed HSV-1 DNA (Miller and Danaher, 2008). Miller and Danaher also showed that HSV-1 shedding can occur at many intraoral sites and that the HSV-1 DNA copy numbers are sufficient to be transmitted even in seronegative individuals. This review highlights two important facts. First, seronegative subjects can shed HSV-1 and second, that a minimum of 70% of all subjects shed HSV-1 DNA at least once in a 30-day period.

Early studies indicating that oral shedding occurs in younger individuals (14 years and younger) (Buddingh et al., 1953; Tateishi et al., 1994) were confirmed and extended to show no statistical difference in gender or age and the detection or copy number of HSV-1 DNA in saliva (Kaufman et al., 2005). While the study by Kaufman et al. (2005) did not contain subjects younger than 21 years of age, PCR analysis detected HSV-1 DNA in approximately 90% of 157 human trigeminal ganglia (TG), with no statistical association found between subject age or gender or the presence or abundance of HSV-1 DNA (Hill et al., 2008). Therefore, HSV-1 reactivation data obtained from the study of tears and saliva are in agreement with the data on HSV-1 latent infection in the human TG.

Further evidence suggesting that HSV-1 reactivation is frequent and independent of age, gender, and HSV-1 serology is the detection of viral DNA an average of four times in 48 of 50 (96%) subjects. The distribution of HSV-1 DNA in the ~ 2700 tear samples was 10.0-14.9 copies (20%), 15.0-239.9 copies (14%); 240-24,000 copies (34%) and >24,000 copies (32%) (Kaufman et al., 2005). A summary of 22 reports (Miller and Danaher, 2008) revealed a great deal of variation in the copy numbers per individual swab and/or per subject thereby confirming the saliva study of Kaufman et al (2005).

Frequent sampling and method of detection are important to obtain an accurate account of subclinical HSV-1 reactivation. When saliva was obtained once daily for 5 months, infectious HSV-1 was detected, on average, 8 times (Spruance et al., 1984). In addition, all 25 subjects whose saliva was tested periodically for 30 days were positive for HSV-1 at least once (Da Silva et al., 2005). Also, HSV-1 detection in saliva is two-fold greater when comparing oral samples taken once [117 of 1861 (6.3%)] to oral samples taken >3 time per individual [212 of 1708 (12.4%)] (Miller and Danaher, 2008). PCR detected HSV-1 in saliva at a rate ~2.5 more frequent that virus isolation. When all available reports are summarized, PCR detected HSV-1 DNA in 1355 of 5315 samples (26%) samples compared to the isolation of HSV-1 in 202 of 1954 (10%) samples.

Finally, the frequency (~100%) and intensity (high copy number) of oral HSV-1 DNA shedding suggest frequent transition from latent to lytic infection in human ganglia; however, more research is needed to decipher the molecular and virological mechanisms that regulate asymptomatic shedding. Also, the clinical studies cited in Tables 2-5 rely on the patients' self reporting. Since the cornea is very sensitive, it is likely that subjects who reported no symptoms are accurate; however, the same may not be true for oral lesions. Thus, self reporting for oral lesions may be less accurate.

3. Human Herpesvirus Type 2 (HSV-2)

Herpes simplex virus type 2 (HSV-2) exhibits the typical alphaherpesvirus dual tropism for epithelial cells and neurons. The most obvious biological difference between HSV-1 and HSV-2 is the clinical predilection of HSV-2 for the anogenital area. It is not yet known precisely which single or ensemble nucleotide or amino acid differences control this anatomical preference, but chimeric viruses have implicated the LAT region in differential reactivation from sacral vs. trigeminal ganglia (Yoshikawa et al., 1996). To date, site-specific behaviors of HSV-2 have mainly been described at the level of reactivation rather than epithelial infection or initiation or maintenance of neuronal latency. As a corollary, peripheral recurrent shedding of virus during the chronic phase of infection, whether symptomatic or asymptomatic, is much greater for established HSV-2 than for HSV-1 infections in the anogenital region (Koelle et al., 1992). There are more descriptive data on human asymptomatic shedding for HSV-2 than for HSV-1, contrasting with lesser knowledge of pathogenesis of viral mutants in animals or cell culture for HSV-2. Mice can be provoked to have at least molecular HSV-1 reactivation with extreme stress (Gebhardt and Halford, 2005), but asymptomatic reactivation and especially HSV-2 detection in the periphery are rarely studied. Guinea pigs spontaneously reactivate genital HSV-2 with lesions and detectable virus (Hoshino et al., 2005), but most work has focused on symptomatic disease in this model. This host-species specific behavior has limited research into asymptomatic shedding in experimental systems.

Clinical Importance of Ssymptomatic HSV-2 Shedding

The majority of HSV-2 infections have no known medically serious consequences. However, since the HSV-2 infection rate of US adults hovers near 20% (Xu et al., 2006) and is higher in many parts of the world (Corey and Wald, 2008), even rare complications such as dissemination in immunocompetent (Czartoski et al., 2006) or immunocompromised (Ramsey et al., 1982) persons, transmission to neonates (Kimberlin, 2005), encephalitis (Tang et al., 2003) and ocular syndromes (Inoda et al., 2001; King et al., 2007) have a significant global disease burden. It is not known if reactivation events are truly pathogenic in the mass of seropositive persons. Recent data detect chronic inflammation in human HSV-1-infected ganglia (Vergans et al., 2007; Theil et al., 2003; Hufner et al., 2006; Derfuss et al., 2007). There is no reason to think that chronic HSV-2 infection of sacral ganglia would be biologically different, but there are not yet studies of ganglionic infiltration or cytokine expression at this site. It is unclear if the ganglia or peripheral nerves are clinically damaged by chronic HSV infection and periodic reactivation. The primary clinical importance of asymptomatic HSV-2 shedding is therefore its contribution to transmission of infection and the maintenance of the worldwide HSV-2 pandemic.

Several recent clinical trials have addressed roles for HSV-2 in HIV transmission (Ouedraogo et al., 2006; Nagot et al., 2007; Celum et al., 2008; Watson-Jones et al., 2008; Zuckerman et al., 2007). The potential role for asymptomatic HSV-2 shedding in HIV transmission is unclear. Symptomatic HSV-2 lesions contain HIV-1 (Schacker et al., 1998), and HSV-2 lesions are rich in CD4 T-cells (Cunningham et al., 1985), but there are no studies concerning HIV shedding specifically from asymptomatic shedding sites, or of the infiltration of CD4 T-cells to such areas.

Epidemiologic studies and case reports concur that the majority of horizontal (sexual) transmission of HSV-2 occurs due to asymptomatic shedding (Mertz et al., 1988, 1992; Rooney et al., 1986). In one study, about a third of probable HSV-2 transmitting partners had no clinical history of genital herpes, even after being educated about signs and symptoms (Metz et al., 1985). The epidemiology and medical consequences of neonatal herpes (vertical transmission) differs from horizontal transmission between adults. The risk per delivery of transmitting HSV is higher for primary genital herpes, likely because there are no pre-formed antibodies to cross the placenta and afford some protection (Brown et al., 1997, 2003). Given the greater number of chronically vs. primarily infected women undergoing labor, and the long-term nature of periodic shedding, there is still a considerable disease burden in neonates due to reactivation disease despite a lower attack rate. In either primary or recurrent infection, the HSV virus shedding responsible for vertical transmission is usually asymptomatic (Brown et al., 2005).

It might be considered surprising that primary genital HSV-2 infection, during which the virus can replicate unchecked by acquired immune responses, could be completely asymptomatic. However, natural history data from the placebo arm of an HSV-2 vaccine trial are available that combine accurate HSV-2 serology to detect new HSV-2 infections, during the observation period, with intensive subject clinical histories. The majority of documented new HSV-2 infections in these adults went unnoticed (Langenberg et al., 1999). These persons contribute to the approximately 75% of HSV-2 seropositive US adults who have no overt clinical history of genital herpes (Corey and Wald, 2008).

Definitions of Asymptomatic HSV-2 Shedding

The strictest definition of asymptomatic HSV-2 shedding is detection of virus in the absence of any abnormality on physical exam with no symptoms. In practice, subtle changes may be noticed on physical examinations that are not classic epithelial defects (Koutsky et al., 1992). These can include erythema, non-inflammed fissures in the skin or mucosa, urethral or vaginal discharge, or tiny lesions only visible with specialized optics. Persons may experience symptoms such as neuropathic pain or dysuria that they do not associate with HSV. People with these signs and symptoms may be considered not to be truly asymptomatic, but to have unrecognized recurrent genital herpes. There have been three longitudinal cohort studies in which HSV-2-seropositive persons without a known clinical history of genital herpes have undergone some combination of subject education, virus detection, and documentation of genital signs and symptoms (Langenberg et al., 1989; Frenkel et al., 1993; Wald et al., 2000). As reviewed elsewhere (Corey and Wald, 2008) the studies agree that about half of such persons do have viral shedding events that correlated in time and place with signs and/or symptoms. Overall, the classification of an HSV-2 shedding event, defined as detection of viral DNA and/or culturable virus from a peripheral site, as either symptomatic or asymptomatic is therefore somewhat colored by the knowledge base of the infected individual and/or the clinician.

The biological differentiation of asymptomatic from symptomatic shedding is surprisingly unclear. In a study of over 31,000 samples obtained in the absence of lesions, the rate of culture positivity was 1.7%, while HSV-2 DNA was detected in 8.4% of specimens. In comparison, among 4,670 specimens obtained from lesions, cultures were positive for 12% and PCR positive for 37%. The mean HSV-2 DNA copy number was slightly lower (4.4 $\log_{10}$ versus 4.9 $\log_{10}$) in specimens from asymptomatic persons compared to symptomatic persons. It is debatable whether this ½ $\log_{10}$ difference accounts for the presence or absence of symptoms and lesions. Lesions were more likely to be culture positive than were specimens from asymptomatic, HSV-2 DNA (+) surfaces. There is a fairly linear relationship between HSV-2 DNA copy number and culture positivity for specimens from asymptomatic persons, with cultures 50% positive at between 10^6 and 10^7 DNA copies. The shape and 50% point of this curve were quite similar for specimens from symptomatic lesions (Wald et al., 2003). We know that infiltration of HSV-specific T-cells is part of the local reaction in both symptomatic and asymptomatic HSV-2 infection (Koelle et al., 1998, 2001; Zhu et al., 2007). The host factors that might decide whether the presence of HSV-2 provokes a lesion are unclear. Recent animal CNS model data suggest that host responses may contribute to HSV disease (Sergerie et al., 2007). The virologic similarity between symptomatic and asymptomatic shedding holds open the possibility that the host response to the presence of HSV-2 could in some way be causative for lesion formation.

Patterns and Rates of Asymptomatic HSV-2 Shedding

Asymptomatic shedding of HSV-2 was noted anecdotally several decades ago using cell culture, but systematic studies are fairly recent. The rate of measured asymptomatic shedding is clearly a function of the frequency of sampling, the number of anatomic sites sampled per person, and, as mentioned above, the detection technology employed. Once daily sampling from genital (internal and multiple external sites) and peri-rectal swabs has been employed in the majority of studies. Several noteworthy conclusions can be abstracted from reviews (Corey and Wald, 2008; Koelle and Wald 2000) and original reports. Almost all HSV-2-seropositive persons have detectable HSV-2 shedding. It is therefore very possible for persons with no clinical history of HSV-2, even after intensive education and correlation of virus detection with subtle signs or symptoms, to transmit HSV-2. The rate of asymptomatic shedding does correlate with the presence or absence of symptomatic disease: persons with typical lesions have about twice as much asymptomatic shedding as do seropositive persons without disease. Women have higher rates of asymptomatic shedding than do men. Immune compromise due to HIV-1 infection correlates with higher rates of HSV-2 shedding (Mostad et al., 2000; Schacker et al., 1998). Among men, the most common site is the penile skin, followed by the perianal area, although the pattern is reversed among men who have sex with men. A variety of temporal patterns are noted, ranging from one-day shedding at low HSV-2 DNA copy numbers to multi-day periods of high titer shedding. Asymptomatic shedding is more frequent during the first year after primary HSV-2 infection but appears to persist for at least 10 years at relatively stable rates thereafter (Corey and Wald, 2008).

Medical Interventions and Asymptomatic HSV-2 Shedding

Recognition of the contribution of asymptomatic shedding to HSV-2 transmission, reviewed above, has increased interest in using HSV-2 shedding, and by hopeful implication, HSV-2 transmission, as a measure of the success or usefulness of treatments for established HSV-2 infection. The nucleoside antiviral drug, acyclovir, and the orally bioavailable prodrugs valacyclovir and famciclovir, have favorable safety profiles suitable for chronic administration. Inhibition of HSV-2 DNA polymerase by activated triphosphate metabolites of these compounds leads to profound reduction of symptomatic HSV but does not remove HSV genomes from infected neurons. The pharmacokinetics of the drugs and their intracellular metabolites require at least daily therapy for clinically significant reductions of recurrences. Attention has recently turned to their effect on asymptomatic shedding and upon transmission.

Each of the licensed systemic nucleosides, mentioned above, results in significant reduction in asymptomatic (as well as symptomatic) HSV-2 shedding (Wald et al., 1996, 1997, 2006; Leone et al., 2007). When the percentage of days with any detection of HSV-2 is used as the primary measure, a 50-75% reduction of shedding rate is observed. Interestingly, on a quantitative basis, the amount of HSV-2 DNA detected during asymptomatic shedding events is not drastically decreased by nucleoside therapy. Average copy number for asymptomatic shedding was reduced from a mean of 4.97 $\log_{10}$ to 4.60 $\log_{10}$ by famciclovir (Leone et al., 2007). The asymptomatic shed geometric mean HSV-2 DNA copy number was reduced somewhat more, by 0.8 and 1.3 $\log_{10}$, by acyclovir and valacylovir, respectively. Because higher DNA levels correlate with culture positivity, the reduction of culture positive shedding as a percent of days is usually more impressive than the reduction of DNA positive days. These studies usually use once daily sampling of the anogenital area. Symptomatic shedding, and by implication, total (symptomatic plus asymptomatic) shedding are also greatly reduced. Crossover study designs, in which each subjects serves as their own control during daily monitoring periods before and during active therapy, add statistical power and reduce the number of persons required to show treatment effects. When therapy ceases, shedding resumes after about 5 days with no detectable change compared to prior to therapy (Leone et al., 2007; Wald et al., 1997; Gupta et al., 2004).

There are relatively few data to rank the effects of antiviral drugs on asymptomatic shedding. Head-to-head comparison of valcyclovir and acyoclovir in a three-period crossover study (including placebo) showed a trend to better suppression of asymptomatic shedding for valacyclovir (Gupta et al., 2004). A head-to-head, non cross-over, and non placebo-controlled trial showed slightly lower shedding rates for valacyclovir than for famciclovir (Wald et al., 2006). It is not clear if these differences have clinical or public health (transmission) significance.

It is not certain if these drugs reduce HSV DNA replication associated with reactivation in neurons, virus DNA replication at the periphery, or both. Reduction of chronic ganglionic inflammation in drug-treated animals indicates at least some activity in the nervous system (Halford et al., 1997). Intracellular nucleoside levels in neurons can influence HSV reactivation and the ability of acyclovir to work (Tenser et al., 1996). Recently, genital asymptomatic HSV-2 shedding was studied in untreated subjects using PCR swabs obtained every 6 hours. The majority of the shedding events were less than 12 hours in duration (Mark et al., 2008). While the biology at the ganglionic and skin levels responsible for these intermittent shedding events is unclear, it is possible the intracellular metabolism of the current nucleosides and cell-type differences place a limit on the ability of clinically rational dosing schedules to limit these brief asymptomatic shedding events.

Attempts to reduce viral shedding have included both innate and acquired immune interventions. These have the possibility of requiring less frequent administration. Early immunotherapy trials of HSV-2 envelope glycoprotein subunits showed variable activity for reduction of symptomatic genital herpes but did not evaluate asymptomatic shedding (Straus et al., 1994, 1997). Topical application of the TLR7 agonist resiquimod was studied using PCR detection of HSV-2 shedding in the weeks after a symptomatic recurrence as the endpoint, with some indication of reduction of asymptomatic (as well as total) HSV-2 shedding (Mark et al., 2007). Administration of a replication-incompetent HSV-2 strain, designed to boost pre-existing acquired immunity, failed to show any reduction in genital HSV-2 shedding (de Bruyn et al., 2006).

It is rational that reduction of asymptomatic shedding should correlate with a reduction of sexual HSV-2 transmission. Daily valacyclovir use by the potential HSV-2 transmitting partner lead to an approximately 50% reduction in HSV-2 acquisition by the susceptible partner (Corey et al., 2004). An embedded shedding sub-study documented about 73% reduction of HSV-2 shedding. As mentioned above, the drop in viral titer (DNA copy number) in residual shedding events during therapy is modest. We don't know the functional inoculum size for HSV-2 genital transmission, but the discrepancy between the reduction in shedding and the lesser reduction in transmission may reflect the ability of residually shed virus to initiate infection. In ongoing studies, the effect of medications on asymptomatic shedding is being studied at higher temporal and spatial resolution to further define residual shedding, and provide a baseline for future drug or immunologic interventions. Ultimately, limitation of asymptomatic shedding, and by implication, HSV-2 transmission, should join reduction of symptomatic HSV-2 disease as criteria for evaluating future HSV-2 therapeutics.

4. Human Herpesvirus Type 3 (VZV)

Varicella zoster virus (VZV) is a highly successful human pathogen, characterized by varicella (chickenpox) on primary infection and zoster (shingles) following virus reactivation from latency. VZV is acquired early in life. Of 3208 children (<5 years) residing in temperate climates, 42% have circulating anti-VZV IgG suggestive of virus exposure (Nardone et al., 2007). While serologic status early in life may be confounded by maternal anti-VZV IgG which has a half-life in infants of 25 days (Der Zwet et al., 2002), successive age groups show an increasing prevalence of circulating anti-VZV antibody such that by age 14, VZV exposure is detected in >90% of subjects (n=4985). In the US, 95% of 1201 military basic trainees had circulating antibodies against VZV (Jerant et al., 1998). VZV is highly contagious with a secondary attack rate approaching 100% (Asano et al., 1977) that can lead to epidemics in places of close confinement such as prisons (Levy et al., 2003), summer camps (Winquist et al., 2001) and day care centers (Galil et al., 2002). VZV is transmitted by direct contact with vesicle fluid or aerosolized respiratory tract secretions (Kavaliotis et al., 1998). VZV DNA is present in the air in hospital rooms of varicella or zoster patients (Sawyer et al., 1994). While the air and even remote surfaces around zoster patients can contain VZV DNA (Yoshikawa et al., 2001), only recently has infectious virus been recovered in saliva from a zoster patent (Mehta et al., 2008). The finding of VZV in saliva suggests that virus spread may not be limited to cutaneous vesicles, and the epidemiological significance of VZV in saliva will be addressed in the modeling scenario (below).

VZV infections are typically benign; however, serious outcomes can occur. Primary VZV infection typically results in varicella which is characterized by malaise, fever and an extensive vesicular rash. Varicella is normally self-limiting and resolves with the development of humoral and cell mediated immunity; however, varicella is not always a mild disease. Varicella associated deaths were reported in otherwise healthy children during a winter epidemic (Blair et al., 1965). Three deaths were reported among 292 varicella cases in a 1994 epidemic (Balraj and John, 1994). While wide spread aggressive vaccination has greatly lessened the morbidity and mortality associated with varicella (Arvin and Gershon, 1996), in countries where vaccination is not mandatory, deaths still occur (Rawson et al., 2001).

During varicella, VZV accesses ganglionic neurons where it becomes latent in multiple cranial nerve, dorsal root and autonomic ganglia (reviewed in Meuller et al., 2008). Like HSV, VZV latency is exclusively in neurons where the endless virus DNA is coated with histones whose modifications reflect transcriptional activity (Clarke et al., 1995; Gary et al., 2006). Unlike HSV, polyadenylated VZV transcripts mapping to numerous genes along with their encoded proteins have been detected in latently infected human ganglia (Cohrs et al., 1994, 1995, 2003, Mahalingam et al., 1996; Theil et al., 2003). VZV gene 63 transcripts are the most prevalent and abundant virus transcript detected during latency (Cohrs and Gilden, 2007), and may serve the same function as HSV LAT. Support for this assertion comes from the finding that both HSV-1 LAT and IE63 (the immediate-early protein encoded by VZV gene 63) are antiapoptotic in infected ganglia (Preng et al., 2000; Hood et al., 2006).

VZV reactivation typically occurs once during life, and is accompanied with a significant burden of illness felt by both the patient and society (reviewed in Quan et al., 2007). The most common clinical outcome of VZV reactivation is zoster (shingles). Zoster, "a belt of roses from Hell" as it is known by the Norwegians (Crow and Ellis, 1979), is characterized by severe, sharp, lancinating, radicular pain and a vesicular eruption on an erythematous base. Annually, over 1 million new cases of zoster are reported in the US, with most patients over age 60 or immunocomprimised (Harnisch, 1984; Donahue et al., 1995). There is no cure for zoster, and treatment is only supportive. In addition, 5.3% of patients over age 64 died of zoster complications during zoster related hospitalizations (Lin and Hadler, 2000). Approximately 40% of elderly zoster patients will experience postherpetic neuralgia where the pain of zoster continues for months to years after resolution of the rash of zoster (Rogeres and Tindall, 1971; Bowsher, 1997).

The severity of VZV zoster with the potential of its accompanying sequellae (postherpetic neuralgia) has overshadowed studies of subacute or asymptomatic VZV reactivation. As molecular detection techniques have advanced, correlations have been found to suggest that VZV reactivation is more frequent and can occur without cutaneous rash (Nagel and Gilden, 2007).

Clinical Importance of Asymptomatic VZV Shedding

The most obvious sign of VZV reactivation is vesicular rash and pain associated with zoster, however in the absence of rash, the virus can also spread to the retina causing blindness (Knox et al., 1998), to the spinal cord causing paralysis and incontinence (Orme et al., 2007), and to cerebral arteries resulting in stroke (Kleinschmidt-DeMasters and Gilden, 2001). While associating VZV with disease is straightforward when rash and vesicles are present, correlating VZV with disease is difficult when the outward signs are absent. For example, when stroke occurs in the elderly, especially many months following zoster, the association with VZV reactivation requires cerebral spinal fluid analysis for VZV antibodies (Nagel et al., 2007). Likewise, detection of asymptomatic VZV reactivation, which often is only seen as an increase in antibody titer against VZV, but may also result in virus transmission is difficult to detect.

Asymptomatic VZV Reactivation and Virus Transmission

Prolonged maintenance of anti-VZV antibodies in small, isolated populations supports the notion of subclincial reactivation; however this finding equally supports periodic boost in anti-VZV titer due to subclinical reactivation of latent VZV (Hope-Simpson, 1965, Black et al., 1974). The eyes are a likely site to demonstrate subclinical VZV reactivation since, both HSV-1 and VZV become latent in trigeminal ganglia (Cohrs et al., 2005) and even within the same neuron (Theil et al., 2003), both viruses cause keratitis following reactivation (Cook et al., 1986; Kayes et al., 2000; Reijo et al., 1983), and HSV-1 DNA can be detected in tears of healthy individuals (Kauffman et al., 2005). However, using equally sensitive PCR technology, VZV DNA was not detected in tear film from 35 normal subjects (Yamamoto et al., 1994; Willoughby et al., 2002) or conjunctival scrapings from 30 individuals with eye trauma or unrelated disease (Lee-Wing et al., 1999). Thus, unlike HSV-1, where asymptomatic virus reactivates often and can be detected frequently in tear film, asymptomatic VZV reactivation is either a rare event or does not progress to yield virus in the eyes.

In an effort to understand the prevalence of virus reactivation in the unique environment of space, DNA extracted form 312 saliva samples were collected from eight astronauts (two short term shuttle missions). VZV DNA was detected in only 1 of 112 saliva samples taken 234-265 days before flight, whereas during and shortly after space flight 61 of 200 saliva samples were positive for the virus DNA (Mehta et al., 2004). No VZV DNA was detected in saliva from 10 age matched control subjects (88 samples). Subsequently, VZV DNA was again detected in saliva samples from 2 of 3 space shuttle astronauts during and within days following space flight, but not before launch (Cohrs et al., 2008). Importantly, infectious VZV was isolated in saliva samples following landing from the 2 astronauts whose saliva contained VZV DNA. These results suggest asymptomatic VZV reactivation does occur, and saliva is a convenient source material for its detection. While it is impossible to determine if the virus in both astronauts resulted from simultaneous reactivation, or if a single reactivation and shed in one subject resulted in asymptomatic infection of the second subject, the presence of a rare restriction endonuclease recognition site in the VZV DNA isolated from both subjects argues for the later case. While PCR-based sequence analysis of all VZV DNA samples obtained from saliva may aid in determining the source of the virus, due to the restrictions associated with space flight, confirmation of asymptomatic VZV reactivation resulting in virus shedding and transmission most likely will require Earth-based analogues to space flight.

Space flight is a unique and stressful environment where astronauts experience isolation, confinement, anxiety, psychosocial stressors, sleep deprivation, increased radiation, and microgravity. Ground-based analogs have been developed to model specific aspects of space flight. NASA's Extreme Environment Operation (NEEMO) is a 14 m 175 m^3 chamber located 4.5 km offshore where "aquanauts" live and work in an atmosphere 2.5 more dense than sea level and experience stress-induced physiologic changes similar to short duration space flight (Smith et al., 2004; Leach, 1992). Asymptomatic VZV reactivation was detected during NEEMO 5. No VZV DNA was found in 98 saliva samples collected prior to the 14 day mission. However, VZV DNA was detected in 12 of 72 saliva samples collected during, and in 11 of 70 saliva samples collected after the mission. A second Earth-based analogue to space flight is the bed rest study. To model cardiovascular and neuron-musculoskeletal changes seen in astronauts, subjects recline for up to 17 weeks in a 6 degrees head-down tilt position (Hargens, 1994). Reactivation of latent VZV is measured by PCR on DNA extracted from the saliva collected from subjects before, during and after the bed rest study. During a 90-day bed rest study, evidence of VZV DNA was detected only in two of the 10 subjects.

In the space analogue studies, VZV DNA was quantitated by real-time PCR using TaqMan technology and showed only trace amounts (<20 VZV copies) in subject saliva. While these studies show that VZV reactivated in subjects participating in Earth-based space analogue studies, the magnitude of reactivation was less than that experienced by astronauts during spaceflight. Thus unique aspects of spaceflight are not yet modeled on Earth. Future studies will determine the effect of increased exposure to cosmic radiations and microgravity on reactivation of human herpesviruses (Mehta et al., 2007).

Asymptomatic VZV Reactivation and Disease Production

Intrauterine transmission of VZV can be life threatening to the infant. Congenital varicella syndrome (CVS) is the serious consequence in infants whose moms developed primary varicella during pregnancy (Daley et al., 2007). Maternal primary varicella within the first 20 weeks of pregnancy may interfere with normal fetal organ development. CVS is characterized (in decreasing frequency) by skin involvement (lesions, local thickening and scarring), underdeveloped limbs, ocular abnormalities, low birth weight, and mental retardation (Sauerbrei and Wutzler, 2000). Severe CVS can result in fetal death (Mazzella et al., 2003). Fortunately, the frequency of CVS in infants born to mothers experiencing primary varicella during pregnancy is low (0.4 – 1.3%; Harger et al., 2002); however, CVS may not be the only outcome associated with VZV infection during pregnancy. Healthy infants born to moms with primary VZV but who do not manifest obvious CVS may develop zoster (Enders et al., 1994) and seizures (Mustonen et al., 1998) early in life. A controversial, but exciting finding is that in the infant both zoster (Dent and Baetz-Greenwalt, 2007) and neuropathology (Mustonen et al., 1998, 2001) can develop from intrauterine VZV transmission from asymptomatic virus reactivation in pregnant moms. Maternal varicella was not reported in either the case study (Dent and Baetz-Greenwalt, 2007) or the large scale screens (Mustonen et al., 1998, 2001). It is difficult to differentiate between maternal subclinical viremia due to recent VZV exposure, or subclinical VZV reactivation due to transient herpesvirus-specific immunosuppression (Kumar et al., 1984) or haemodilution of maternal anti-VZV antibodies (Baboonian and Griffiths, 1983) experienced during pregnancy. In either event, VZV associated disease in infants is rare and further studies are required to determine if maternal subclinical VZV reactivation and intrauterine transmission occurs.

Asymptomatic VZV Shedding and Epidemiology

Currently, VZV epidemiology is based on the paradigm that virus transmission occurs only during varicella or zoster. To test the hypothesis whether subclinical VZV reactivation is a viable component of VZV epidemiology, a mathematical model describing VZV transmission (Schuette and Hethcote, 1999; Schuette, 2003) was modified to include shed of infectious virus. The model (Figure 2) describes a population of constant size that is divided into nine epidemiological classes. To describe the model, we shall follow a hypothetical individual as he ages through the various epidemiological classes. Our subject enters the model as an infant protected by maternal anti-VZV antibodies (**M**). As time progresses, the infant looses passive immunity and becomes susceptible to primary VZV infection (**S**). Exposure to VZV moves our subject out of population **S** and into the exposed (**E**) population. If VZV exposure results in varicella, our subject becomes infectious and moves into population **I**. Following varicella resolution, the individual is no longer infectious, but has robust anti-VZV immunity, and consequently moves out of population **I** and into population $\mathbf{R_V}$. With age, immunity to VZV wanes and our subject moves out of population $\mathbf{R_V}$ and into population (**W**). Within population **W**, our subject has three viable alternatives. Contact with an infectious individual (varicella or zoster) can boost the waning anti-VZV immunity resulting in a movement from population **W** into population $\mathbf{R_B}$. If no exposure to external virus occurs, age related decrease in anti-VZV immunity continues which may result in subclinical VZV reactivation ($\mathbf{Z_S}$) or zoster ($\mathbf{Z_C}$). Within each population, an individual may exit due to death. This is shown by an exiting arrow that does not lead to a subsequent population, where μ is the per capita death rate.

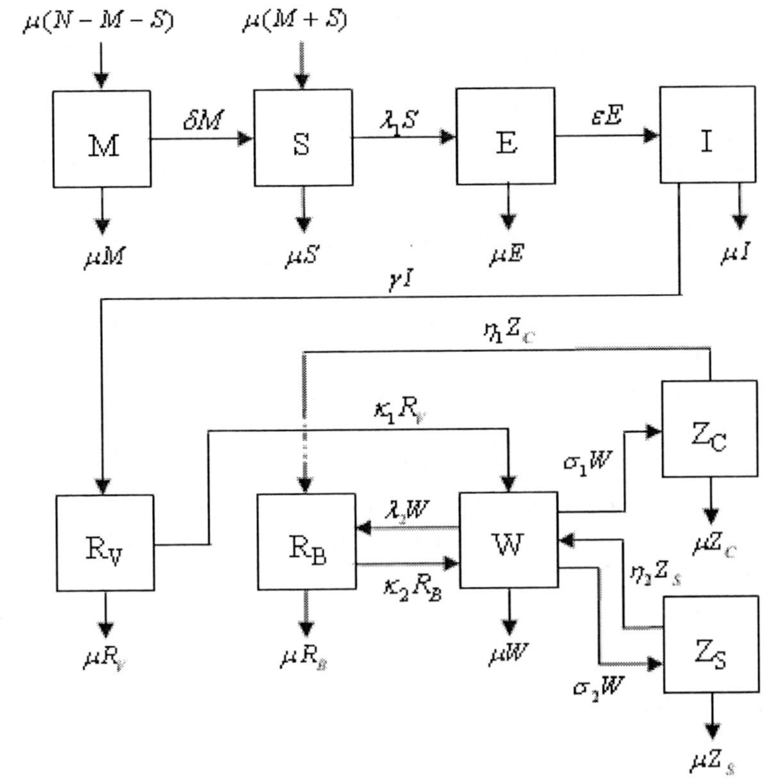

Figure 2. Compartmental Model for Varicella-Zoster Virus with Subclinical Reactivation of Zoster. A hypothetical person either enters the model as an infant protected by maternal anti-VZV antibodies (**M**) or enters the model with susceptibility (**S**) to VZV. As time progresses, the infant loses passive immunity and becomes susceptible to primary VZV infection (**S**). Exposure to VZV moves our subject out of population **S** and into the exposed (**E**) population. If VZV exposure results in varicella, our subject becomes infectious and moves into population **I**. Following varicella resolution, the individual is no longer infectious, but has robust anti-VZV immunity, and consequently moves out of population **I** and into population $\mathbf{R_V}$. With age, immunity to VZV wanes and our subject moves out of population $\mathbf{R_V}$ and into population (**W**). Within population **W**, our subject has three viable alternatives. Contact with an infectious individual (varicella or zoster) can boost the waning anti-VZV immunity resulting in a movement from population **W** into population $\mathbf{R_B}$. If no exposure to external virus occurs, age related decrease in anti-VZV immunity continues which leads to subclinical VZV reactivation ($\mathbf{Z_S}$) or zoster ($\mathbf{Z_C}$). Within each population, an individual may exit due to death. This is shown by an exiting arrow that does not lead to a subsequent population, where μ is the per capita death rate.

At the heart of the model is a system of differential equations (appendix) based on the transfer rates between the epidemiological classes. The transfers out of many of the classes are assumed proportional to the class sizes, hence waiting times due to each term have negative exponential distributions, and therefore the average waiting times are the reciprocals of the rate parameters. Of special interest are the variable parameters λ_1 and λ_2.

$\lambda_1(t) = \beta[I(t) + \rho_1 Z_C(t) + \rho_2 Z_S(t)]$ is the ***force of infection***, which is the number of personal contacts required to produce an infection. The varicella incidence is the product of the force of infection and the number of susceptible individuals, $\lambda_1(t)S(t)$.

$\lambda_2(t) = \beta[I(t) + \rho_1 Z_C(t)]$ estimates the ***force of boosting*** of cell-mediated immunity due to exposure to VZV.

Immunity to VZV receives a boost in individuals following exposure to varicella or zoster. Mothers exposed to children with varicella have increased anti-VZV antibody titers (Arvin et al., 1983), and the incidence of zoster is lower in adults who have greater contact with children (Brisson et al., 2002; Thomas et al., 2002). Cell-mediated immunity to VZV is also enhanced following zoster (Hayward, 1990). In addition, VZV immunity may be maintained by subclinical reactivation of latent virus (Arvin and Gershon, 1996). Reactivation of latent VZV accounts for recovery of cell-mediated immunity to VZV in following bone marrow transplant in recipients (Wilson et al., 1992).

Our model is designed to determine the influence of subclinical VZV reactivation on the occurrence of zoster. Therefore, two alternative models are considered. In Model **B** (boost), anti-VZV immunity receives a boost by exposure to individuals in class ***W***, to individuals with varicella or clinical zoster, and the number of new zoster cases per unit time is given by $\lambda_2(t)W(t)$. In model **NB** (no boost), anti-VZV immunity is not increased by contact individuals with varicella or zoster, and $\lambda_2(t) = 0$.

Simulations were run in *Mathematica* (Ver 5.2.0.0, Wolfram Research, Inc.) using the differential equation solver NDSolve. Initial parameters were determined from published (prevaccine) observations (Table 6). Four parameters ($1/\square_1$, $1/\square_2$, $1/\square_1$, and $1/\square_1$) were adjusted to achieve realistic zoster incidence values (Figure 3). The average zoster incidence of 5.7 per 1,000 person-years was used (Insinga et al., 2005; Chaves et al. 2007). In the simulations, the contact number, β, was determined by setting the basic reproductive number (appendix) to 12 (Anderson and May, 1991).

Each simulation began with 100% of the population divided into the following initial conditions: 0.5% in class **M**, 10% in class **S**, 0.1% in class **E**, 0.5% in class **I**, 50% in class $\mathbf{R_V}$, 33.3% in class $\mathbf{R_B}$, 5% in class **W**, 0.2% in class $\mathbf{Z_C}$, and 0.4% in class $\mathbf{Z_S}$. The choice of these values is somewhat arbitrary. However, the long-term dynamics most likely end up the same for any choice of initial values, as models similar to the one presented here have a unique equilibrium.

Zoster incidence at time *t* (beginning in year 1) was calculated by first estimating the daily prevalence at time *t*. This was done by averaging the daily number of zoster cases per 1,000 people over the previous 365 days. Since incidence equals the ratio of prevalence to average duration, zoster incidence rates per 1,000 persons per year were calculated at time *t* by multiplying the daily prevalence by 365 days and dividing by the average duration of zoster.

Simulations were performed using baseline conditions presented in Table 6, and repeated iterations of the adjustable parameters. Figure 3 shows the incidence of subclinical VZV reactivation and zoster predicted over a simulated 150-year time period. Figure 3 shows the oscillations in subclinical VZV reactivation incidence over the first two simulated decades.

Although oscillations in zoster do occur in the simulation, they are difficult to observe under the selected initial conditions.

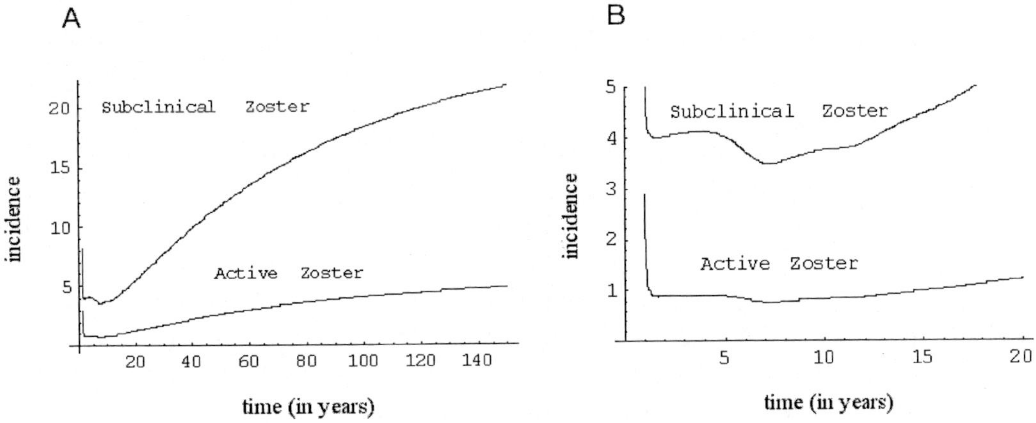

Figure 3. Zoster incidence over time using model **B** (boosting of anti-VZV immunity for individuals with waned immunity by exposure to varicella or clinical zoster). The vertical axis is the incidence rate per 1,000 person-years. Baseline parameter set used (Table 6) with adjustable parameters as follows: $1/\kappa_1 = 20$ years, $1/\kappa_2 = 15$ years, $1/\sigma_1 = 40$ years, and $1/\sigma_2 = 10$ years. Contact number is $\beta = 1.319$ to achieve a basic reproduction number of 12. Active zoster incidence at equilibrium is 5.7. Varicella incidence at equilibrium is 11.5.

Table 6. Parameter Values for VZV Models

Parameter	Explanation	Baseline Value
$1/\delta$	Avg. period of passive immunity	6 months
$1/\varepsilon$	Avg. latent period	14 days
$1/\gamma$	Avg. infectious period with varicella	7 days
$1/\eta_1$	Avg. length of clinical zoster	28 days
$1/\eta_2$	Avg. length of subclinical zoster	14 days
$1/\mu$	Avg. life expectancy	78 years
ρ_1	Relative infectivity of people with clinical zoster	0.07
ρ_2	Relative infectivity of people with subclinical zoster	$\rho_1/1000$
$1/\kappa_1$	Avg. period of high immunity after varicella	adjustable
$1/\kappa_2$	Avg. period of high immunity after boosting	adjustable
$1/\sigma_1$	Avg. period of waned immunity until clinical zoster	adjustable
$1/\sigma_2$	Avg. period of waned immunity until subclinical zoster	adjustable

When model **NB** was simulated, the predicted incidence of zoster was significantly higher than expected, unless average waiting times in $\mathbf{R_B}$ and **W** were increased beyond values appropriate for a human lifespan. For example, to obtain a simulated equilibrium zoster incidence of 6.2 per 1,000 person-yrs, $1/\kappa_1 = 60$ yrs, $1/\kappa_2 = 25$ yrs, $1/\sigma_1 = 64$ years, and $1/\sigma_2 = 15$ yrs. The equilibrium varicella incidence under these conditions is 11.68 per 1,000 person-yrs, which is consistent with the value in model **B**. However, the average waiting times are much too high to achieve the zoster and varicella incidences. Therefore, model **NB** does not simulate nature, indicating boosting of anti-VZV immunity by subacute virus reactivation is an important factor.

A second result of the simulations is the prediction that the incidence of zoster oscillates with time. Although seasonal variations in the incidence of varicella have been noticed with major peaks in the spring in the United States (Shah et al., 2006), summer in Australia (Miller and Kelly, 2008) and autumn in Taiwan (Liu et al., 1998), it is generally accepted that the incidence of zoster does not oscillate (Mazur and Dolin, 1978). Using the baseline parameter set (Table 6) and choosing the variable parameters to match observed overall zoster and varicella rates, model **B** simulations suggest that oscillations in the incidences of zoster do occur. However, the oscillations in zoster are masked by much larger oscillations in subclinical VZV reactivation (Figure 3). Thus, simulations performed on model **B** would predict that subclinical VZV reactivation may obscure detection of oscillations in the natural incidence of zoster. It is interesting that slight variations in the rate of zoster are observed (Glynn et al., 1990).

Our model may seem simplistic, since it does not include an age-structure, and assumes equal birth and death rates. In doing so, however, the model features VZV transmission and focuses more on epidemiological rather than demography. Adjusting the average period of waned immunity until subclinical zoster, while maintaining the basic reproduction number, did not significantly alter the clinical zoster incidence or varicella incidence as equilibrium is approached (>150 simulated years). As equilibrium is approached (>150 simulated years), the incidence of zoster predicted from the model is in line with the average reported zoster incidence of 5.7 per 1,000 person-years (Insinga et al., 2005; Chaves et al. 2007). Therefore, the simulations of the model suggest that including subclinical zoster is a feasible epidemiological feature.

5. Summary of Asymptomatic Alphaherpesvirus Shedding

By the second generation of life, most individuals (>90%) have been exposed to and harbor at least one latent alphaherpesvirus. Subsequent asymptomatic shedding of HSV-1, HSV-2, and VZV most likely involves reactivation of the viruses from their neuronal site of latency. Almost all HSV-1 and HSV-2-infected persons shed HSV from mucosal if sampled using frequent specimens and sensitive technologies. Current work supports the concept that HSV-1 can reactivate and shed infectious virus in individuals containing detectable amounts of anti-HSV-1 antibody as well as individuals with undetectable amounts of anti-HSV-1 antibody. In addition, neither age, gender, nor ethnicity is correlated with the frequency, duration, or intensity of asymptomatic HSV-1 shedding. HSV-2 asymptomatic shedding appears, for unknown reasons, to decrease with time after primary infection. Asymptomatic shedding of HSV-2 is clinically important because it is responsible for the majority of cases of horizontal and vertical transmission.

Studies investigating asymptomatic VZV reactivation have lagged behind those of HSV-1 and HSV-2. VZV DNA is present in saliva of individuals undergoing physical (astronaut/aquanaut) and physiological (bed rest) stress. In one case where infectious VZV was assayed, virus was retrieved from 2 of 3 individuals in the absence of clinical disease. Addition of asymptomatic virus shedding to an existing model of VZV epidemiology predicts the occurrence of subclinical VZV reactivation is greater than the number of zoster cases. Future studies are required to determine the prevalence of asymptomatic VZV shedding in the normal population and its possible contribution to VZV epidemiology.

Acknowledgments

The authors thank Drs. Anne Gershon and Arlene Dent for helpful discussions. This work is supported in part by Public Health Service grants AG 06127 (D.H.G) and NS 32623 (R.J.C)) and AI50132 (D.M.K.) from the National Institutes of Health. This research was made possible in part by National Eye Institute Grants NIH AG02085 (JMH) and EY006311 (JMH), also supported in part by Research to Prevent Blindness, Senior Scientific Investigator Award (JMH) and the LSUHSC Core Grant for Vision Research NIH EY002377. The LSUHSC Department of Ophthalmology has an unrestricted grant from Research to Prevent Blindness, New York, New York. We wish to thank Trisha Chiasson for editorial assistance.

Appendix

From the compartmental diagram shown in Figure 2, the differential equations for the class sizes are given below. The solutions to the differential equations are restricted by the population constraint: $N = M + S + E + I + R_V + R_B + W + Z_C + Z_S$.

The equation for S' is redundant. We reformulated the model in terms of fractional sizes in each class by dividing all rate equations by the population size N. For example, $i = I / N$ represents the infectious fraction. For convenience, we also defined mortality adjusted parameters, $\overline{\delta} = \delta + \mu$, $\overline{\varepsilon} = \varepsilon + \mu$, etc. These changes led to a system of eight differential equations in terms of the fractional sizes.

$$M' = \mu(N - M - S) - \delta M - \mu M$$
$$S' = \mu(M + S) + \delta M - \beta \frac{I + \rho_1 Z_C + \rho_2 Z_S}{N} S - \mu S$$
$$E' = \beta \frac{I + \rho_1 Z_C + \rho_2 Z_S}{N} S - \varepsilon E - \mu E$$
$$I' = \varepsilon E - \gamma I - \mu I$$
$$R_V' = \gamma I - \kappa_1 R_V - \mu R_V$$
$$R_B' = \eta_1 Z_C + \beta \frac{I + \rho_1 Z_C}{N} W - \kappa_2 R_B - \mu R_B$$
$$W' = \kappa_1 R_V + \kappa_2 R_B + \eta_2 Z_S - \beta \frac{I + \rho_1 Z_C}{N} W - \sigma_1 W - \sigma_2 W - \mu W$$
$$Z_C' = \sigma_1 W - \eta_1 Z_C - \mu Z_C$$
$$Z_S' = \sigma_2 W - \eta_2 Z_S - \mu Z_S$$

$$m' = \mu(e + i + r_V + r_B + w + z_C + z_S) - \overline{\delta} m$$
$$e' = \beta(i + \rho_1 z_C + \rho_2 z_S)(1 - m - e - i - r_V - r_B - w - z_C - z_S) - \overline{\varepsilon} e$$
$$i' = \varepsilon e - \overline{\gamma} i$$
$$r_V' = \gamma i - \overline{\kappa_1} r_V$$
$$r_B' = \eta_1 z_C + \beta(i + \rho_1 z_C) w - \overline{\kappa_2} r_B$$
$$w' = \kappa_1 r_V + \kappa_2 r_B + \eta_2 z_S - \beta(i + \rho_1 z_C) w - \sigma_1 w - \overline{\sigma_2} w$$
$$z_C' = \sigma_1 w - \overline{\eta_1} z_C$$
$$z_S' = \sigma_2 w - \overline{\eta_2} z_S$$

The basic reproductive number R_0 was found by a local stability analysis of the disease-free equilibrium. A value of $R_0 > 1$ leads to a stable endemic equilibrium in the simulations.

$$R_0 = \frac{\beta}{\overline{\gamma}} \frac{\varepsilon}{\overline{\varepsilon}} \left[1 + \frac{\gamma \kappa_1 \overline{\kappa_2} \left(\rho_1 \sigma_1 \overline{\eta_2} + \rho_2 \sigma_2 \overline{\eta_1} \right)}{\overline{\kappa_1}\,\overline{\kappa_2}\,\overline{\eta_1}\,\overline{\eta_2} \left(\sigma_1 + \overline{\sigma_2} \right) - \left(\overline{\kappa_1} \kappa_2 \sigma_1 \eta_1 \overline{\eta_2} + \overline{\kappa_1}\,\overline{\kappa_2} \sigma_2 \overline{\eta_1} \eta_2 \right)} \right]$$

References

[1] Anderson RM and May RM. 1991. *Infectious Diseases of Humans*. Oxford University Press.

[2] Arvin, A. M., C. M. Koropchak, and A. E. Wittek. 1983. Immunologic evidence of reinfection with varicella-zoster virus. *J. Infect. Dis*. 148:200-205.

[3] Arvin, A. M. and A. A. Gershon. 1996. Live attenuated varicella vaccine. *Annu. Rev. Microbiol*. 50:59-100.

[4] Asano, Y., H. Nakayama, T. Yazaki, R. Kato, and S. Hirose. 1977. Protection against varicella in family contacts by immediate inoculation with live varicella vaccine. *Pediatrics,* 59:3-7.

[5] Baboonian, C. and P. Griffiths. 1983. Is pregnancy immunosuppressive? Humoral immunity against viruses. *Br. J. Obstet. Gynaecol.* 90:1168-1175.

[6] Balraj, V. and T. J. John. 1994. An epidemic of varicella in rural southern India. *J Trop. Med. Hyg.* 97:113-116.

[7] Black, F. L., W. J. Hierholzer, F. Pinheiro, A. S. Evans, J. P. Woodall, E. M. Opton, J. E. Emmons, B. S. West, G. Edsall, W. G. Downs, and G. D. Wallace. 1974. Evidence for persistence of infectious agents in isolated human populations. *Am. J Epidemiol.* 100:230-250.

[8] Blair, A. W., W. M. Jamieson, and G. H. Smith. 1965. Complications and death in chicken-pox. *Br. Med. J.* 2:981-983.

[9] Branco, F. J. and N. W. Fraser. 2005. Herpes simplex virus type 1 latency-associated transcript expression protects trigeminal ganglion neurons from apoptosis. *J Virol.* 79:9019-9025.

[10] Brisson, M., N. J. Gay, W. J. Edmunds, and N. J. Andrews. 2002. Exposure to varicella boosts immunity to herpes-zoster: implications for mass vaccination against chickenpox. *Vaccine*, 20:2500-2507.

[11] Brown, Z. A., S. Selke, J. Zeh, J. Kopelman, A. Maslow, R. L. Ashley, D. H. Watts, S. Berry, M. Herd, and L. Corey. 1997. The acquisition of herpes simplex virus during pregnancy. *N. Engl. J. Med.* 337:509-515.

[12] Brown, Z. A., A. Wald, R. A. Morrow, S. Selke, J. Zeh, and L. Corey. 2003. Effect of serologic status and cesarean delivery on transmission rates of herpes simplex virus from mother to infant. *JAMA*, 289:203-209.

[13] Brown, Z. A., C. Gardella, A. Wald, R. A. Morrow, and L. Corey. 2005. Genital herpes complicating pregnancy. *Obstet. Gynecol.* 106:845-856.

[14] Buddingh, G. J., D. I. Schrum, J. Lanier, and D. Guidry. 1953. Studies of the natural history of herpes simplex infections. *Pediatrics,* 11:595-610.

[15] Celum, C., A. Wald, J. Hughes, J. Sanchez, S. Reid, S. Delany-Moretlwe, F. Cowan, M. Casapia, A. Ortiz, J. Fuchs, S. Buchbinder, B. Koblin, S. Zwerski, S. Rose, J. Wang, and L. Corey. 2008. Effect of aciclovir on HIV-1 acquisition in herpes simplex virus 2 seropositive women and men who have sex with men: a randomised, double-blind, placebo-controlled trial. *Lancet,* 371:2109-2119.

[16] Chaves SS, Santibanez TA, Gargiullo P, and Guris D. 2007. Chickenpox exposure and herpes zoster disease incidence in older adults in the U.S. *Public Health Reports.* 122:155-59.

[17] Clarke, P., T. Beer, R. Cohrs, and D. H. Gilden. 1995. Configuration of latent varicella-zoster virus DNA. *J. Virol.* 69:8151-8154.

[18] Cohrs, R. J., K. Srock, M. B. Barbour, G. Owens, R. Mahalingam, M. E. Devlin, M. Wellish, and D. H. Gilden. 1994. Varicella-zoster virus (VZV) transcription during latency in human ganglia: construction of a cDNA library from latently infected human trigeminal ganglia and detection of a VZV transcript. *J Virol.* 68:7900-7908.

[19] Cohrs, R. J., M. B. Barbour, R. Mahalingam, M. Wellish, and D. H. Gilden. 1995. Varicella-zoster virus (VZV) transcription during latency in human ganglia: prevalence of VZV gene 21 transcripts in latently infected human ganglia. *J Virol*. 69:2674-2678.

[20] Cohrs, R. J. and D. H. Gilden. 2003. Varicella zoster virus transcription in latently-infected human ganglia. *Anticancer Res*. 23:2063-2069.

[21] Cohrs, R. J., J. J. Laguardia, and D. Gilden. 2005. Distribution of latent herpes simplex virus type-1 and varicella zoster virus DNA in human trigeminal Ganglia. *Virus Genes*, 31:223-227.

[22] Cohrs, R. J. and D. H. Gilden. 2007. Prevalence and abundance of latently transcribed varicella-zoster virus genes in human ganglia. *J Virol*. 81:2950-2956.

[23] Cohrs, R. J., S. K. Mehta, D. S. Schmid, D. H. Gilden, and D. L. Pierson. 2008. Asymptomatic reactivation and shed of infectious varicella zoster virus in astronauts. *J. Med. Virol*. 80:1116-1122.

[24] Cook, S. D., D. A. Aitken, K. U. Loeffler, and S. M. Brown. 1986. Herpes simplex virus in the cornea; an ultrastructural study on viral reactivation. Trans. Ophthalmol. Soc. U. K. 105 (Pt 6):634-641.

[25] Corey, L. and A. Wald. 2008. Genital Herpes, p. 399-437. *In* K.K.Holmes, P. F. Sparling, W. E. Stamm, P. Piot, J. N. Wasserheit, L. Corey, M. S. Cohen, and D. H. Watts (eds.), *Sex. Trans. Dis.* McGraw Hill Medical, New York.

[26] Corey, L., A. Wald, R. Patel, S. L. Sacks, S. K. Tyring, T. Warren, J. M. Douglas, Jr., J. Paavonen, R. A. Morrow, K. R. Beutner, L. S. Stratchounsky, G. Mertz, O. N. Keene, H. A. Watson, D. Tait, and M. Vargas-Cortes. 2004. Once-daily valacyclovir to reduce the risk of transmission of genital herpes. *N. Engl. J. Med*. 350:11-20.

[27] Crow, K. D. and J. P. Ellis. 1979. Shingles: a belt of roses from Hell. *Br. Med. J.* 1:5.

[28] Cunningham, A. L., R. R. Turner, A. C. Miller, M. F. Para, and T. C. Merigan. 1985. Evolution of recurrent herpes simplex lesions. An immunohistologic study. *J. Clin. Invest*. 75:226-233.

[29] Czartoski, T., C. Liu, D. M. Koelle, S. Schmechel, A. Kalus, and A. Wald. 2006. Fulminant, acyclovir-resistant, herpes simplex virus type 2 hepatitis in an immunocompetent woman. *J. Clin. Microbiol*. 44:1584-1586.

[30] da Silva, L. M., A. L. Guimaraes, J. M. Victoria, C. C. Gomes, and R. S. Gomez. 2005. Herpes simplex virus type 1 shedding in the oral cavity of seropositive patients. *Oral Dis*. 11:13-16.

[31] Daley, A. J., S. Thorpe, and S. M. Garland. 2008. Varicella and the pregnant woman: prevention and management. *Aust. N. Z. J. Obstet. Gynaecol*. 48:26-33.

[32] de Bruyn, G., M. Vargas-Cortez, T. Warren, S. K. Tyring, K. H. Fife, J. Lalezari, R. C. Brady, M. Shahmanesh, G. Kinghorn, K. R. Beutner, R. Patel, M. A. Drehobl, P. Horner, T. O. Kurtz, S. McDermott, A. Wald, and L. Corey. 2006. A randomized controlled trial of a replication defective (gH deletion) herpes simplex virus vaccine for the treatment of recurrent genital herpes among immunocompetent subjects. *Vaccine*, 24:914-920.

[33] Dent, A. E. and B. A. Baetz-Greenwalt. 2007. Herpes zoster in an infant. *Clin. Pediatr.* (Phila) 46:646-649.

[34] Der Zwet, W. C., C. M. Vandenbroucke-Grauls, R. M. Van Elburg, A. Cranendonk, and H. L. Zaaijer. 2002. Neonatal antibody titers against varicella-zoster virus in relation to gestational age, birth weight, and maternal titer. *Pediatrics,* 109:79-85.

[35] Derfuss, T., S. Segerer, S. Herberger, I. Sinicina, K. Hufner, K. Ebelt, H. G. Knaus, I. Steiner, E. Meinl, K. Dornmair, V. Arbusow, M. Strupp, T. Brandt, and D. Theil. 2007. Presence of HSV-1 immediate early genes and clonally expanded T-cells with a memory effector phenotype in human trigeminal ganglia. *Brain Pathol.* 17:389-398.

[36] Enders, G., E. Miller, J. Cradock-Watson, I. Bolley, and M. Ridehalgh. 1994. Consequences of varicella and herpes zoster in pregnancy: prospective study of 1739 cases. *Lancet,* 343:1548-1551.

[37] Frenkel, L. M., E. M. Garratty, J. P. Shen, N. Wheeler, O. Clark, and Y. J. Bryson. 1993. Clinical reactivation of herpes simplex virus type 2 infection in seropositive pregnant women with no history of genital herpes. *Ann. Intern. Med.* 118:414-418.

[38] Galil, K., B. Lee, T. Strine, C. Carraher, A. L. Baughman, M. Eaton, J. Montero, and J. Seward. 2002. Outbreak of varicella at a day-care center despite vaccination. N. Engl. *J. Med.* 347:1909-1915.

[39] Gary, L., D. H. Gilden, and R. J. Cohrs. 2006. Epigenetic regulation of varicella-zoster virus open reading frames 62 and 63 in latently infected human trigeminal ganglia. *J. Virol.* 80:4921-4926.

[40] Gebhardt, B. M. and W. P. Halford . 2005. Evidence that spontaneous reactivation of herpes virus does not occur in mice. *Virol. J.* 2:67.

[41] Glynn, C., G. Crockford, D. Gavaghan, P. Cardno, D. Price, and J. Miller. 1990. Epidemiology of shingles. *J. R. Soc. Med.* 83:617-619.

[42] Gupta, R., A. Wald, E. Krantz, S. Selke, T. Warren, M. Vargas-Cortes, G. Miller, and L. Corey. 2004. Valacyclovir and acyclovir for suppression of shedding of herpes simplex virus in the genital tract. *J. Infect. Dis.* 190:1374-1381.

[43] Halford, W. P., B. M. Gebhardt, and D. J. Carr. 1997. Acyclovir blocks cytokine gene expression in trigeminal ganglia latently infected with herpes simplex virus type 1. *Virology,* 238:53-63.

[44] Hargens, A. R. 1994. Recent bed rest results and countermeasure development at NASA. *Acta Physiol Scand. Suppl.* 616:103-114.

[45] Harger, J. H., J. M. Ernest, G. R. Thurnau, A. Moawad, E. Thom, M. B. Landon, R. Paul, M. Miodovnik, M. Dombrowski, B. Sibai, P. Van Dorsten, and D. McNellis. 2002. Frequency of congenital varicella syndrome in a prospective cohort of 347 pregnant women. *Obstet. Gynecol.* 100:260-265.

[46] Hayward, A. R. 1990. T-cell responses to predicted amphipathic peptides of varicella-zoster virus glycoproteins II and IV. *J. Virol.* 64:651-655.

[47] Hill, J. M., M. Ball, D. Neumann, A. Azcuy, P. Bhattacharjee, S. Bouhanik, C. Clement, W. J. Lukiw, T. Foster, M. Kumar, H. Kaufman, and H. Thompson. 2008. The high prevalence of HSV-1 DNA in human trigeminal ganglia is not a function of age or gender. *J. Virol.* 82:8230-8234.

[48] Hobbs, M. R., B. B. Jones, B. E. Otterud, M. Leppert, and J. D. Kriesel. 2008. Identification of a herpes simplex labialis susceptibility region on human chromosome 21. *J. Infect. Dis.* 197:340-346.

[49] Hood, C., A. L. Cunningham, B. Slobedman, A. M. Arvin, M. H. Sommer, P. R. Kinchington, and A. Abendroth. 2006. Varicella-zoster virus ORF63 inhibits apoptosis of primary human neurons. *J Virol.* 80:1025-1031.

[50] Hope-Simpson R. E. 1965. The Nature of Herpes Zoster: A Long-Term Study And A New Hypothesis. *Proc. R. Soc. Med.* 58:9-20.

[51] Hoshino, Y., S. K. Dalai, K. Wang, L. Pesnicak, T. Y. Lau, D. M. Knipe, J. I. Cohen, and S. E. Straus. 2005. Comparative efficacy and immunogenicity of replication-defective, recombinant glycoprotein, and DNA vaccines for herpes simplex virus 2 infections in mice and guinea pigs. *J. Virol.* 79:410-418.

[52] Hufner, K., T. Derfuss, S. Herberger, K. Sunami, S. Russell, I. Sinicina, V. Arbusow, M. Strupp, T. Brandt, and D. Theil. 2006. Latency of alpha-herpes viruses is accompanied by a chronic inflammation in human trigeminal ganglia but not in dorsal root ganglia. *J. Neuropathol. Exp. Neurol.* 65:1022-1030.

[53] Inoda, S., M. Wakakura, J. Hirata, N. Nakazato, and Y. Toyo-Oka. 2001. Stromal keratitis and anterior uveitis due to herpes simplex virus-2 in a young child. *Jpn. J. Ophthalmol.* 45:618-621.

[54] Insinga, R. P., R. F. Itzler, J. M. Pellissier, P. Saddier, and A. A. Nikas. 2005. The incidence of herpes zoster in a United States administrative database. *J Gen. Intern. Med.* 20:748-753.

[55] Jerant, A. F., J. S. DeGaetano, T. D. Epperly, A. C. Hannapel, D. R. Miller, and A. J. Lloyd. 1998. Varicella susceptibility and vaccination strategies in young adults. *J. Am. Board Fam. Pract.* 11:296-306.

[56] Kaufman, H. E., D. C. Brown, and E. M. Ellison. 1967. Recurrent herpes in the rabbit and man. *Science*, 156:1628-1629.

[57] Kaufman, H. E., A. M. Azcuy, E. D. Varnell, G. D. Sloop, H. W. Thompson, and J. M. Hill. 2005. HSV-1 DNA in tears and saliva of normal adults. *Invest. Ophthalmol. Vis. Sci.* 46:241-247.

[58] Kavaliotis, J., I. Loukou, M. Trachana, N. Gombakis, H. Tsagaropoulou-Stigga, and D. Koliouskas. 1998. Outbreak of varicella in a pediatric oncology unit. *Med. Pediatr. Oncol.* 31:166-169.

[59] Kaye, S. and A. Choudhary. 2006. Herpes simplex keratitis. *Prog. Retin. Eye Res.* 25:355-380.

[60] Kaye, S. B., K. Baker, R. Bonshek, H. Maseruka, E. Grinfeld, A. Tullo, D. L. Easty, and C. A. Hart. 2000. Human herpesviruses in the cornea. *Br. J. Ophthalmol.* 84:563-571.

[61] Kimberlin, D. W. 2005. Herpes simplex virus infections in neonates and early childhood. *Semin. Pediatr. Infect. Dis.* 16:271-281.

[62] King, J., M. Chung, and D. A. DiLoreto, Jr. 2007. A 9 year-old girl with herpes simplex virus type 2 acute retinal necrosis treated with intravitreal foscarnet. Ocul. Immunol. *Inflamm.* 15:395-398.

[63] Koelle, D. M., J. Benedetti, A. Langenberg, and L. Corey. 1992. Asymptomatic reactivation of herpes simplex virus in women after the first episode of genital herpes. *Ann. Intern. Med.* 116:433-437.

[64] Koelle, D. M., J. M. Frank, M. L. Johnson, and W. W. Kwok. 1998. Recognition of herpes simplex virus type 2 tegument proteins by CD4 T cells infiltrating human genital herpes lesions. *J. Virol.* 72:7476-7483.

[65] Koelle, D. M. and A. Wald. 2000. Herpes simplex virus: the importance of asymptomatic shedding. *J. Antimicrob. Chemother.* 45 Suppl T3:1-8.

[66] Koelle, D. M., H. B. Chen, M. A. Gavin, A. Wald, W. W. Kwok, and L. Corey. 2001. CD8 CTL from genital herpes simplex lesions: recognition of viral tegument and immediate early proteins and lysis of infected cutaneous cells. *J. Immunol.* 166:4049-4058.

[67] Koutsky, L. A., C. E. Stevens, K. K. Holmes, R. L. Ashley, N. B. Kiviat, C. W. Critchlow, and L. Corey. 1992. Underdiagnosis of genital herpes by current clinical and viral-isolation procedures. *N. Engl. J. Med.* 326:1533-1539.

[68] Kumar, A., D. L. Madden, and G. A. Nankervis. 1984. Humoral and cell-mediated immune responses to herpesvirus antigens during pregnancy--a longitudinal study. *J. Clin. Immunol.* 4:12-17.

[69] A. Langenberg, A., J. Benedetti, J. Jenkins, R. Ashley, C. Winter, and L. Corey. 1989. Development of clinically recognizable genital lesions among women previously identified as having "asymptomatic" herpes simplex virus type 2 infection. *Ann. Intern. Med.* 110:882-887.

[70] Langenberg, A. G., L. Corey, R. L. Ashley, W. P. Leong, and S. E. Straus. 1999. A prospective study of new infections with herpes simplex virus type 1 and type 2. Chiron HSV Vaccine Study Group. *N. Engl. J. Med.* 341:1432-1438.

[71] Leach, C. S. 1992. Biochemical and hematologic changes after short-term space flight. *Microgravity. Q.* 2:69-75.

[72] Lee-Wing, M. W., W. G. Hodge, and F. Diaz-Mitoma. 1999. The prevalence of herpes family virus DNA in the conjunctiva of patients positive and negative for human immunodeficiency virus using the polymerase chain reaction. *Ophthalmology*, 106:350-354.

[73] Leone, P., T. Warren, K. Hamed, K. Fife, and A. Wald. 2007. Famciclovir reduces viral mucosal shedding in HSV-seropositive persons. *Sex Transm. Dis.* 34:900-907.

[74] Levy, M. H., S. Quilty, L. C. Young, W. Hunt, R. Matthews, and P. W. Robertson. 2003. Pox in the docks: varicella outbreak in an Australian prison system. *Public Health*, 117:446-451.

[75] Liesegang, T. J. 2001. Herpes simplex virus epidemiology and ocular importance. *Cornea*, 20 :1-13.

[76] Liu, S. C., J. D. Wang, C. Y. Lee, and M. C. Chou. 1998. Seasonal variation of chickenpox, mumps and rubella in Taiwanese children estimated by pediatric clinics. *J. Microbiol. Immunol. Infect.* 31:217-224.

[77] Mahalingam, R., M. Wellish, R. Cohrs, S. Debrus, J. Piette, B. Rentier, and D. H. Gilden. 1996. Expression of protein encoded by varicella-zoster virus open reading frame 63 in latently infected human ganglionic neurons. *Proc. Natl. Acad. Sci. U. S. A*, 93:2122-2124.

[78] Mark, K. E., L. Corey, T. C. Meng, A. S. Magaret, M. L. Huang, S. Selke, H. B. Slade, S. K. Tyring, T. Warren, S. L. Sacks, P. Leone, V. A. Bergland, and A. Wald. 2007.

Topical resiquimod 0.01% gel decreases herpes simplex virus type 2 genital shedding: a randomized, controlled trial. *J. Infect. Dis.* 195:1324-1331.

[79] Mark, K. E., A. Wald, A. S. Magaret, S. Selke, L. Olin, M. L. Huang, and L. Corey. 2008. Rapidly cleared episodes of herpes simplex virus reactivation in immunocompetent adults. *J Infect. Dis.* 198:1141-1149.

[80] Mazur, M. H. and R. Dolin. 1978. Herpes zoster at the NIH: a 20 year experience. *Am. J. Med.* 65:738-744.

[81] Mazzella, M., C. Arioni, C. Bellini, A. E. Allegri, C. Savioli, and G. Serra. 2003. Severe hydrocephalus associated with congenital varicella syndrome. *CMAJ.* 168:561-563.

[82] Mehta, S. K., R. J. Cohrs, B. Forghani, G. Zerbe, D. H. Gilden, and D. L. Pierson. 2004. Stress-induced subclinical reactivation of varicella zoster virus in astronauts. *J. Med. Virol.* 72:174-179.

[83] Mehta, S. K., B. Crucian, D. L. Pierson, C. Sams, and R. P. Stowe. 2007. Monitoring immune system function and reactivation of latent viruses in the Artificial Gravity Pilot Study. *J Gravit Physiol.* 14:21-25.

[84] Mehta, S. K., S. K. Tyring, D. H. Gilden, R. J. Cohrs, M. J. Leal, V. A. Castro, A. H. Feiveson, C. M. Ott, and D. L. Pierson. 2008. Varicella-zoster virus in the saliva of patients with herpes zoster. *J Infect. Dis.* 197:654-657.

[85] Mertz, G. J., O. Schmidt, J. L. Jourden, M. E. Guinan, M. L. Remington, A. Fahnlander, C. Winter, K. K. Holmes, and L. Corey. 1985. Frequency of acquisition of first-episode genital infection with herpes simplex virus from symptomatic and asymptomatic source contacts. *Sex Transm. Dis.* 12:33-39.

[86] Mertz, G. J., R. W. Coombs, R. Ashley, J. Jourden, M. Remington, C. Winter, A. Fahnlander, M. Guinan, H. Ducey, and L. Corey. 1988. Transmission of genital herpes in couples with one symptomatic and one asymptomatic partner: a prospective study. *J. Infect. Dis.* 157:1169-1177.

[87] Mertz, G. J., J. Benedetti, R. Ashley, S. A. Selke, and L. Corey. 1992. Risk factors for the sexual transmission of genital herpes. *Ann. Intern. Med.* 116:197-202.

[88] Miller, C. S., L. L. Cunningham, J. E. Lindroth, and S. A. Avdiushko. 2004. The efficacy of valacyclovir in preventing recurrent herpes simplex virus infections associated with dental procedures. *J. Am. Dent. Assoc.* 135:1311-1318.

[89] Miller, C. S. and R. J. Danaher. 2008. Asymptomatic shedding of herpes simplex virus (HSV) in the oral cavity. *Oral Surg. Oral Med. Oral Pathol. Oral Radiol. Endod.* 105:43-50.

[90] Miller, E. R. and H. A. Kelly. 2008. Varicella infection--evidence for peak activity in summer months. *J. Infect.* 56:360-365.

[91] Mostad, S. B., J. K. Kreiss, A. J. Ryncarz, K. Mandaliya, B. Chohan, J. Ndinya-Achola, J. J. Bwayo, and L. Corey. 2000. Cervical shedding of herpes simplex virus in human immunodeficiency virus-infected women: effects of hormonal contraception, pregnancy, and vitamin A deficiency. *J. Infect. Dis.* 181:58-63.

[92] Mueller, N. H., D. H. Gilden, R. J. Cohrs, R. Mahalingam, and M. A. Nagel. 2008. Varicella zoster virus infection: clinical features, molecular pathogenesis of disease, and latency. *Neurol. Clin.* 26:675-97, viii.

[93] Mustonen, K., P. Mustakangas, M. Smeds, L. Mannonen, L. Uotila, A. Vaheri, and M. Koskiniemi. 1998. Antibodies to varicella zoster virus in the cerebrospinal fluid of neonates with seizures. *Arch. Dis. Child Fetal Neonatal Ed.* 78:F57-F61.

[94] Mustonen, K., P. Mustakangas, L. Valanne, M. H. Professor, and M. Koskiniemi. 2001. Congenital varicella-zoster virus infection after maternal subclinical infection: clinical and neuropathological findings. *J. Perinatol.* 21:141-146.

[95] Nagot, N., A. Ouedraogo, V. Foulongne, I. Konate, H. A. Weiss, L. Vergne, M. C. Defer, D. Djagbare, A. Sanon, J. B. Andonaba, P. Becquart, M. Segondy, R. Vallo, A. Sawadogo, P. P. Van de, and P. Mayaud. 2007. Reduction of HIV-1 RNA levels with therapy to suppress herpes simplex virus. *N. Engl. J. Med.* 356:790-799.

[96] Nardone, A., F. de Ory, M. Carton, D. Cohen, P. van Damme, I. Davidkin, M. C. Rota, H. de Melker, J. Mossong, M. Slacikova, A. Tischer, N. Andrews, G. Berbers, G. Gabutti, N. Gay, L. Jones, S. Jokinen, G. Kafatos, M. V. de Aragon, F. Schneider, Z. Smetana, B. Vargova, R. Vranckx, and E. Miller. 2007. The comparative sero-epidemiology of varicella zoster virus in 11 countries in the European region. V*accine*, 25:7866-7872.

[97] Ouedraogo, A., N. Nagot, L. Vergne, I. Konate, H. A. Weiss, M. C. Defer, V. Foulongne, A. Sanon, J. B. Andonaba, M. Segondy, P. Mayaud, and P. P. Van de. 2006. Impact of suppressive herpes therapy on genital HIV-1 RNA among women taking antiretroviral therapy: a randomized controlled trial. *AIDS*, 20:2305-2313.

[98] Perng, G. C., C. Jones, J. Ciacci-Zanella, M. Stone, G. Henderson, A. Yukht, S. M. Slanina, F. M. Hofman, H. Ghiasi, A. B. Nesburn, and S. L. Wechsler. 2000. Virus-induced neuronal apoptosis blocked by the herpes simplex virus latency-associated transcript. *Science*, 287:1500-1503.

[99] Quan, D., R. J. Cohrs, R. Mahalingam, and D. H. Gilden. 2007. Prevention of shingles: safety and efficacy of live zoster vaccine. *Ther. Clin. Risk Manag.* 3:633-639.

[100] Ramsey, P. G., K. H. Fife, R. C. Hackman, J. D. Meyers, and L. Corey. 1982. Herpes simplex virus pneumonia: clinical, virologic, and pathologic features in 20 patients. *Ann. Intern. Med.* 97:813-820.

[101] Rawson, H., A. Crampin, and N. Noah. 2001. Deaths from chickenpox in England and Wales 1995-7: analysis of routine mortality data. *BMJ*, 323:1091-1093.

[102] Reijo, A., V. Antti, and M. Jukka. 1983. Endothelial cell loss in herpes zoster keratouveitis. *Br. J. Ophthalmol.* 67:751-754.

[103] Roizman, B. 1978. Provisional classification of herpesviruses, p. 1079-1082. *In* B. dt The and F. Rapp (eds.), Oncogenesis and herpesviruses III. International agency for research on cancer, Lyon, France.

[104] Roizman, B. and R. J. Whitley. 2001. The nine ages of herpes simplex virus. *Herpes.* 8:23-27.

[105] Rooney, J. F., J. M. Felser, J. M. Ostrove, and S. E. Straus. 1986. Acquisition of genital herpes from an asymptomatic sexual partner. *N. Engl. J. Med.* 314:1561-1564.

[106] Sauerbrei, A. and P. Wutzler. 2000. The congenital varicella syndrome. *J. Perinatol.* 20:548-554.

[107] Sawyer, M. H., C. J. Chamberlin, Y. N. Wu, N. Aintablian, and M. R. Wallace. 1994. Detection of varicella-zoster virus DNA in air samples from hospital rooms. *J. Infect. Dis*. 169:91-94.

[108] Schacker, T., A. J. Ryncarz, J. Goddard, K. Diem, M. Shaughnessy, and L. Corey. 1998. Frequent recovery of HIV-1 from genital herpes simplex virus lesions in HIV-1-infected men. *JAMA,* 280:61-66.

[109] Schacker, T., J. Zeh, H. L. Hu, E. Hill, and L. Corey. 1998. Frequency of symptomatic and asymptomatic herpes simplex virus type 2 reactivations among human immunodeficiency virus-infected men. *J. Infect. Dis*. 178:1616-1622.

[110] Schuette, M. C. and H. W. Hethcote. 1999. Modeling the effects of varicella vaccination programs on the incidence of chickenpox and shingles. *Bull. Math. Biol.* 61:1031-1064.

[111] Schuette, M. C. 2003. A qualitative analysis of a model for the transmission of varicella-zoster virus. *Math. Biosci*. 182:113-126.

[112] Sergerie, Y., G. Boivin, D. Gosselin, and S. Rivest. 2007. Delayed but not early glucocorticoid treatment protects the host during experimental herpes simplex virus encephalitis in mice. *J. Infect. Dis*. 195:817-825.

[113] Shah, A. P., M. H. Smolensky, K. D. Burau, I. M. Cech, and D. Lai. 2006. Seasonality of primarily childhood and young adult infectious diseases in the United States. *Chronobiol. Int.* 23:1065-1082.

[114] Smith, S. M., J. E. Davis-Street, J. V. Fesperman, M. D. Smith, B. L. Rice, and S. R. Zwart. 2004. Nutritional status changes in humans during a 14-day saturation dive: the NASA Extreme Environment Mission Operations V project. *J. Nutr.* 134:1765-1771.

[115] Spruance SL. 1984. Pathogenesis of herpes simplex labialis: excretion of virus in the oral cavity. *J. Clin. Microbiol.* 19:675-679.

[116] Spruance, S. L., J. C. Overall, E. R. Kern, G. G. Krueger, V. Pliam, and W. Miller. 1977. The natural history of recurrent herpes simplex labialis: implications for antiviral therapy. *N. Engl. J. Med.* 297:69-75.

[117] Stevens, J. G. and M. L. Cook. 1971. Latent herpes simplex virus in spinal ganglia of mice. *Science,* 173:843-845.

[118] Straus, S. E., L. Corey, R. L. Burke, B. Savarese, G. Barnum, P. R. Krause, R. G. Kost, J. L. Meier, R. Sekulovich, S. F. Adair, and . 1994. Placebo-controlled trial of vaccination with recombinant glycoprotein D of herpes simplex virus type 2 for immunotherapy of genital herpes. *Lancet*, 343:1460-1463.

[119] Straus, S. E., A. Wald, R. G. Kost, R. McKenzie, A. G. Langenberg, P. Hohman, J. Lekstrom, E. Cox, M. Nakamura, R. Sekulovich, A. Izu, C. Dekker, and L. Corey. 1997. Immunotherapy of recurrent genital herpes with recombinant herpes simplex virus type 2 glycoproteins D and B: results of a placebo-controlled vaccine trial. *J. Infect. Dis*. 176:1129-1134.

[120] Tang, J. W., L. J. Coward, N. W. Davies, A. M. Geretti, R. S. Howard, N. P. Hirsch, and K. N. Ward. 2003. Brain stem encephalitis caused by primary herpes simplex 2 infection in a young woman. *J. Neurol. Neurosurg. Psychiatry*, 74:1323-1325.

[121] Tateishi, K., Y. Toh, H. Minagawa, and H. Tashiro. 1994. Detection of herpes simplex virus (HSV) in the saliva from 1,000 oral surgery outpatients by the polymerase chain reaction (PCR) and virus isolation. *J. Oral Pathol. Med.* 23:80-84.

[122] Taylor, G. R. and R. P. Janney. 1992. In vivo testing confirms a blunting of the human cell-mediated immune mechanism during space flight. *J Leukoc. Biol.* 51:129-132.

[123] Tenser, R. B., A. Gaydos, and K. A. Hay. 1996. Reactivation of thymidine kinase-defective herpes simplex virus is enhanced by nucleoside. *J. Virol.* 70:1271-1276.

[124] Theil, D., I. Paripovic, T. Derfuss, S. Herberger, M. Strupp, V. Arbusow, and T. Brandt. 2003. Dually infected (HSV-1/VZV) single neurons in human trigeminal ganglia. *Ann. Neurol.* 54:678-682.

[125] Theil, D., T. Derfuss, I. Paripovic, S. Herberger, E. Meinl, O. Schueler, M. Strupp, V. Arbusow, and T. Brandt. 2003. Latent herpesvirus infection in human trigeminal ganglia causes chronic immune response. *Am. J. Pathol.* 163:2179-2184.

[126] Thomas, S. L., J. G. Wheeler, and A. J. Hall. 2002. Contacts with varicella or with children and protection against herpes zoster in adults: a case-control study. *Lancet,* 360:678-682.

[127] Verjans, G. M., R. Q. Hintzen, J. M. van Dun, A. Poot, J. C. Milikan, J. D. Laman, A. W. Langerak, P. R. Kinchington, and A. D. Osterhaus. 2007. Selective retention of herpes simplex virus-specific T cells in latently infected human trigeminal ganglia. *Proc. Natl. Acad. Sci. U. S. A,* 104:3496-3501.

[128] Wald, A., J. Zeh, G. Barnum, L. G. Davis, and L. Corey. 1996. Suppression of subclinical shedding of herpes simplex virus type 2 with acyclovir. *Ann. Intern. Med.* 124:8-15.

[129] Wald, A., L. Corey, R. Cone, A. Hobson, G. Davis, and J. Zeh. 1997. Frequent genital herpes simplex virus 2 shedding in immunocompetent women. Effect of acyclovir treatment. *J. Clin. Invest.* 99:1092-1097.

[130] Wald, A., J. Zeh, S. Selke, T. Warren, A. J. Ryncarz, R. Ashley, J. N. Krieger, and L. Corey. 2000. Reactivation of genital herpes simplex virus type 2 infection in asymptomatic seropositive persons. *N. Engl. J. Med.* 342:844-850.

[131] Wald, A., M. L. Huang, D. Carrell, S. Selke, and L. Corey. 2003. Polymerase chain reaction for detection of herpes simplex virus (HSV) DNA on mucosal surfaces: comparison with HSV isolation in cell culture. *J. Infect. Dis.* 188:1345-1351.

[132] Wald, A., S. Selke, T. Warren, F. Y. Aoki, S. Sacks, F. Diaz-Mitoma, and L. Corey. 2006. Comparative efficacy of famciclovir and valacyclovir for suppression of recurrent genital herpes and viral shedding. *Sex Transm. Dis.* 33:529-533.

[133] Watson-Jones, D., H. A. Weiss, M. Rusizoka, J. Changalucha, K. Baisley, K. Mugeye, C. Tanton, D. Ross, D. Everett, T. Clayton, R. Balira, L. Knight, I. Hambleton, J. Le Goff, L. Belec, and R. Hayes. 2008. Effect of herpes simplex suppression on incidence of HIV among women in Tanzania. *N. Engl. J. Med.* 358:1560-1571.

[134] White, R. J. and M. Averner. 2001. Humans in space. *Nature,* 409:1115-1118.

[135] Williams, D. R. 2003. The biomedical challenges of space flight. *Annu. Rev. Med.* 54:245-256.

[136] Willoughby, C. E., K. Baker, S. B. Kaye, P. Carey, N. O'Donnell, A. Field, L. Longman, R. Bucknall, and C. A. Hart. 2002. Epstein-Barr virus (types 1 and 2) in the tear film in Sjogren's syndrome and HIV infection. *J. Med. Virol.* 68:378-383.

[137] Wilson, A., M. Sharp, C. M. Koropchak, S. F. Ting, and A. M. Arvin. 1992. Subclinical varicella-zoster virus viremia, herpes zoster, and T lymphocyte immunity to varicella-zoster viral antigens after bone marrow transplantation. *J. Infect. Dis.* 165 :119-126.

[138] Winquist, A. G., A. Roome, and J. Hadler. 2001. Varicella outbreak at a summer camp for human immunodeficiency virus-infected children. *Pediatrics,* 107:67-72.

[139] Xu, F., M. R. Sternberg, B. J. Kottiri, G. M. McQuillan, F. K. Lee, A. J. Nahmias, S. M. Berman, and L. E. Markowitz. 2006. Trends in herpes simplex virus type 1 and type 2 seroprevalence in the United States. *JAMA*, 296:964-973.

[140] Yamamoto, S., Y. Shimomura, S. Kinoshita, K. Nishida, R. Yamamoto, and Y. Tano. 1994. Detection of herpes simplex virus DNA in human tear film by the polymerase chain reaction. *Am. J. Ophthalmol.* 117:160-163.

[141] Yoshikawa, T., J. M. Hill, L. R. Stanberry, N. Bourne, J. F. Kurawadwala, and P. R. Krause. 1996. The characteristic site-specific reactivation phenotypes of HSV-1 and HSV-2 depend upon the latency-associated transcript region. *J. Exp. Med.* 184:659-664.

[142] Yoshikawa, T., M. Ihira, K. Suzuki, S. Suga, A. Tomitaka, H. Ueda, and Y. Asano. 2001. Rapid contamination of the environments with varicella-zoster virus DNA from a patient with herpes zoster. *J. Med. Virol.* 63:64-66.

[143] Zhu, J., D. M. Koelle, J. Cao, J. Vazquez, M. L. Huang, F. Hladik, A. Wald, and L. Corey. 2007. Virus-specific CD8+ T cells accumulate near sensory nerve endings in genital skin during subclinical HSV-2 reactivation. *J. Exp. Med.* 204:595-603.

In: Herpesviridae Viral Structure, Life Cycle and Infections
Editor: Toma R. Gluckman
ISBN 978-1-60692-947-6

Chapter 6

Do Cytomegalovirus or Epstein-Barr Virus Play a Role in Periodontitis?

Bjørn Grinde[1,2*] and Ingar Olsen[2]
[1]Norwegian Institute of Public Health, Oslo
[2]Institute of Oral Biology, University of Oslo, Oslo

Abstract

Periodontitis has traditionally been ascribed to bacterial activity. However, herpesviruses, particularly Epstein-Barr virus (EBV) and cytomegalovirus (CMV), are found in clinical samples from both apical and marginal periodontitis. Reported prevalence are typically in the range 30-70 % while the viruses are found more sporadically in material taken from healthy sites in the mouth. These observations have led some scientists to suggest that the viruses play a role in the etiology of periodontitis. Several lines of investigation have been pursued in an attempt to clarify the issue: Quantification of viruses in clinical samples, methods suggesting local viral activity, associations between virus and bacteria to indicate possible synergism, and the treatment of patients with antiviral medication to see whether a subsequent decrease in viral titer may impact on the periodontitis. The conclusion based on the present review of the literature is that these viruses can in some cases impact on the pathogenesis, but that in the majority of patients their detection probably does not reflect any clinical role. Yet, particularly in cases with advanced or chronic periodontitis, viral analysis is called for. If there are signs of local viral activity, for example a high viral load, antiviral therapy may be tried as an adjunct to conventional periodontal treatment.

---

* Corresponding address: Bjørn Grinde, Norwegian Institute of Public Health, PO Box 4404 Nydalen, NO-0403 Oslo; Phone +47 2107 6420, FAX +47 2107 6447, Cell: +47 9970 8805; E-mail: bjgr@fhi.no; grinde10@hotmail.com

Introduction

There are several examples of diseases in which both bacteria and viruses contribute to the etiology. A well documented case is the bacterial complications associated with an influenza virus infection: Deaths, or severe affliction, are often attributed to secondary bacterial pneumonia, typically caused by *Haemophilus influenzae*, *Staphylococcus aureus*, or *Streptococcus pneumoniae* [Cate, 1998; Sethi, 2002]. A combined etiology of bacteria and viruses has also been discussed in connection with other respiratory tract infections [Bakaletz et al., 1995], and in otitis media [Heikkinen and Chonmaitree, 2000]. In these cases, there appear to be a form of synergy between bacteria and viruses, in that one of the agents may pave the way for the other. This effect could be due to reduced immune competence as a consequence of the stress associated with the original infection, or there may be more specific mechanisms by which one or both of the agents have adapted to particular conditions caused by the other.

Herpesviruses are particularly interesting in this respect. They are known to modulate the host immune response, for example, by producing cytokine mimics. The modulation may lead to an inadequate immune response towards both the herpesviruses and other microbial agents present, and a concomitant increase in severity of the clinical condition.

It is well documented that both gingivitis (inflammation of the gums), as well as apical and marginal periodontitis (inflammation of the tissue surrounding respectively the root tip and the part of teeth protruding into the oral cavity) are associated with bacteria colonizing the gingiva and tooth surfaces [Kakehashi et al., 1965; Socransky and Haffajee 2002]. When somebody abstains from the cleaning of teeth, clinical signs of gingivitis tend to appear reasonably fast, but normally the inflammatory alterations are resolved or reversed when the bacterial deposits are removed from the tooth surfaces [Löe et al., 1965]. Antiseptic agents, for example chlorhexidine, can suppress bacterial colonization and the development of gingivitis [Löe et al., 1965; Corbet et al., 1997]. Moreover, the use of antibiotics can reduce bacterial plaque and improve periodontal problems in patients with severe disease [Ciancio et al., 1982]. In other words, it has been taken for granted that bacteria are the major initiators of periodontal inflammation and tissue destruction.

Recently, however, several laboratories have shown that these lesions often contain viruses of the herpes family, particularly human cytomegalovirus (CMV), Epstein-Barr virus (EBV), and herpes simplex viruses (HSV) [Slots, 2004; Cappuyns et al., 2005; Sunde et al., 2008a]. Some authors, e.g., Slots et al. [2006], suggest that these viruses can influence the development and course of periodontitis, while others, such as Cappuyns et al. [2005], are skeptical. In the present chapter, the case for and against a role of herpesviruses in the pathology of periodontitis is reviewed.

Bacteria Only Hypothesis Seems Insufficient

It seems reasonably obvious that bacteria do contribute to the inflammation and periodontal tissue damage associated with periodontitis, yet bacteria alone cannot easily account for all the observations related to the disease: Although most subjects with inadequate oral hygiene may develop gingivitis, not every case of gingivitis leads to the more severe forms of periodontitis or loss of tooth attachment. Despite considerable variation as to oral hygiene, and consequently gingivitis, in different societies, and a high prevalence of potential bacterial pathogens in most populations [McNabb et al., 1992; Al-Yahfoufi et al., 1994; Gmür and Guggenheim, 1994], periodontal destruction seems to be limited to some 10 % worldwide [Schürch et al., 1988; Baelum et al., 1996]. Moreover, epidemiological data suggest that the progression of destructive periodontitis is associated with the vulnerability of certain individuals [Papapanou, 1996].

Furthermore, periodontitis has a tendency to be periodic, i.e., the condition worsens and improve at more or less regular intervals [Goodson et al., 1982]. This observation suggests that if the bacteria represent the underlying cause, then some other factor influences their activity. The relevant factor could, for example, be the typical variations in herpes viral activity, shifting between prolonged periods of latency interrupted by periods of activation.

The above observations strongly suggest that other factors than the actual presence of particular species of bacteria impact on the etiology of periodontitis. Certain exogenous factors, such as tobacco smoking [Bergström, 1989], as well as endogenous factors, such as genetic constitution [Kornman, 2001], apparently do influence periodontal pathology. It would not be surprising if viruses were found to constitute additional factors.

Viruses Associated with Periodontitis

Besides viruses of the herpes family, several other viruses are known to be capable of causing lesions in the gingiva, including papillomaviruses, enteroviruses and HIV (reviewed in Cappuyns et al. [2005]). HIV has been directly linked to the prevalence of periodontitis [Patton et al., 2002], however, the role of HIV may be more in terms of a decrease in general immune competence, rather than a specific effect on gingival tissue.

The more interesting viruses in connection with periodontitis are the herpesviruses. Of the eight herpesviruses associated with humans, four in particular have been investigated as to a role in periodontitis: herpes simplex 1 and 2 (HSV-1 and HSV-2), Epstein-Barr virus (EBV), and cytomegalovirus (CMV).

Most people are infected with herpesviruses as infants. Once contracted, the viruses tend to be chronically present. EBV and CMV, for example, are harbored by some 70 – 90 % of the adult population. Once infected, herpesviruses may remain as inactive forms in various cells for the rest of the individual's life, but they are also likely to be activated for various reasons. Upon activation, viral replication may be asymptomatic, or cause clinical symptoms, such as cold sores (HSV) or cancer (EBV).

The main routes of infection for all these viruses are presumably either directly through sputum, i.e., by kissing or drinking from the same bottle, or by aerosols released from the mouth. Thus a viral presence in saliva should be expected, and is occasionally observed even in healthy individuals [Sixbey et al., 1984; Roizman and Pellett, 2001; Rickinson and Kieff, 2001]. For the present discussion, however, the pertinent point is that these viruses are found considerably more frequently in samples taken from tooth pockets at sites with periodontitis compared to the pockets of healthy teeth or sites with gingivitis (see Table 1 for an overview of literature). The question is, do their presence there reflect a role in the etiology of periodontitis?

Of the relevant herpesviruses, the simplex viruses are the ones least commonly observed (Table 1). As to EBV and CMV, their prevalence varies considerably in clinical samples. The variations may be partly due to geographic location, or to other factors influencing the selection of patients examined, but is also most likely a question of the sensitivity of the methods used for detection. If a virus is typically present at levels close to the detection limit, minor variations in sensitivity will have considerable impact on the prevalence obtained.

Most studies are done with samples from marginal periodontitis. In the case of apical periodontitis, surgical operation is required to obtain relevant samples, and there will necessarily be a more massive contamination with blood. While control samples in the case of apical periodontitis are not easily obtained, several laboratories have reported that the prevalence of viruses correlates with the severity of the condition [Contreras and Slots, 1998; Ting et al., 2000; Sabeti et al., 2003; Sunde et al., 2008a]. In the case of apical samples, EBV appears to be more common than CMV.

Arguments Against a Role in Periodontitis

The herpesviruses most commonly found in periodontitis samples are EBV and CMV. These viruses are transmitted by saliva and their presence in saliva and oral tissue is well documented, i.e., they frequently reach sufficient concentrations to be within the detection limits [Sixbey et al., 1984; Roizman and Pellett, 2001; Rickinson and Kieff, 2001].

In connection with marginal periodontitis, samples are usually taken by either a curette, or paper points, which respectively physically remove or suck up material from the pocket between the tooth and the periodontium. The teeth affected with periodontitis have wider and deeper pockets. As a consequence, more material is typically obtained from diseased sites compared to healthy ones. Moreover, the inflamed sites are more likely to contain cellular material and to be contaminated with blood. These factors are generally not compensated for when comparing the prevalence of virus between samples from diseased or healthy sites.

EBV is primarily harbored in B cells and in epithelial cells of the oropharynx, while CMV is present in a greater variety of cells, including various epithelial cells, endothelial cells and leukocytes. The number of lymphocytes, which may carry latent viruses, is significantly higher in sites with active periodontitis compared with stable sites [Zappa et al., 1991]. In other words, the presence of viruses in clinical samples may reflect the amount of blood and cells included in the material analyzed. Viruses present in these cells are not necessarily active, and, if not, they are unlikely to contribute to the etiology.

Most of the reports associating herpesviruses with periodontitis used non-quantitative PCR (Table 1). In cases where quantitative methods are employed, the level of virus is typically reported to be low [Kubar et al., 2005; Sunde et al., 2008a]. If the quantity present is close to the detection limit, but slightly higher in clinical samples, it is to be expected that a non-quantitative diagnostics will tend to report a distinct discrepancy in the prevalence when

Table 1. Typical reports on the prevalence of herpesviruses in samples from periodontitis. Viral prevalence (%) in either samples from periodontitic pockets or controls (gingivitis or healthy pockets) are presented

Virus	Periodontitis %	Controls %	Subjects (*N*)	Method	Reference
EBV CMV HSV	30 59 26	20 18 7	Chronic periodontitis (27), same subject controls	Nested PCR	Contreras and Slots, 1996
EBV CMV HSV	59 60 20	0 31 0	Advanced periodontitis (30), controls (26) with gingivitis	Nested PCR	Parra and Slots, 1996
EBV CMV HSV	73 72 54	18 18 9	Juvenile periodontitis (11), same subject controls	Nested PCR	Ting et al., 2000
EBV CMV HSV	18 44 7	14 14 0	Chronic periodontitis (30), healthy controls (21)	Nested PCR	Saygun et al., 2002
EBV CMV	71 65	6 0	Aggressive periodontitis (17), healthy controls (16)	Single PCR	Yapar et al., 2003
CMV	69	0	Aggressive periodontitis (16), healthy controls (15)	Real-time PCR	Kubar et al., 2005
EBV CMV	44 3	0 0	Periodontitis (66 samples), healthy controls (30 samples)	Single PCR	Klemenc et al., 2005
EBV CMV	31 23		Apical periodontitis (35), mostly HIV positive	Immunohisto-chemistry	Saboia-Dantas et al., 2007
EBV CMV	57 7	30 0	Aggressive periodontitis (30), same subject controls	Single PCR	Watanabe et al., 2007
EBV CMV	40 12	7 0	Chronic periodontitis (25), healthy controls (15)	Real-time PCR	Sunde et al., 2008a
EBV CMV	50 0		Apical periodontitis (40)	Real-time PCR	Sunde et al., 2008a

comparing clinical samples with controls. Thus the association of EBV and CMV with periodontitis reported by several authors may be artifactual, even if it is statistically highly significant.

Several authors point to the immunomodulating potential of herpesviruses as having a possible impact on bacterial replication. It is, however, also conceivable that the microbiota may impact on the activity of the viruses. It has recently been shown, for example, that malaria can induce the replication of EBV [Chêne et al., 2007]. If periodontitis is caused by bacteria that for some reason activate latent viruses, this offers an alternative explanation as to why samples typically contain EBV or CMV. A local stimulation of viral replication does not necessarily mean that the viruses play a role in the pathogenesis.

Quantity and Activity of Virus

Theoretically, herpesviruses may impact on the pathogenesis of periodontitis even if present at modest quantities, e.g., by producing cytokine mimics. One would, however, expect that in order to have an impact the virus must be active at the site, not just present as viral particles produced elsewhere, or as latent virus harbored in some of the cells included in the material analyzed. If present only at a low level, it is, at the least, difficult to distinguish between a clinical relevant observation, and the detection of agents commonly present in oral samples.

Several studies have quantified the levels of EBV and/or CMV in blood from patients with various virus-associated clinical symptoms [Hakim et al., 2007; Gouarin et al., 2007]. It should be noted that even in these cases, the viral loads differ considerably. Thus one cannot exclude that even a low level of virus may be clinically relevant.

The levels of EBV and CMV in saliva appear to be associated with periodontal status, i.e., their concentration are higher in affected individuals, and decrease upon treatment of the condition [Idesawa et al., 2004; Saygun et al., 2005].

Most reports on herpesviruses in periodontitis have used non-quantitative PCR (see Table 1). However, where quantitative methods are employed, the virus concentration is generally found to be low, although it may reach significant quantities in select patients. These patients tend to have particularly aggressive and troublesome conditions [Kubar et al., 2005; Sunde et al., 2008b].

It is possible to approach the question as to whether the viruses are active at the site. As a single viral genome can produce a large number of transcripts and proteins, the detection of these products not only suggests viral activity, but can actually offer a more sensitive diagnostic tool than genomic PCR.

Activation of CMV has been studied by RT-PCR designed at detecting viral RNA transcripts. Although active CMV has been indicated, it is typically observed only in a subset of patients for which CMV was found by genomic PCR in periodontal samples [Contreras and Slots, 1998; Ting et al., 2000]. The more interesting data came from 10-14 year olds with localized juvenile periodontitis [Ting et al., 2000]. In this case, all the five patients, out of the six for which CMV was detected, also appeared to have an active infection.

In the case of EBV and CMV in apical periodontitis, viral activity was assessed by respectively in situ hybridization and immunohistochemistry [Sunde et al., 2008a]. In this case, no signs of viral activity were demonstrated, suggesting that the viral genomes detected in the apical samples may reflect either free viral particles or cells containing dormant viruses.

Synergy between Viruses and Bacteria

If the herpesviruses in any way impact on the conditions for bacterial growth on or around the teeth, one would expect some correlation between the presence of virus and the bacterial species present in the local microbiota.

The presence of EBV and CMV in periodontal samples have indeed been reported to correlate with the occurrence of specific periodontopathic bacteria. In a study on gingivitis and periodontitis, virus was associated with an increased occurrence of *Porphyromonas gingivalis, Tannerella forsythia, Prevotella intermedia, Prevotella nigrescens* and *Treponema denticola* [Contreras et al., 1999]. Another study compared samples from two disease-active and two disease-stable periodontitis sites in each of 16 patients [Kamma et al., 2001]. They found that EBV and HCMV were associated with the disease-active sites, as well as with *Dialister pneumosintes* and *P. gingivalis*. CMV-associated localized juvenile periodontitis lesions also exhibit elevated levels of *P. gingivalis* [Michalowicz et al., 2000] and *Aggregatibacter actinomycetemcomitans* [Contreras et al., 1999, Ting et al., 2000]. A more recent study [Sunde et al., 2008a] found significant associations between EBV and the latter two bacterial species, but not the other 18 species tested, which included the species mentioned above with the exception of *D. pneumosintes.*

Overall the results do indicate a correlation between the presence of virus and particular species of bacteria. However, the associations are not extensive, and they may be due to confounding factors.

Antiviral Treatment of Periodontitis

A pertinent question is: If herpesviruses play a role in periodontitis, should antiviral treatment be included in the intervention? There are medications available that restrain the relevant viruses, mostly in the form of nucleoside analogs designed to inhibit viral polymerase activity. For example, acyclovir and valacyklovir have proven to be both efficient and well tolerated by most patients. The risk of side-effects due to the use of these inhibitors seems minor compared to the morbidity of severe periodontitis. Moreover, the administration of antiviral medicine offers the best strategy for elucidating the actual role of these viruses in the individual patient.

To our knowledge, antiviral medication has only been applied to one case [Sunde et al., 2008b]. The patient had a particularly troublesome and chronic marginal periodontitis, which had proven refractory for conventional treatment. Moreover, the patient had a very high level of EBV in the pockets of affected teeth (Table 2). A ten day cure of Valtrex® (500 mg of valaciklovir taken orally twice daily) not only reduced the viral load down to the detection limit, but within approximately a month the clinical condition was drastically improved. The patient was followed for another year in which the condition remained stable and the viral load remained insignificant.

Table 2. EBV quantity in subgingival samples taken before and after antiviral therapy. Viral load was measured by real-time PCR and the actual number of viral genomes in the complete sample calculated. (ND = not determined)

	Before Therapy	After Therapy (weeks)			
		1	5	8	12
Tooth 26	353 000	70	50	50	
Tooth 27	926 000	0	50	50	
Tooth 33	ND	50	0	0	32

Adapted from Sunde et al. [2008b]

Conclusion

A variety of viruses are present and replicate in the human body without causing any symptoms [Roizman and Pellett, 2001; Grinde, 2003; Witsø et al., 2006]. Various factors, including stress and loss of immune competence, will tend to enhance the replication of these viruses. One should therefore be careful when considering the clinical relevance of an association between virus and a pathological condition. The virus may simply be an opportunist that thrives in patients with a range of diseases, for example, as a consequence of reduced immune competence. On the other hand, evidence is accumulating that viruses do play a role in several conditions previously thought to be solely of bacterial origin, including otitis media and respiratory tract infections [Bakaletz et al., 1995; Heikkinen et al., 2000; Cappuyns et al., 2005].

In the case of herpesviruses, even low levels of viral activity can theoretically aggravate bacterial infections, for instance by the release of cytokine mimics. Moreover, herpesviral-bacterial interactions can help explain various, otherwise puzzling clinical observation as to periodontitis: The alteration between prolonged periods of virus latency interrupted by periods of activation may be responsible for the typical flare-ups observed in patients with periodontal problems.

Several recognized risk factors for periodontal disease, including HIV infection, emotional and physical stress, pregnancy and hormonal changes [Salvi et al., 1997] also have the potential to reactivate herpesviruses [Croen, 1991]. Thus, the initial trigger of periodontal disease could actually be the activation of latent herpesviruses in periodontal tissue.

On the other hand, one should be careful when evaluating the presence of low levels of viral genomes in clinical samples as an indication of a viral role in pathogenesis. EBV and CMV are expected to be occasionally present in any mouth if a sufficiently sized and relevant sample is analyzed by a sensitive technique. Thus the mere presence of virus, in the absence of signs of local viral activity, either in the form of high viral titers or detection of viral RNA or proteins, probably do not constitute any appreciable impact on the etiology.

Moreover, associations such as between viruses and particular bacterial species, or between viruses and the severity of the condition, may be explained by confounding factors. A more active inflammation would be expected to correspond to the presence of particular bacteria, and cause more pain, but also to contain more lymphoid cells and/or more bodily fluids. The latter factors could explain the association with herpesviruses.

The observation that a patient recovered from a chronic and highly treatment refractory periodontal condition upon antiviral treatment may be the single most relevant data suggesting a clinical role for these viruses [Sunde et al., 2008b]. Moreover, both the clinical condition and the viral load remained stable during a one year follow up period. Hopefully, in the future more cases will be administered antiviral treatment, thus adding statistical weight to this observation.

Antiviral treatment seems to be the best test to shed light on the actual role of EBV or CMV in periodontitis. Moreover, if successful, it may save the patients from considerable pain and agony. We therefore believe that quantitative antiviral tests, such as real-time PCR, is highly relevant in the management of these patients, maybe particularly in juvenile and/or chronic and aggressive cases for which other therapy fails. If the tests find reasonable amounts of virus, or other signs of local viral activity, antiviral treatment should be considered as an adjunct to conventional periodontal therapy.

References

Al-Yahfoufi Z, Mombelli A, Wicki A, Lang NP. 1994. The occurrence of Actinobacillus actinomycetemcomitans, Porphyromonas gingivalis and Prevotella intermedia in an Arabic population with minimal periodontal disease. *Microb Ecol Health Dis* 7:217-224.

Baelum V, Chen X, Manji F, Luan W-M, Fejerskov O. 1996. Profiles of destructive periodontal disease in different populations. *J Periodontal Res* 31:17-26.

Bakaletz LO. 1995. Viral potentiation of bacterial superinfection of the respiratory tract. *Trends Microbiol* 3:110-114.

Bergström J. 1989. Cigarette smoking as a risk factor in chronic periodontal disease. *Community Dent Oral Epidemiol* 17:245-247.

Cappuyns I, Gugerli P, Mombelli A. 2005. Viruses in periodontal disease – a review. *Oral Dis* 11:219-229.

Cate TR. 1998. Impact of influenza and other community-acquired viruses. *Semin Respir Infect* 13:17-23.

Chêne A, Donati D, Guerreiro-Cacais AO, Levitsky V, Chen O, Falk KI, Orem J, Kironde F, Wahlgren M, Bejarano MT. 2007. Molecular link between malaria and Epstein-Barr virus reactivation. *PLoS Pathog* 3:e80.

Ciancio SG, Slots J, Reynolds HS, Zambon JJ, McKenna JD. 1982. The effect of short term administration of minocycline HCl on gingival inflammation and subgingival microflora. *J Periodontol* 53:557-561.

Contreras A, Slots J. 1998. Active cytomegalovirus infection in human periodontitis. *Oral Microbiol Immunol* 13:225-230.

Contreras A, Umeda M, Chen C, Bakker I, Morrison JL, Slots J. 1999. Relationship between herpesviruses and adult periodontitis and periodontopathic bacteria. *J Periodontol* 70:478-484.

Corbet EF, Tam JOW, Zee KY, Wong MC, Lo EC, Mombelli AW, Lang NP. 1997. Therapeutic effects of supervised chlorhexidine mouthrinses on untreated gingivitis. *Oral Dis* 3:9-18.

Croen KD. 1991. Latency of the human herpesviruses. *Annu Rev Med* 42:61-67.

Gmür R, Guggenheim B. 1994. Interdental supragingival plaque – a natural habitat of Actinobacillus actinomycetemcomitans, Bacteroides forsythus, Campylobacter rectus and Prevotella nigrescens. *J Dent Res* 73:1421-1428.

Goodson JM, Tanner ACR, Haffajee AD, Sornberger GC, Socransky SS. 1982. Patterns of progression and regression of destructive periodontal disease. *J Clin Periodontol* 9: 472-481.

Gouarin S, Vabret A, Scieux C, Agbalika F, Cherot J, Mengelle C, Deback C, Petitjean J, Dina J, Freymuth F. 2007. Multicentric evalutaion of a new commercial cytomegalovirus real-time PCR quantitation assay. *J Virol Meth* 146:147-154.

Grinde B. 2003. Human circoviruses: clinical and applied perspectives. *Cur Top Virol* 3:81-90.

Hakim H, Gibson C, Pan J, Srivastava K, Gu Z, Bankowski MJ, Hayden RT. 2007. Comparison of various blood compartments and reporting units for the detection and quantification of Epstein-Barr virus in peripheral blood. *J Clin Microbiol* 45:2151-2155.

Heikkinen T, Chonmaitree T. 2000. Viral-bacterial synergy in otitis media: implications for management. *Curr Infect Dis Rep* 2:154-159.

Idesawa M, Sugano N, Ikeda K, Oshikawa M, Takane M, Seki K, Ito K. 2004. Detection of Epstein-Barr virus in saliva by real-time PCR. *Oral Microbiol Immunol* 19:230-232.

Kakehaski S, Stanley HR, Fitzgerald RJ. 1965. The effect of surgical exposures of dental pulps in germ-free and conventional laboratory rats. *Oral Surg Oral Med Oral Pathol* 20:340-349.

Kamma JJ, Contreras A, Slots J. 2001. Herpes viruses and periodontopathic bacteria in early-onset periodontitis. *J Clin Periodontol* 28:879-885.

Klemenc P, Skaleric U, Artnik B, Nograsek P, Marin J. 2005. Prevalence of some herpesviruses in gingival crevicular fluid. *J Clin Virol* 34:147-152.

Kornman KS. 2001. Patients are not equally susceptible to periodontitis: does this change dental practice and the dental curriculum? *J Dent Educ* 65:777-784.

Kubar A, Saygun I, Ozdemir A, Yapar M, Slots J. 2005. Real-time polymerase chain reaction quantification of human cytomegalovirus and Epstein-Barr virus in periodontal pockets and the adjacent gingiva of periodontitis lesions. *J Periodontal Res* 40:97-104.

Löe H, Theilade E, Jensen SB. 1965. Experimental gingivitis in man. *J Periodontol* 36:177-187.

McNabb H, Mombelli A, Gmür R, Mathey-Dinç S, Lang NP. 1992. Periodontal pathogens in shallow pockets in immigrants from developing countries. *Oral Microbiol Immunol* 7:267-272.

Michalowicz BS, Ronderos M, Camara-Silva R, Contreras A, Slots J. 2000. Human herpesviruses and Porphyromonas gingivalis are associated with early-onset periodontitis. *J Periodontol* 71:981-988.

Papapanou PN. 1996. Periodontal diseases: epidemiology. *Ann Periodontol* 1:1-36.

Patton LL, Phelan JA, Ramos-Gomez FJ, Nittayananta W, Shiboski CH, Mbuguye TL. 2002. Prevalence and classification of HIV-associated oral lesions. *Oral Dis* 8:98-109.

Parra B, Slots J. 1996. Detection of human viruses in periodontal pockets using polymerase chain reaction. *Oral Microbiol Immunol* 11:289-293.

Rickinson E, Kieff E. 2001. Epstein-Barr virus P2575-2627. In: Knipe DM, Howley PM, editors. *Fields Virology*, 4th edition. Philadelphia, PA: Lippincott/Williams & Wilkins Co.

Roizman R, Pellett PE. 2001. The family Herpesviridae: A brief introduction P2381-2397. In: Knipe DM, Howley PM, editors. *Fields Virology*, 4th edition. Philadelphia; PA: Lippincott/ Williams & Wilkins Co.

Sabeti M, Simon JH, Slots J. 2003. Cytomegalovirus and Epstein-Barr virus are associated with symptomatic periapical pathosis. *Oral Microbiol Immunol* 18:327-328.

Saboia-Dantas CJ, Coutrin de Toledo LF, Sampaio-Filho HR, Siqueira JF. 2007. Herpesviruses in asymptomatic apical periodontitis lesions: an immunohistochemical approach. *Oral Microbiol Immunol* 22:320-325

Salvi GE, Lawrence HP, Offenbacher S, Beck JD. 1997. Influence of risk factors on the pathogenesis of periodontitis. *Periodontol 2000* 14:173-201.

Saygun I, Sahin S, Ozdemir A, Kurtis B, Yapar M, Kubar A, Ozcan G. 2002. Detection of human viruses in patients with chronic periodontitis and the relationship between viruses and clinical parameters. *J Periodontol* 73:1437-1443.

Saygun I, Kubar A, Özdemir A, Slots J. 2005. Periodontitis lesions are a source of salivary cytomegalovirus and Epstein-Barr virus. *J Periodontal Res* 40:187-191.

Schürch E Jr, Minder CE, Lang NP, Geering AH. 1988. Periodontal conditions in a randomly selected population in Switzerland. *Community Dent Oral Epidemiol* 16:181-186.

Sethi S. 2002. Bacterial pneumonia. Managing a deadly complication of influenza in older adults with comorbid disease. *Geriatrics* 57:56-61.

Sixbey JW, Nedrud JG, Raab-Traub N, Hanes RA, Pagano JS. 1984. Epstein-Barr virus replication in oropharyngeal epithelial cells. *N Engl J Med* 310:1225-1230.

Slots J. 2004. Update on human cytomegalovirus in destructive periodontal disease. *Oral Microbiol Immunol* 19:217-223.

Slots J, Saygun M, Sabeti M, Kubar A. 2006. Epstein-Barr virus in oral diseases. *J Periodontal Res* 41:234-244.

Socransky SS, Haffajee AD. 2002. Dental biofilms: difficult therapeutic targets. *Periodontol 2000*, 28:12-55.

Sunde PT, Olsen I, Enersen M, Beiske K, Grinde B. 2008a. Human cytomegalovirus and Epstein-Barr virus in apical and marginal periodontitis: a role in pathology? *J Med Virol* 80:1007-1011.

Sunde PT, Olsen I, Enersen M, Grinde B. 2008b. Patient with severe periodontitis and subgingival Epstein-Barr virus treated with antiviral therapy. *J Clin Virol* 42:176-178.

Ting M, Contreras A, Slots J. 2000. Herpesvirus in localized juvenile periodontitis. *J Periodontal Res* 35:17-25.

Watanabe SA, de Fátima Correia-Silva J, Horta MC, da Costa JE, Gomez RS. 2007. EBV-1 and HCMV in aggressive periodontitis in Brazilian patients. *Braz Oral Res* 21:336-341.

Witsø E, Palacios G, Cinek O, Stene LC, Grinde B, Janowitz D, Lipkin WI, Rønningen KS. 2006. High prevalence of human enterovirus a infections in natural circulation of human enteroviruses. *J Clin Microbiol* 44:4095-4100.

Yapar M, Saygun I, Ozdemir A, Kubar A, Sahin S. 2003. Prevalence of human herpesviruses in patients with aggressive periodontitis. *J Periodontol* 74:1634-1640.

Zappa U, Reinking-Zappa M, Graf H, Espeland M. 1991. Cell populations and episodic periodontal attachment loss in humans. *J Clin Periodontol* 18:508-515.

In: Herpesviridae Viral Structure, Life Cycle and Infections ISBN 978-1-60692-947-6
Editor: Toma R. Gluckman

Chapter 7

Human Herpesvirus-6 in Transplant Organ Recipients*

Bartłomiej Matłosz, Dominika Dęborska-Materkowska and Magdalena Durlik[†]
Medical University of Warsaw; Ul.Nowogrodzka 59, 02 006 Warsaw, Poland

Abstract

Human herpesvirus-6 (HHV-6) is a β-herpesvirus first recognized in 1986. Recent studies have shown a pathogenic role for HHV-6 in immunosuppressed patients, including transplant recipients. HHV-6 latently infects the body after the primary infection and reactivates after introduction of immunosuppressive therapy or another form of stimulation. The clinical sequelae of HHV-6 may range from asymptomatic infection, febrile illness to tissue-invasive, life-threatening disseminated disease. Several severe complications of viral infection in transplant recipients have been reported including encephalitis, interstitial pneumonitis, bone marrow suppression and hepatitis. Prospective studies suggest, however, disease associations are rare. HHV-6 infection has been documented in 31-66% of kidney transplant recipients. The clinical impact of HHV-6 is being investigated. The role of HHV-6 as an immunomodulatory virus that may facilitate acute rejection episodes and chronic nephropathy is discussed. According to DNA sequence homology and similar clinical features between cytomegalovirus and human herpesvirus-6, the association and correlation in both CMV and HHV-6 activity is also discussed.

* A version of this chapter was also published in *Kidney Transplantation: New Research,* edited by Judith Fox, published by Nova Science Publishers, Inc. It was submitted for appropriate modifications in an effort to encourage wider dissemination of research.

[†] Medical University of Warsaw; Ul.Nowogrodzka 59, 02 006 Warsaw, Poland; Email: durlikmj@amwaw.edu.pl

Introduction

Human herpes virus type 6 (HHV-6) is a β-herpesvirus first isolated from the peripheral blood of patients with lymphoproliferative disorders and AIDS [1]. In 1988 it was demonstrated that HHV-6 is the agent of *Exantema subitum*, a common rash illness of infants [2]. Although originally named *human β-lymphotropic virus,* subsequent studies established that the virus was primarily T-cell lymphotropic, causing it to be classified as HHV-6 [3]. HHV-6 belongs to the family *Herpesviridae*, subfamily *Betaherpesvirinae,* the genus *Roseolovirus.* It shares many properties with other β-herpesvirinae subfamily members, such as human herpesvirus type 7 (HHV-7) and cytomegalovirus (CMV), including virion structure and the ability to establish latent infection in mononuclear cells. Seroepidemiologic studies show that HHV-6 infection is common in the healthy adult population. Similarly to other human herpesviruses the majority of clinical syndromes in immunocompromised hosts are due to viral reactivation.

Biologic Features

Human herpesvirus 6 is an enveloped virion with an icosahedral nucleocapsid of 162 capsomers, enclosing a double- stranded DNA genome. HHV-6 genome vary in length from 160 to 170 kb [4]. Two distinct variants of HHV-6 have been described; the variants are designated as variant A and variant B. The two variants are closely related but show consistent differences in molecular, immunologic, biologic and epidemiologic properties [5]. HHV-6 is a powerful inducer of inucer of IL 1β, IL 15, TNF α and IFN α [6,7]. HHV-6 infection of PBMCs results in CD4 T-lymphocytes depletion (down-regulation of IL2, inducer of CD46-mediated cell fusion, inducer of apoptosis in the CD4 T-cell line) [8]. HHV-6 has been associated with inhibition of p53-activated transcription [9]. The results of several studies have suggested that possible mechanisms for causing HHV-6 associated clinical events include its suppressive effect on haematopoietic progenitor cells [10, 11]. HHV-6 and HIV can coinfect and simultaneously replicate within the same CD4+. Indeed, HHV-6 has been proposed as a cofactor in the acceleration of HIV infection [12]

Pathogenesis and Epidemiology

HHV-6 is characterized by broad tropism for human cell types. The primary target cell for HHV-6 is CD4+ T lymphocytes what differentiates it from other DNA viruses [13]. HHV-6 can also infect CD8 T lymphocytes and natural killer cells resulting in the induction of surface CD4 expression. The cellular receptor for HHV-6 entry is CD46, ubiquitous type-1glycoprotein that is a member of a family of regulators of complement activation [14]. This protein is expressed on the surface of all nucleated human cells.

Primary infection occurs in early childchood so by 3 years of age almost all children have been infected with HHV-6[15]. It remains latent in monocytes/macrophages, early bone marrow progenitor cells and persists in a variety of tissues. The mode of transmission is unclear, but the virus is present in saliva and replicates in epithelial cells, suggesting that oral secretions contribute to transmission [16]. The donor tissue is also belived to be the site where HHV-6 may be transmitted. Superinfection with a donor strain distinct from the strain latent in the recipient may occur [17].

Most of the subjects in studies of HHV-6 infection in solid organ transplant recipients are adults patients. Because of the highly prevalent nature of HHV-6 infection it is assumed that the majority of HHV-6 infection in transplant recipients is the result of endogenous viral reactivation upon host immunosuppression. The virus infection occurs mainly between 2 and 4 weeks after transplantation [18]. In bone marrow transplant recipients the frequency of the virus infection ranges from 28-75% whereas in solid organ transplant recipients 0-82% [19]. However, the frequency and time course of the virus infection in the posttransplant period are affected by the procedures used to monitor the virus infection.

Clinical Features of HHV-6 Infection in Transplant Recipients

The prospective studies of transplant recipients have demonstrated that HHV-6 reactivation, although frequent, is usually asymptomatic. Infection with HHV-6 in the post-transplant period is common with predominantly, but not exclusively, variant B detected [20, 21]. The majority of studies concerning the association between viral infection and post-transplant disease have been made in bone marrow transplant recipients. The clinical impact of HHV-6 infection after solid organ transplantation has been mostly supported by anecdotal and observational studies. The most well documented clinical manifestation of HHV-6 in transplant recipients is bone marrow suppression. In those cases without other etiological agents identified, HHV-6 was cultured in the bone marrow. The most common cell lineage suppressed are leukocytes, followed by platelets and erythrocytes [22, 23]. HHV-6 has been implicated as the most frequently reported viral cause of undifferentiated febrile illness in organ transplant recipients [24], Individual cases of severe disease caused by HHV-6 in posttransplant period are reported, particularly: encephalitis [25], pneumonitis [26] and hepatitis [27]. It has been recently reported that HHV-6 seronegativity before transplantation was associated with an increased risk of fungal infection [28]. The timing of HHV-6 infection, at 2-4 weeks post-transplantation and before CMV infection develops (6-12 weeks), would allow for interaction to occur. HHV-6 infection, in association with CMV infection, has been linked to graft dysfunction, biopsy- proven acute and chronic graft rejection post-transplantation [29,30,31]. Hepatitis is associated in particular with OLT recipients [27]. Skin rash association with acute graft versus host disease and thrombotic microangiopathy were reported in bone marrow recipients [32,33]. The majority of HHV-6 infections in transplant recipients are due to reactivation of HHV-6B [18] but case reports with HHV-6 variant A infection has been recently reported [34,35].

Indirect Clinical Sequelae of HHV-6 in Transplant Recipients

The indirect clinical sequelae of HHV-6 include altering the net state of immunosuppression that may facilitate superinfections wth other opportunistic pathogens after transplantation. HHV-6 infection has been linked with severe clinical symptoms if concominant CMV infection occurs. HHV-6 infection was identified as a significant risk factor for the development of CMV disease with organ involvement [36].

Fatal myocarditis associated with acute parvovirus B19 and human herpesvirus 6 coinfection was reported [37]. HHV-6 infection and the degree of HHV-6 replication were found to be significantly associated with the development of Epstein-Barr virus-associated posttransplantation lymphoproliferative disorder, multidermatomal zoster, invasive pneumococcal disease and myobacterial disease [27]. HHV-6 viraemia modifies the natural history of hepatitis C virus infection post-transplantation [38].

Diagnosis

The method of virus isolation from peripheral blood lymphocytes prepared by IL-2 and phytohemagglutinin was firstly described by Salahuddin [1]. PBL from the patient may be used directly to produce lymphoblasts. Low level of HHV-6 replication is also observed in other cell lines e.g: megacariocytes (HEL), glioblastoma or astrocytes [39, 40]. The culture method used for HHV-6 detection is labour intensive and may take up to 3 weeks. A rapid shell vial assay has been developed that can detect HHV-6 within 72 hours.

Several serologic assays are available for HHV-6 studies including immunofluorescence, neutralization, radioimmunoprecipitation and enzyme immunoassays. The prsesnce of anti-HHV-6 IgM or a fourfold rise in anti-HHV-6 IgG supports a clinical diagnosis of active infection. Detection of anti-HHV-6 IgG is useful for epidemiological studies. As with other herpesviruses IgM antibodies to HHV-6 per se are not unique markers of primary infection because most cases confirmed by culture or seroconversion have no detectable IgM.

Virus antigens can be detected using immunohistochemical stains detecting HHV-6 in formalin-fixed, paraffin-embedded tissues. The monoclonal antibodies reactive against the structural protein p101 of variant B [41] and structural protein gp 82 of variant A detect cells productively infected with HHV-6[18].

Viral DNA can be detected using polymerase chain reaction (PCR) methods. These techniques are rapid, utilize samples obtained by noninvasive techniques and are sensitive in immunocompromised populations. Qualitative PCR for the diagnosis of HHV-6 is limited by the fact thatit can detect latent virus and is not able to distinguish between latent and active infection. Thus, the recent availability of quantitative PCR assays with real-time detection may offer the advantage of correlating HHV-6 load with clinical disease [42,43]. Quantifiable PCR utilizing a Taq-Man system has been demonstrated to be useful for monitoring active HHV-6 infection in organ transplant recipients [44].

Treatment

Although some reports have documented the successful treatment of transplant recipients with HHV-6 infection, the indications for therapy, the drug choice, and the efficacy of antiviral therapy for HHV-6 have not been adequately assessed in transplant patients. *In vitro* data indicate greater susceptibility of HHV-6 to ganciclovir and foscarnet than to aciclovir, which inhibited viral replication only at high concentrations [45, 46]. Cidofovir has the best inhibitory activity *in vitro* [47]. Successful use of ganciclovir and foscarnet for serious disease in immunocompromised and transplant patients has been reported with clearance of virus [48,49], but no randomized studies comparing the activity of antiviral agents against HHV-6 *in vivo* have been reported to date.

References

[1] Salahuddin S.Z., Ablashi D.V., Markham P.D., Josephs S.F., Sturzenegger S., Kaplan M., Halligan G., Biberfeld P., Wong-Staal F., Kramarsky B.,Gallo R.C. "Isolation of a new virus, HBLV, in patients with lymphoproliferative disorders." *Science* 1986; 234:596-601

[2] Yamanishi K, Okuno T, Shiraki K, Takahashi M, Kondo T, Asano Y, Kurata T. "Identification of human herpesvirus -6 as a casual agent for exanthema subitum." *Lancet* 1988; 1(8594):1065-67

[3] Lusso P, Markham PD, Tschachler E, di Marzo Veronese F, Salahuddin SZ, Ablashi DV, Pahwa S, Krohn K, Gallo RC. "In vitro cellular tropism of human B-lymphotropic virus (human herpesvirus-6)" *J Exp Med.* 1988; 167(5), 1659-70

[4] Biberfeld P, Kramarsky B, Salahuddin Sz, Gallo RC. "Ultrastructural characterization of a new human B lymphotropic DNA virus (human herpesvirus 6) and human cytomegalovirus." *J Natl Cancer Inst 1987*, 79:933-941

[5] Schrimer EC, Wyatt LS, Yamanishi K, Rodriquez WJ, Frenkel N. "Differentiation between two distinct classes of viruses now classified as human herpesvirus 6." *Proc. Natl. Acad. Sci. USA* 1991; 88: 5922-5926

[6] Burd EM, Knox KK, Carrigan DR. "Human herpesvirus-6 associated suppression of growth factor-induced macrophage maturation in human bone marrow cultures." *Blood.*1993 15; 81(6):1645-50

[7] Flammand L, Gosselin J, D'Addario M, Hiscott J, Ablashi DV, Gallo RC, Menezes J. "Human herpesvirus 6 induces interleukin-1 beta and tumor necrosis factor alpha, but not interleukin-6, in peripheral mononuclear cell cultures." *J Virol* 1991;65: 5105-10

[8] Flamand L, Gosselin J, Stefanescu I, Ablashi D, Menezes J. "Immunosupressive effect of human herpesvirus 6 on T-cell functions: suppression of interleukin-2 synthesis and cell proliferation." *Blood 1995*; 85 (5):1263-71

[9] Doniger J, Muralidhar S, Rosenthal LJ. "Human cytomegalovirus and human herpesvirus 6 genes that transform and tranactivate." *Clin. Microbiol. Rev.*1999; 12: 367-82.

[10] Isomura H, Yamada M, Yoshida M, Tanaka H, Kitamura T, Oda M, Nii S, SeinoY. "Suppressive effects of human herpesvirus 6 on In vitro colony formation of hematopoietic progenitor cells." *J. Med. Virol.* 1997; 52 (4): 406-12

[11] Isomura H, Yoshida M, Namba H, Fujiwara N, Ohuchi R, Uno F, Oda M, Seino Y,Yamada M."Suppressive effects of human herpesvirus-6 on thrombopoietin-inducible megakaryocytic colony formation in vitro." *J. Gen Virol* 2000; 81 (Pt3): 663-73

[12] Lusso P, Gallo RC. "Human herpesvirus-6 in AIDS" *Immunol. Today* 1995; 16 (2): 67-71

[13] Lusso P, Malnati M, De Maria A, Balotta C, DeRocco SE, Markham PD, Gallo RC "Productive infection of CD4+ and CD8+ mature human T cell populations and clones by human herpesvirus 6. Transcriptional down regulation of CD3." *J Immunol* 1991; 147 92):685-691

[14] Santoro F, Kennedy P, Locatelli G, Malnati M, Berger E, Lusso P. "CD46 is a cellular receptor for human herpesvirus 6." *Cell.* 1999; 99, 817-27

[15] Brown NA, Sumaya CV, Liu G-R, Ench Y, Kovacs A, Coronesi M, Kaplan MH. "Fall in human herpesvirus 6 seropositivity with age." *Lancet* 1988; 2:396

[16] Robinson WS. "Human herpesvirus type 6." *Curr Clin.Top Infect. Dis* 1994; 14: 159-69

[17] Levy J, Greenspan D, Ferro F, Lennette ET. "Frequent isolation of HHV-6 from saliva and high seroprevalence of the virus in the population." *Lancet* 1990; 335:1047-1050

[18] Yoshikawa T, Nakashima T, Asano Y, Suga S, Yazaki T, Kojima S, Mukai T, Yamanishi K." Endonuclease analyses of DNA of human herpesvirus-6 isolated from blood before and after bone marrow transplantation." *J Med Virol* 1992; 37 (3): 228-31

[19] Singh N, Donald R, Carrigan. "Human herpesvirus-6 in Transplantation: An Emerging Pathogen." *Ann of Internal Med.* 1996; 124:1065-1071

[20] Dockrell DH, Paya CV. "Human herpesvirus 6 and 7 in transplantation " *Rev Med Virol* 2001; 11:23-36

[21] Hall CB, Long CE, Schnabel KC, Caserta MT, Mcintyre KM, Costanzo MA, Knott A, Dewhurst S, Insel RA, Epstein LG. "Human herpesvirus -6 in children: a prospective study of complications and reactivation." *N.Engl J Med* 1994; 331 (7) :432-438

[22] Lautenschlager I, H□ckerstedt K, Linnavuori K, Taskinen E. "Human herpesvirus-6 after liver transplantation." *Clin Infect Dis* 1998;26 (3): 702-7

[23] Carrigan DR, Knox KK. "Human herpesvirus -6 (HHV-6) isolation from bone marrow: HHV-6 associated bone marrow suppression in bone marrow transplant patients." *Blood* 1994; 84: 3307-3310.

[24] Benito N, Ricart MJ, Pumarola T, Marcos MA, Oppenheimer F, Camacho AM. "Infection with human herpesvirus 6 after kidney-pancreas transplant." *Amer. J* Transpl. 2004; 4: 1197-99

[25] Chang FY, Singh N, Gayowski T, Wagener MM, Marino IR. "Fever in liver transplant recipients: changing spectrum of etiologic agents" *Clin Infect Dis* 1998;26: 59-65

[26] Singh N, Paterson D. "Encephalitis caused by human herpesvirus-6 in transplant recipients." *Transplantation* 2000;69: 2474-79

[27] Singh N, Paterson D. "Encephalitis caused by human herpesvirus-6 in transplant recipients." *Transplantation* 2000;69: 2474-79

[28] Humar A, Kumar D, Caliendo AM, Moussa G, Ashi-Sulaiman A, Levy G, Mazzulli T. "Clinical impact of human herpesvirus-6 infection after liver transplantation." *Transplantation* 2002;73: 599-604

[29] Dockrell DH, Mendez JC, Jones M, Harmsen WS, Ilstrup DM, Smith TF, Wiesner RH, Krom RAF, Paya CV. "Human herpesvirus 6 seronegativity before transplantation predicts the occurance of fungal infection in liver transplant recipients." *Transplantation* 1999; 67:399-403

[30] Acott PD, Lee SH, Bitter Suermann H, Lawen JG, Crocker JF. "Infection concomitant with pediatric renal allograft rejection"*Transplantation* 1996;62 (5), 689-691

[31] Tong CY, Bakran A, Peiris JS, Muir P, Herrington CS. "The association of viral infection and chronic allograft nephropathy with graft dysfunction after renal transplantation." *Transplantation* 2002; 74(4): 576-8

[32] Tong CY, Bakran A, Peiris JS, Muir P, Herrington CS. "The association of viral infection and chronic allograft nephropathy with graft dysfunction after renal transplantation." *Transplantation* 2002; 74(4): 576-8

[33] Belford A, Myles O, Magill A, Wang J, Myhand RC, Waselenko JK. "Thrombotic microangiopathy (TMA) and stroke due to human herpesvirus – 6 (HHV-6) reactivation in an adult receiving high – dose melphalan with autologous peripheral stem cell transplantation." *Am J Hematol* 2004;76:156-162

[34] Wilborn F, Brinkmann V, Schmidt CA, Neipel F, Gelderblom H, Siegert W. " Herpesvirus type 6 in patients undergoing bone marrow transplantation: serologic features and detection by polymerase chain reaction." *Blood* 1994; 83(10):3052-8

[35] Rossi C, Delforge ML, Jacobs F, Wissing M, Pradier O, Remmelink M, Byl B, Thys JP, Liesnard C. "Fatal primary infection due to human herpesvirus 6 variant A in a renal transplant recipient." *Transplantation* 2001; 71:288-292

[36] Deborska-Materkowska D, Sadowska A, Wesolowska A, Perkowska-Ptasinska A, Durlik M. "Human herpesvirus variant A infection in renal transplant recipient" *Nephrol. Dial. Transplant.* 2005 Oct; 20 (10):2294

[37] DesJardin JA, Cho E, Supran S, Gibbons L, Werner BG, Snydman DR. "Association of Human Herpesvirus 6 reactivation with severe Cytomegalovirus-associated disease in orthotopic liver transplant recipients." *Clin Infect Diseas.* 2001;33:1358-62

[38] Rohayem J, Dinger J, Fisher R, Klingel K, Kandolf R, Rethwilm A. "Fatal myocarditis associated with acute parvovirus B19 and human herpesvirus 6 coinfection." *J of Clin Microbiol.* 2001;12:4585-4587

[39] Singh N, Husain S, Carrigan DR, Knox KK, Weck KE, Wagener MM, Gayowski T. " Impact of human herpesvirus -6 on the frequency and severity of recurrent hepatitis C virus hepatitis in liver transplant recipients." *Clin Transplant* 2002;16: 92-96

[40] Ablashi DV, Salahuddin SZ, Josephs SF, Imama F, Lusso P, Gallo RC, Hung C, Lemp J, Markham PD. "HBLV (or HHV6) in human cell lines." *Nature* 1987;329 (6136): 207

[41] He J, McCarthy M, Zhou Y, Chandran B, Wood C. "Infection of primary human fetal astrocytes by human herpesvirus6." *J Virol* 1996; 70(2): 1296-1300

[42] Drobyski WR, Knox KK, Majewski K, and Carrigan DR. "Brief report: fatal encephalitis due to variant B human herpesvirus-6 infection in bone marrow transplant recipient." *New Engl. J. Med.* 1994; 330 (19):1356-60

[43] Secchiero P, Carrigan DR, Asano Y, Benedetti L, Crowley RW, Komaroff A, Gallo RC, Lusso P."Detection of human herpesvirus 6 in plasma of children with primary infection and immunosupressed patients by polymerase chain reaction" *J Infect Dis* 1995;171: 273-280

[44] Van den Bosh G, Locatelli G, Geerts L, Faga G, Ieven M, Goossens H, Bottiger D, Oberg B, Lusso P, Berneman ZN. "Development of reverse transcriptase PCR assays for detection of active human herpesvirus 6." *J Clin Microbiol.* 2001;39(6): 2308-10

[45] Gautheret-Dejean A, Manichanh Ch,Thien-Ah-Koon F, Fillet AM, Mangeney N, Vidaud M, Dhedin N, Vernant JP, Agut H."Development of real-time polymerase chain reaction assay for the diagnosis of human herpesvirus-6 infection and application to bone marrow transplant patients." *J Virol Meth* 2002;100: 27-35 45 Burns WH, Sandford GR. "Susceptibility of human herpesvirus 6 to antivirals in vitro." *J Infect Dis* 1990;162: 634-37

[46] Russler SK, Tapper MA, Carrigan DR. "Susceptibility of human herpesvirus 6 to acyclovir and ganciclovir." *Lancet.* 1989;2(8659): 382

[47] Yoshida M, Yamada M, Tsakuzaki T, Chatterjee S, Lakeman FD, Nii S, Whitley RJ. "Comparison of antiviral compounds against human herpesvirus 6 and 7." *Antiviral Res* 1998; 40:73-84

[48] Drobyski WR, Dunne WM, Burd EM, Knox KK, Ash RC, Horowitz MM, Flomenberg N, Carrigan DR. "Human herpesvirus -6 (HHV6) infection in allogenic bone marrow transplant recipients: evidence of a marrow-suppressive role for HHV6 in vivo." *J Infect Dis.* 1993; 167: 735-9

[49] Bethge W, Beck R, Jahn G, Mundinger P, Kanz L, Einsele H. "Successful treatment of human herpesvirus-6 encephalitis after bone marrow transplantation". *Bone Marrow Transpl* 1999; 24:1245- 48

In: Herpesviridae Viral Structure, Life Cycle and Infections ISBN 978-1-60692-947-6
Editor: Toma R. Gluckman

Chapter 8

Gammaherpesviruses and Oncogenesis*

M. Kúdelová and J. Rajčáni
Institute of Virology, Slovak Academy of Sciences,
845 05 Bratislava, Slovak Republic

Abstract

Gammaherpesviruses comprise a subfamily (*Gammaherpesvirinae*) of the *Herpesviridae* genus; they fall into two genera: Rhadinovirus and Lymphocryptovirus. Human gammaherpesviruses encompass the Epstein-Barr virus (EBV, HHV-4) and the Kaposi´s sarcoma herpesvirus (KSHV, HHV-8). Their genomes as well as the genomes of several mammalian gammaherpesviruses were fully sequenced. The gammaherpesvirus genes may be grouped according to several criteria. As a rule, non-structural and structural genes can be distinguished. Another commonly used classification is related to transcription kinetics, distinguishing immediate-early, early, early-late and late genes. Genes which expression is inevitable for productive virus replication *in vitro* are usually referred to as essential ones. The non-structural early gammaherpesvirus genes encode enzymes for viral DNA synthesis and specify polypeptides involved in immune evasion and in complement regulation. These also modulate or hamper the effects of cytokines and/or disregulate interferon action. During latency, which can be defined as non-productive maintenance of the circularized episomal dsDNA genome, a few (or at least one) latency-associated gene(s) are (is) expressed. Comparative sequence analysis of herpesvirus genomes throughout all subfamilies revealed the group of herpesvirus common genes (showing relatively wide sequence homologies), which encode structural as well as non-structural proteins with related functions. An important group of genes was found gammaherpesvirus specific (γ-specific). Finally, about 10 – 15 genes may be unic for each gammaherpesvirus. Such

* A version of this chapter was also published *in Oncogenic Viruses Research Trends*, edited by Lilian T. Johannes, published by Nova Science Publishers, Inc. It was submitted for appropriate modifications in an effort to encourage wider dissemination of research.

genes, present in the given gammaherpesviruses only, may encode proteins, which act in analogical manner though being different in their sequence. The products of gammaherpesvirus specific genes are often virus-coded counterparts of cellular genes; such proteins usually promote cell division and/or cause false intracellular signaling. The latter are believed to represent pirated cellular genes, which have been modified by evolution when becoming virus genome components. Viral oncogenes and virus-coded immune regulation proteins act in accord with infected lymphocytes. Since gammaherpesviruses remain latent in lymphatic tissues and may be associated with lymphoproliferation, comparison of their DNA sequences and functional analysis of corresponding proteins are of special interest.

Keywords: gammaherpesvirus, oncogenesis, genome, gene, intracellular signaling, lymphoproliferation, latent infection.

Abbreviations

aa	amino acid
AIDS	acquired immunodeficiency syndroma
AlHV-1	Alcelaphine herpesvirus 1
AP1	activator protein 1
AtHV-2	Ateles herpesvirus 2
Apo1	Apoptosis receptor 1 (*Fas*-receptor)
Bcl-2	B cell leukemia 2
BCR	B cell receptor
BH	*Bcl-2* homolog
BoHV-4	Bovine herpesvirus 4
bp	base pair
BRLF	*Bam*HI R leftward fragment (EBV DNA)
BZLF	*Bam*HI Z leftward fragment (EBV DNA)
CCP	complement control protein
CD	cluster of differiantion (leukocyte marker)
Cdk	cyclin dependent kinase
CIP	cyclin/*cdk* inhibitor protein
c-jun	cellular ju-nana (japanese expression for 17 from sarcoma virus 17)
CMV	Cytomegalovirus
c-myc	cellular myelocytoma
CNS	central nervous system
DD	death domain
EBV	Epstein-Barr virus
EBNA	Epstein-Barr nuclear antigen
ERK	extracellular signal-regulated kinase
FGARAT	N-formyl glycinamid ribotide aminotransferase
FGF	fibroblast growth factor
FLICE	FADD like ICE (interleukin-1β converting enzyme)

FR	family of repeats (EBV DNA region)
GPCR	G-protein coupled receptor
HIV	Human immunodeficiency virus
HLA	human leukocyte antigen
HSV	Herpes simplex virus
HVS	Herpesvirus saimiri
ICAM	intercellular adhesion molecule
IE proteins	immediate early proteins
IFN	interferon
IKK	inhibitor kinase kinase
IL	interleukin
IRF	interferon regulatory factor
IS	immunosuppression
ITAM	immunoreceptor tyrosine based activation motif
K-βZIP	KSHV analog of the EBV-specified *Zta*
KIP	kinase inhibitor protein
KS	Kaposi's sarcoma
KSHV	Kaposi's sarcoma herpesvirus
LCL	lymphoblastoid cell line
LMP	latent membrane protein
MAK	mitogen activated kinase
MAPK	mitogen activated phosphokinase
MIP	macrophage inflammatory protein
MuHV-4	Murid herpesvirus 4
NFAT	nuclear factor of activated T-cells
NFκB	nuclar factor kappa B
NIK	NFκB inactivator kinase
Ori	origin of replication
ORF	open reading frame
PDGF	platelet derived growth factor
Pi3K	phosphoinositol 3 kinase
PCR	polymerase chain reaction
Ras	Rous associated sarcoma
Rta	R transactivator protein (R fragment encoded)
Sos	son of sevenless (protein)
STAT	signal transcription and transduction
STP	saimiri transformation (associated) protein
TCR	T cell receptor
TIP	tyrosine-kinase interacting protein
TNF	tumor necrosis factor
TNFR	tumor necrosis factor receptor
TRAF	TNF receptor associated factor
TRADD	TNF receptor associated death domain
VEGF	vascular endothelial growth factor

vFLIP	viral FLICE (caspase 1) inhibitor protein
vGPCR	viral G-protein coupled receptor
vMIP	viral macrophage inflammatory protein
VZV	Varicella zoster virus
w.t.	wild type
Zta	zipper transactivator (Z fragment encoded)

1. Biological Properties of Gammaherpesviruses

Gammaherpesviruses comprise a subfamily, which members by tradition have been regarded for lymphotropic. The most widespread human gammaherpesvirus, the Epstein-Barr virus (EBV/HHV-4), belongs to the Lymphocryptovirus genus (γ-1 herpesviruses). The majority of gammaherpesvirus subfamily members belong to the Rhadinovirus genus (γ-2 herpesviruses), which human representative is the Kaposi's sarcoma herpesvirus (KSHV/HHV-8). Productive replication of EBV starts easier in epithelium cells than in B cells [166]. In contrast to EBV, which at primoinfection causes infectious mononucleosis (IM), primary infection with Rhadinoviruses (such as KSHV) is clinically silent. Gammaherpesviruses persist in host lymphocytes for lifelong. The latent KSHV reactivates in immunosuppressed (IS) subjects (in association with HIV-1 infection or after organ transplantation). During latency, gammaherpesviruses express non-transforming latency-associated proteins (such as EBNA-1), which help to maintain the latent genome within dividing cells. The viral circularized plasmid-like dsDNA duplicates together with the host cell DNA and gets separated into progeny cells by a special mechanism [119]. In addition to the basic latency-associated protein expressed in EBV latency I, a few genome carrier cells may express further latency associated proteins (EBV latency II and/or III), which induce proliferation and immortalization of host cells.

Due to the close relationship between the viral and cellular DNA replication, non-lytic infection of lymphocytes with gammaherpesviruses may cause lymphoproliferative disorders in man as well as in mammals (Table 1).Several gammaherpesviruses (such as EBV and possibly the murid herpesvirus 4, MuHV-4) promote development of malignant disease in the natural host. The non-human primate and ungulate gammaherpesviruses (such as herpesvirus saimiri 2, HVS-2) are usually non-pathogenic in their natural hosts, but cause lymphoproliferation in other related or even unrelated monkey species. Several latency-associated viral gene products (latent membrane proteins - LMPs, nuclear proteins such as EBNA-2, viral cyclins), immortalize the gammaherpesvirus carrier cells by inducing transcription of cellular genes participating in host DNA synthesis. Viral cyclins activate the cellular cyclin dependent kinases (*Cdks*), which, in turn, phosphorylate (and inactivate) the retinoblastoma (*Rb*) protein(s). Activated transcription factors, released from phosphorylated Rb protein(s) drive cells into the S phase of division cycle. Other latency-associated oncogenic proteins constitutively produce false stimuli which phosporylate the proteins of intracellular signaling pathways. These are either analogs of extracellular cellular signal transduction proteins (LMP/LAMP, vFLIP) or anti-apoptotic proteins (v*Bcl-2)*. In addition, γ-herpesvirus coded interleukin analogs (vIL-6, vIL-10) or cytokine receptor analogs (vIL-

8R/GPCR) may contribute to proliferation of non-productively infected carrier lymphocytes continuously activating the natural immune response mechanisms.

Table 1. Gammaherpesviruses and lymphoproliferative disorders*

Virus	Abbreviation	Natural host	Disorders	Ref
Genus *Lymphocryptovirus*				
Epstein–Barr virus/ Human herpesvirus 4	EBV/ HHV-4	man	lymphomas in natural host	† [10]
Cercopithecine herpesvirus 12**/Herpesvirus papio 1/		baboon	EBV-like	[67]
Cercopithecine herpesvirus 14**	CeHV-14	African green monkey	EBV-like	
Cercopithecine herpesvirus 15**	CeHV-15	rhesus monkey	EBV-like	
Genus Rhadinovirus				
Kaposi's sarcoma herpesvirus/ Human herpesvirus 8	KSHV/ HHV-8	man	tumors at conditions of immunodeficiency	† [172]
Rhesus rhadinovirus/ Cercopithecine herpesvirus 17	RRV/ CeHV-17	rhesus monkey	KSHV-like	[53]
Pongine herpesvirus 1 Pongine herpesvirus 2 Pongine herpesvirus 3	PoHV-1 PoHV-2 PoHV-2	chimpanzee orangutan gorilla	KSHV-like	
Herpesvirus ateles/ Ateline herpesvirus 2	AtHV-2	spider monkey	tumors in marmosets	† [2]
Herpesvirus saimiri/ Saimiriine herpesvirus (2)***	HVS (-2)***	squirrel monkey	tumors in owl and marmoset monkeys	† [1]
Bovine herpesvirus 4	BoHV-4	cattle	occasional malignant lymphoma	† [26]
Alcephaline herpesvirus 1 Alcephaline herpesvirus 2	AlHV-1 AlHV-2	wildebeest, wild ruminants bartebeest	acute malignant lymphoproliferation (malignant catarrhal fever) in cattle and captive ruminants	[63]
Ovine herpesvirus 2	OvHV-2	sheep, cattle		
Hippotragine herpesvirus 1	HiHV-1	antelope		
Equid herpesvirus 2 Equid herpesvirus 5	EHV-2 EHV-5	horse		† [188]

Table 1. Continued

Virus	Abbreviation	Natural host	Disorders	Ref
Leporid herpesvirus 1 Leporid herpesvirus 2 Leporid herpesvirus 3/ Herpesvirus sylvilagus	LeHV-1 LeHV-2 LeHV-3	cottontail rabbit		[132]
Murid herpesvirus 4/ Murine herpesvirus 68	MuHV-4/ MHV-68	bank vole	occasional tumors in laboratory mice	† [196]
Marmomid herpesvirus 1	MarHV-1	woodchuck		

*according to Roizman and Pellet [170].

** Closely related to lymphocryptoviruses of non-human primates and closely related to simian EBV homologs [200].

***suggested for this review only.

† the genome was fully sequenced.

When comparing genes encoding the above mentioned oncogenic proteins, our interest will be focused on two human γ-herpesviruses (EBV and KSHV), on the murid herpesvirus MuHV-4 isolated nearly 30 years ago [22], and on HVS-2, the frequently studied oncogenic monkey herpesvirus [134].

These non-human rhadinoviruses specify proteins homologous to LMP-1/LMP-2, ORF73/LANA, ORF72/vCyclin and ORF73/vGPCR of human gammaherpesviruses. The proteins in question mediate transformation by mechanisms, resembling to those associated with KSHV and/or EBV infections. Therefore, animal models of MuHV-4 and/or HVS-2 infections might be useful for studying the pathogenesis of Kaposi's sarcoma (KS) but also of EBV-related lymphomas.

2. Gammaherpesvirus Genomes as Related to Other Subfamily Members

Analysis of the genomes of the gammaherpesviruses sequenced so far (Table 1) showed that they possess genes common for many (probably all) representatives of three (α, β and γ) herpesvirus subfamilies [170]. Table 2 list the genes common for any herpesvirus. The total length of homologous sequences comprises at least 25% of the total herpesvirus DNA genomes. As expected, the sequences of individual herpesvirus family-common genes, when compared to their homologous counterparts, are not fully identical; they usually reveal co-linear stretches, which may be longer among viral DNAs coming from the same subfamily than among the DNAs coming from members of different subfamilies [154, 46]. For example, variations of the herpes family-common gB gene sequence within the gammaherpesvirus subfamily confirmed the subdivision into two genera, termed γ-1 and γ-2. On the other hand, comparison of the DNA polymerase gene sequences, contributed to refine the position of lymphotropic HHV-6 and HHV-7, which are now classified as betaherpesviruses. These novel human herpesviruses were originally isolated from T lymphocytes, where they reside in a latent state. Further genome analyses showed that they comprise the separate Roseolovirus genus [77].

Unlike to genes, which are common for all herpesviruses (Figure 1), some genes may be found in homologous members of at least two subfamilies. As an example, the thymidinkinase (TK) gene was found in alpha and gammaherpesviruses (the UL23 in HSV-1/2 and the BXLF1 in EBV). Since the TK gene is absent within cytomegalovirus (CMV) genomes and not identified in roseoloviruses, it is regarded as a α/γ subfamily common gene. Alternatively, the *ori*-binding protein (OBP) encoded by the UL9 gene of HSV-1/2, can be found in cytomegaloviruses only, but not in gammaherpesviruses. Thus, the OBP encoding gene is an example of α/β subfamily common genes. The gene encoding the viral G-protein coupled receptor (vGPCR) is present in many gamma- as well as betaherpesviruses. In the former it functions as interleukin-8 receptor (IL-8R) homolog. Its equivalent in the human CMV (HCMV) is UL78, while in HHV-6/HHV-7 the corresponding equivalents are UL51 and UL85, respectively. Thus, vGPCR is an example of β/γ subfamily genes. Finally, the gene encoding protein *Ox-2* (N-CAM homolog) can be found in KSHV (K14 gene) and in RRV (R15 gene), as well as in the HCMV genome. Therefore, the latter is a further example of "cross-subfamily" gene, common for several (but not each) members of at least two subfamilies [154].

According to the position of unic and repetitive sequences, the herpesvirus genomes can be classified into 6 categories, termed A to F [169]. The F category genome has no terminal repetitions (TR), while the category A and B genomes possess TRs at their both ends. While TRs are within the DNA class A symmetric in their orientation, the TRs of DNA class B are asymmetrical, when consisting of short repetitive units. The TRs of DNA class C genomes consist of short repetitive units, which are also located within the unic sequence, and called internal repetitions (IR). The sequenced rhadinoviruses revealed class B genomes, while the Lymphocryptoviruses sequenced so far showed a class C genome. The HSV-1/2 genomes have the up most complex structure comprising class E. Their DNAs possess terminal (TR) as well as internal repetitions (IR). The IRs meet at a joint located in asymmetric position, flanking the unic long (UL) and unic short (US) sequences.

The family-common genes of HSV-1 and/or 2 are located within the UL segment. The homologous (conservative) gene regions, which start at the UL1 (gL) gene and end in the UL54 (IE63/ICP27) gene, are clustered into into 7 blocks [173] ordered as follows: VII/VI/V/IV/II/I/III (Figure 1A). The homologous regions of the γ-2 herpesvirus DNAs (Figure 1C) form 4 blocks labeled II–V. As compared with the HSV genomes, the conservative blocks within the EBV genome are located in-between of the terminal and multiple internal repeats starting from blocks III and I, followed by blocks II, IV, V, VI and VII in reversed order (Figure 1B). The order of conservative gene blocks within the MuHV-4 genome (Rhadinovirus) is even more complicated due to several transpositions. The block II of the HSV genome in the MuHV-4 DNA corresponds to block I.

The next conservative cluster in the MuHV-4 DNA is designated II/III. It contains genes of HSV blocks VII to IV in reversed order. Finally, the HSV blocks III and I (again in reversed order) from a cluster designated block IV (Figure 1C).

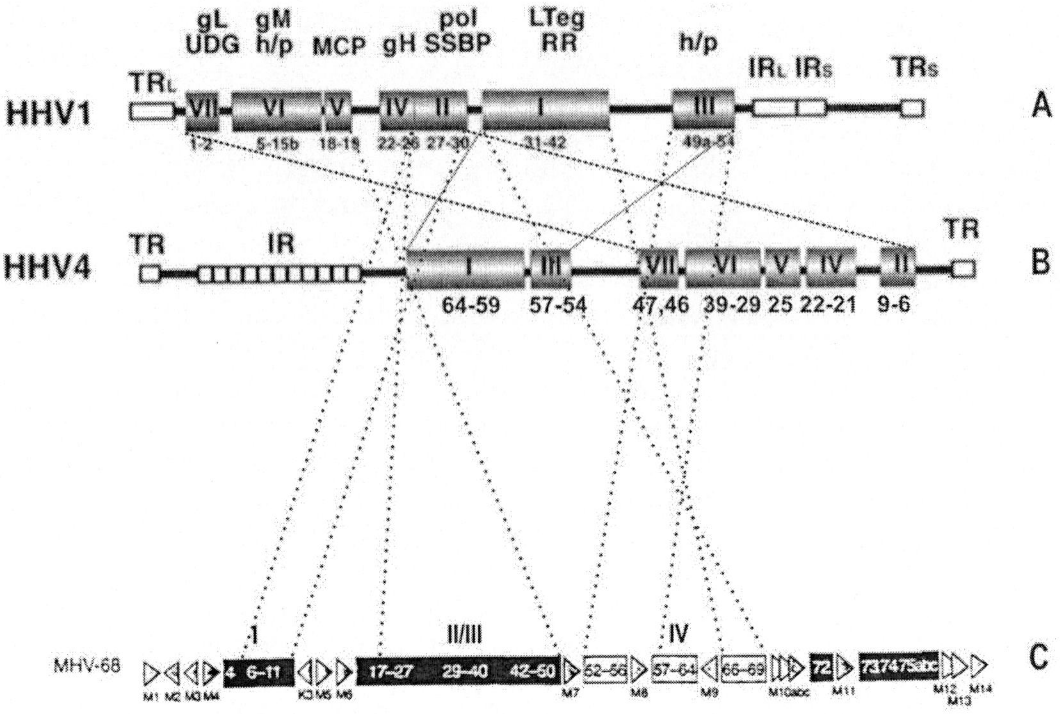

Figure l. Comparison of the conservative gene blocks of herpesviruses (based on Nicholas [154], vanRegenmortel et al. [173]. Arrangement of conservative gene blocks in the HSV-l/HHV-1 genome (A), EBV/HHV-4 genome (B) and in the MuHV-4 genome (C). The blocks are arranged either in parallel and/or reversed directions (compare Table 2).

The herpes family common genes occur in all three kinetic classes (non-structural immediate early, non-structural and structural early genes as well as late structural genes). Table 2 lists the marker genes (in bold type), which are up most typical for the individual conservative blocks.

Table 2. Conservative gammaherpesvirus genes and function of their corresponding proteins common for all herpesviruses (α,βand γ

γ-subfamily gene block	EBV ORF	KSHV ORF	MHV-68 ORF	protein /function[a]	HSV-1/2 ORF/ gene block
I	BALF5	9	9	DNA-polymerase	UL30 / II
I	BALF2[a]	6	6	ssDNA binding protein	UL29 / II
I	BALF3	7	7	transport protein	UL28/ II
I	BALF4	8	8	Glycoprotein B	UL27 / II
I	BVRF3	17	17	Capsid protein	UL26 / II
I	BVRF1	19	19	Tegument protein	UL25 / II
I	BXRF1	20	20	Virion fusion protein	UL24 / IV
II	BXLF2	22	22	Glycoprotein H	UL22 / IV
II	BcLF1	25	25	Major capsid protein	UL19 / V

Table 2. Continued

γ-subfamily gene block	EBV ORF	KSHV ORF	MHV-68 ORF	protein /function[a]	HSV-1/2 ORF/ gene block
III	BDLF1	26	26	Capsid protein triplex-2	UL18 / V
III	BDRF1	29b	29b	Terminase, DNA packaging	UL 15 / V
III	BGLF2	33	33	unknown	UL 16 / V
III	BGLF4	36	36	Phosphotransferase	UL13 / VI
III	BGLF5	37	37	Alkaline exonuclease	UL12 / VI
III	BBRF3	39	39	Glycoprotein M	UL10 / VI
III	BBRF2	42	42	unknown	UL 7 / VI
III	BBRF1	43	43	Capsid protein	UL 6 / VI
III	BBLF4	44	44	Helicase-primase	UL 5 / VI
III	BKRF3	46	46	Uracyl DNA glycosylase	UL 2/ VII
III	BKRF2	47	47	Glycoprotein L	UL 1/ VII
IV	BSLF1	56	56	Helicase-primase	UL52 / III
IV	BMLF1	57	57	Posttranscriptional regulator	UL54 / III
IV	BMRF1	59	59	Processivity factor	UL42 / I
IV	BARF1	60	60	Ribonucleotide reductase	UL40 / I
IV	BORF2	61	61	Ribonucleotide reductase	UL39 / I
IV	BPLF1	64	64	Large tegument protein	UL36 / I
IV	BFLF1	68	68	Glycoprotein	UL32 / I
IV	BFLF2	69	69	unknown	UL 31 / I

a common proteins typical for each gene block in bold.

These are the glycoprotein L and uracil DNA glycosylase (gL/UDG) from block VII, the glycoprotein M and two genes of the helicase/primase complex (gM, h/p) from block VI, the major capsid protein (MCP) from block V, the gH gene from block IV, the DNA-polymerase and the ssDNA binding protein genes (pol/ssBP) from block II, the large tegument protein and ribonucleotide reductase genes (LT/RR) from block I, and finally, the genes encoding the helper proteins of primase/helicase (h/p) from block III. It comes from this list that herpes common genes encode proteins fulfilling important basic functions. These are: 1) Regulation of posttranscriptional viral mRNA transport from nuclei to cytoplasm (the IE gene ICP27 and its homologs); 2) Nucleotide metabolism (RR reductase, uracyl DNA glycosylase, dUTPase); 3) DNA replication (DNA polymerase, ssDNA binding protein, helicase/primase, alkaline exonuclease); 4) Capsid components (major and minor capsid protein); 5) Capsid maturation proteins (DNA packaging protein and terminase); 6) A large tegument protein; 7) Envelope glycoproteins (gB, gH, gM and gL). At least four herpesvirus family-common genes encode envelope glycoproteins, while three encode capsid and/or tegument structural components (all these structural proteins belong to kinetic class-γ). Another 11 proteins are either enzymes and/or regulatory proteins involved in the synthesis of inevitable nucleotides, or polypeptides directly participating in DNA synthesis and capsid maturation (mainly non-structural kinetic class-β proteins). One common protein belonging to immediate early class-α (IE63/UL54) is the post-transcriptional mRNA regulator [159]. At least 4 conservative ORFs encode proteins of unknown function (not listed in Table 2).

The rhadinovirus genomes contain a set of gamma-common and/or rhadinovirus-common genes (Table 3).

Table 3. Examples of γ2 (rhadinovirus) common genes, corresponding proteins and their γ–1 homologs

KSHV ORF	HVS-2 ORF	MuHV-4 ORF	EBV ORF	Protein	Function
4	4	4		CCP	Complement control (regulatory) protein
16	16	M11	BHRF1/ BALF1	v*Bcl*-2	B cell leukemia-2 (anti-apoptotic) protein, *Bax*-inhibitor.
31		31			Required for lytic replication
50	50	50	BRLF1	Rta	Replication transactivator, IE protein (different from Zta)
52	52	52	BLRF2	ORF52	Putative capsid protein
71	71	none		vFLIP	viral FLICE[a] inhibitory protein
72	72	72		vCyclin	Analog of cellular cyclin D
73	73	73	BKRF1	EBNA-1 LANA	EB (or Latent) nuclear antigen KSHV (Latent nuclear antigen)
74	74	74	BLR1	vGPCR	Viral G-protein coupled receptor (Interleukin-8 receptor) homolog
75	3/75	75abc	BNRF1	FGARAT	N-formyl-glycinamide ribotide amino-transferase (tegument protein)

aFLICE = FADD-like ICE (ICE = interleukin-1-beta converting enzyme; FADD = Fas-associated death domain).
EBV = Epstein-Barr virus;
KSHV = Kaposi's sarcoma herpesvirus;
MuHV-4 = murid herpesvirus 4;
HVS-2 = Herpesvirus saimiri 2.

Finally, the individual gammaherpesviruses contain genes specific for that virus only. Some of the latter encode proteins, the functions of which are analogous to those encoded by other gammaherpesviruses. For example, the KHSV genome contains a bulk of gamma common and/or Rhadinovirus common genes and at least 15 largely unic KHSV genes, designated K1-K15 (Table 4). Alternatively, at least 14 MuHV-4 unic genes, termed M1-M14 have described (Table 5) along with at least 11 HVS-2 unic genes, termed S1-S3, S12-S16, S51, S70-S71 [196].

Table 4. KSHV unic genes encoding specific proteins and functionally analogous genes identified within other gammaherpesviruses

KSHV ORF	protein/Function	gammaherpesvirus analogous gene
K1	LMP-1/ STP/Tio/ Latent membrane protein 1/ *saimiri* transformation protein/ two in one (protein)	EBV ORF BNLF1 and HVS ORF 1
K2	vIL-6/viral Interleukin 6 /Interleukin-6 analog	
K3	IE1B/immediate early (protein) HLA class I inhibitor	MHV-68 MK3; BoHV-4 IE Bo5b analog (zinc finger motif)*
	Chemokine/ macrophage inflammatory protein 1	
K5	Immediate early (protein)	BoHV-4 ORF Bo5 analog*
K6 (MIP3)	Chemokine/ macrophage inflammatory protein 3	
K8	b-ZIP/ transactivator protein	EBV ORF BZLF1
K9, K10, K11	vIRFs/interferon regulating factors	
K12	Kaposin/ transformation protein, latency associated	
K14	Ox-2/N-CAM homolog	
K15	Tip/LMP-2/tyrosine kinase interacting protein/latent membrane protein 2	EBV ORF BARF1/BNRFl

analogs of cellular proteins and/or chemokines.
*Zimmerman et al. [209].

Table 5. MuHV-4 unic genes encoding specific proteins and functional analogous genes identified in other gammaherpesviruses #

MuHV- 4 ORF	protein/function	Gammaherpesvirus analogous gene
M1	Serpin/caspase 1 inhibitor, anti-apoptotic protein	
M2	Latency associated protein, an IFN type I antagonist	
M3	Soluble chemokine antagonist, binds several chemokines (receptor-like binding)	
M4	Function unknown	
MK3	IE1B/ immediate early protein, HLA class I synthesis inhibitor, immune response modulator (evasion mediator)	KSHV ORF K3
M5	Function unknown	
M6	Cluster of differentiation (CD) marker, function unknown	HVS ORF 15

Table 5. Continued

MuHV- 4 ORF	protein/function	Gammaherpesvirus analogous gene
M7	Glycoprotein 150/gp150/ surface glycoprotein, interacts with the CD21/CR2 co-receptor on the surface of B-lymphocytes	EBV ORF BLLF1/ BPRF1 codes for gp350/220 (gp340/220)
M8	Function unknown	
M9	Small capsid protein	
ORF45	vIRFs/ interferon regulating factor (vIRF-7) binding protein	KSHV ORF 45
M11	v*Bcl*-2/ B cell leukemia-2 analog, anti-apoptotic protein, *Bax*-inhibitor.	EBV ORF BHRF1/ BALF1 and HVS ORF 16
M12	Function unknown	

cellular protein and/or chemokine analogs.

3. Genes Associated with EBV Malignancies

Several lymphoproliferative disorders (Burkitt´s lymphoma endemic or sporadic, B cell non-Hodgkin lymphomas in immunosuppressed patients, T/NK cell lymphomas and Hodgkin's disease), anaplastic nasopharyngeal carcinoma (NC) as well as gastric tumors (lymphoepithelioma, undifferentiated carcinoma) and salivary gland tumors were associated with Epstein-Barr virus (EBV) at various rates, ranging from 15 to nearly 100% [44]. The mechanisms driving EBV DNA-positive carrier cells to immortalization are different. Essentially, all EBV-infected cells express the EBNA-1 protein and a specific population of small early RNAs, called EBERs (short polynucleotides probably functioning as silencer RNA). The state of non-productive latency I within infected B cells expressing EBNA-1 is controlled by the activity of cytotoxic T cells, which induce apoptosis and/or cytotoxic killing of any other EBV DNA carrier B cells, expressing additional latency II/III antigens such as LMP-1. However this balance can be broken under special conditions, including pathologic stimulation and/or failing cell mediated immune response. A good example of the latter are severe combined immunodeficient (*scid*) mice, which were successfully used to address several aspects of B cell lymphoproliferative disease [96]. Here we shall consider the mechanisms of pathological overstimulation of infected B cells, which may break the immune surveillance provided by T cells.

The EBNA-1 (Epstein-Barr nuclear antigen), when present in B cells in the absence of other latency associated proteins, has no oncogenic properties [119]. EBNA-1 protein is a transcriptional regulator and serves for replication and maintenance of the extrachromosomal circularized EBV DNA plasmid within carrier cells exhibiting type I latency [203]. The EBNA-1 molecule has a C-terminal domain for direct EBV DNA binding [8], an N-terminal domain inhibiting ubiquitin/proteasome degradation and blocking antigen presentation via the MHC I glycoprotein, a signal peptide for nuclear transfer and a domain which binds the virus specific EBERs [105]. It binds specifically to a 30-bp element in the family of repeat (FR) region of the *OriP* EBV DNA sequence [7]. Another region of *OriP*, the dyad symmetry (DS) sequence, consists of two 65 bp palindromes, at which the EBV DNA synthesis starts and terminates [74]. The EBNA-1/*OriP* complex has four sites for binding a cellular kinesin-like protein, linking the EBV plasmid to the cellular spindle apparatus [189]. Since EBNA-1 has no helicase activity, it cannot support the copying of DNA template, i.e. it would not replicate the EBV plasmid in the resting (phase G0) carrier cells. The replication of EBV plasmid occurs only during the S phase of host cell division [207]. Summing up, EBNA-l itself does not promote immortalization. In cells derived from BL, which express neither EBNA-2 nor LMP-1 proteins (see below), immortalization develops due to chromosomal translocations, causing enhanced *c-myc* expression [125].

The chromosomal translocations involving the immunoglobulin genes are a hallmark for B cell lymphomas and play an important role in blastic transformation together with the expression of viral *Bcl-2* (v*Bcl-2*). In addition, antigen driven activation through BCR signaling represents a significant cofactor [112]. The cytogenetic and karyotype changes are present not only in cells, derived from endemic BL cases occurring in Central Africa. They can be also seen in rare sporadic BLs and/or in AIDS-associated cases related to severe immunosuppression. Nevertheless, the major cofactor for occurrence of endemic BL is chronic malaria [14]. The cellular *Bcl-2* (B cell leukemia/lymphoma) protein inhibits apoptosis and interacts with the *Ras*-related protein R-Ras/p23 [85]. Its EBV coded analog v*Bcl-2* specified by the BHRF1 gene, has a significant effect even at low concentrations, since it prevents immortalized cells from undergoing apoptosis [87]. While members of the gammaherpesvirus family in general carry one v*Bcl-2* gene, EBV possibly encodes two *Bcl-2* homologs, namely BHRF3 and BALF1 [128]. However, the significance of the latter is still controversial [16]. In transformed cells v*Bcl-2* expression prevents apoptosis and prolongs the life span of immortalized cells even under conditions of impaired nutrition [90]. Anti-apoptotic proteins also play an important role immediately after B cell infection, i.e. at the initiation of non-productive interaction with the host cell. In the EBV-infected B cells apoptosis is abrogated during the first 24 h indicating a role for v*Bcl-2* immediately post-inoculation. Once latency has been established, the persistence of the EBV genome is not related to the expression of v*Bcl-2* gene. Primary B cells infected with a mutant, having BALF1 and BHRF1 ORFs deleted, undergo immediate apoptosis [6].

Early studies have already identified a transformation deficient, but replication competent EBV strain (designated P3HR), with DNA fragments Y and H missing, thus encoding a protein critical for immortalization [180]. Later on, this protein specified by the BYFR1 gene, was designated EBNA-2. The N-terminus of this polypeptide contains an acidic domain (AD) alike to the immunoreceptor tyrosine-based activation motif (ITAM). The AD can substitute for the HSV-1 VP16 transcriptional activator [41, 42] and shows affinity to cellular transcription factors such as TFIIB, TFIIH [190]. Another important domain of EBNA-2 binds the cellular DNA binding protein RBP-Jκ (recombination signal binding protein J kappa), also known as CBFl [83]. Since RBP-Jκ has intrinsic repressive activity blocking transcription, EBNA-2 may activate transcription from RBP-Jκ-responsive promoters. The third domain that is important for the primary growth of B lymphocytes, appears to flank the polyprolin repeat at the C-terminus of EBNA-2 polypeptide; this domain promotes oligomerization of EBNA-2 polypeptide into larger homotypic complexes [192]. Finally, the EBNA-2 region within aa 337-354 binds to the histone Hl; in consequence of this, it probably mediates chromatin interactions and facilitates gene expression. The EBV-immortalized B lymphocytes expressing EBNA-2 are nearly indistinguishable from naturally proliferating B cells. However, they are larger (LCL, lymphoblastoid cell lines), since they are metabolically very active and display an altered cell phenotype with molecular markers for cell adhesion and dedifferentiation (CD21, CD23, CD11a/LFA-1, CD58/LFA-2 and CD54/ICAM-1).

In EBV immortalized B lymphocytes, the permanent growth is promoted by constitutive presence of a set of non-structural proteins typical for latency II/III (LMP-1, EBNA-2 and the EBNA-3 protein family) in combination with expression of anti-apoptotic *vBcl-2* and cellular *c-myc*. The latent membrane protein 1 (LMP-1) encoded by the BNLFl gene of the EBV genome, is a key molecule activating the cellular signaling pathways [11]. LMP-1 is inserted into the plasma membrane by means of several hydrophobic transmembrane domains. It can form aggregates visible by immunofluorescence (IF) as cap-like patchy structures [84, 121]. Regardless of the presence extracellular growth factors, LMP-1 targets the intracellular signaling cascade activating the NFκB activator kinase (NIK), and a series of inactivator kinases (IKK), which bind to the transcription activator complex NFκB. If NIK is phosphorylated due to extracellular stimuli, the transcription factor NFκB is released from the complex with IKK (inactivator kinase kinase) and translocated into nucleus. Here it serves as transcription factor promoting the transcription of genes needed for B cell proliferation [33]. Under immune signaling within any target cell, the NIK protein is phosphorylated by several adaptor proteins such as TRADD (TNFR associated death domain) or TRAF (TNFR associated factor). These attach to the cytoplasmic domain of corresponding surface receptors, such as TNFR (TNF receptor) and/or CD40. If the TNF (tumor necrosis factor) interacts with the TNFR, a series of intracellular phosphorylation events is triggered, as result of which the transcription factor AP 1 (activator protein 1) is translocated into nucleus [181]. During latency II, which is characterized by expression of LMP-1 within the EBV DNA carrier cells, constitutive false positive signaling occurs through the NIK directed signaling pathway [79, 91]. When LMP-1 is expressed, the EBV carrier B cells undergo transcription, mimicking events similar to their activation by cytokine receptors (TNFR, IL-1R) and/or by antibody receptors (BCR, CD40) resulting in clonal proliferation. As result, LMP-1 positive cells express vimentin, additional CD markers (CD10, CD20, CD39, CD44, CD70, CD77), IL-10, and adhesion molecules [104]. Due to parallel activation of the anti-apoptotic protein(s) v*Bcl-2*, the immortalization of the LMP-1 positive cells becomes more efficient.

Cloning and sequencing of EBV cDNA corresponding to mRNA from latency II/III cells provided evidence for transcripts encoding additional LMPs, designated LMP-2A and LMP2B [175]. In LMP-2, the twelve transmembrane hydrophobic sequences are interrupted by short reverse turns. The C-terminus and the N-terminus form hydrophilic cytoplasmic ends, which are the sites of constitutive tyrosine phosphorylation when associated with tyrosine kinases of the *src*-family [27]. The LMP-2A blocks intracellular signal transduction following cross-linking of IgM receptors and CD19 co-stimulation. On other hand, in latency II cells expressing LMP-2A, the evoked anti-differentiation signals enhance survival in the absence of natural receptor signals [30]. EBNA-3A, 3B and 3C are similar to EBNA-2 in their property to interact with the cellular transcription inhibitor RBP-Jk. EBNA-3C up-regulates the expression of many lymphocyte markers, abundantly expressed on the surface of LCLs. It also co-activates LMP-1 transcription and inhibits p27/KIP [127]. The hydrophilic soluble protein EBNA-3C protein increases transcription despite of growth arrest signaling occurred at contact inhibition [5]. Finally, EBNA-3A represses the activity of the Cp promoter, where the transcription of *Zta/Rta* mRNA starts at initiation of productive replication.

4. Genes Associated with Kaposi's Sarcoma and Related Malignancies

KS (Kaposi's sarcoma) was described over 100 years ago as a rare idiopathic pigmented sarcoma-like skin disease. During the last decades, KS became more frequently associated with HIV-1 infection. Some cases appeared as consequence of radical immunosuppression therapy in allotransplant recipients. Endemic KS unrelated to AIDS was described in Central African countries [142]. The immmunosuppression-related KS consists of nondifferentiated spindle cells resembling fibroblasts (KS cells), believed to originate from blood endothelium precursors [45]. The Kaposi´s sarcoma herpesvirus (KSHV) DNA was identified in skin lesions of AIDS patients by a PCR-based subtractive hybridization procedure [34]. The KS cells were found positive for the DNA [182] and for a latent nuclear antigen, termed LANA [12].

LANA-1 is encoded by ORF73 of the KSHV genome [102]. At first it was regarded for an EBNA-1 analog, because it cooperates to maintain the KSHV genome in dividing KS cells at the episomal state. For example, through its C-terminal domain it was found to bind to H1 histones of mitotic chromosomes [111]. It can repress the transcription of *Rta*, a pivotal regulator for switching to productive KSHV replication [114]. It should be mentioned that LANA-1 is a very large molecule (220-233 kDa), consisting of 1162 amino acids, which has a long acidic domain (AD), a leucin-zipper domain and a basic polypeptide domain [143]. The first 22-23 amino acids hairpin peptide at its N-terminus binds to the folded region of H2A-H2B core histones [13]. In this way it docks to chromosomes, not only by previously proposed H1 histone binding. The H2A-H2B histone interaction may represent an important and more specific mechanism for latency maintenance mediated by the LANA molecule. Due its complex structure, LANA also provides some effects reminding of LMP-l functions. Its striking feature is the binding to anti-oncogen p53 [73]. Elimination of the cell division regulator p53 makes LANA-1 into a leading candidate, which lifts the cell cycle arrest and removes the apoptosis blockade. Namely under physiological conditions, p53 promotes apoptosis and inhibits progression to cell division regulating the S-phase entry and/or progression to mitosis. In uninfected cells, via activation of the p21 inhibitor kinase (KIP) transcription, p53 blocks the mitogenic pathway, which is driven by cellular regulatory cyclins A or D/E and their kinases *cdk 2, 4* or *cdk6* (cyclin dependent kinase 4 or 6). LANA-l was also found to interact with the retinoblastoma (Rb) phosphoprotein; this interaction stimulates transcription from the cellular cyclin E regulated promoter via the E2F transcription factor [160]. Furthermore, it interacts with another cyclin inhibitor, called INK (inhibitory kinase), namely with the p16INK4-A polypeptide [9]. Finally, LANA-1 interacts with several cellular transcription regulators, when activating CREB (c-AMP response element binding) protein-2 [122] and abolishing the transcription corepressor complex mSin3A [110]. In HeLa and Rat1 cells transfected with plasmids carrying ORF73/LANA and *c-myc* genes, their continuous expression promoted chromosomal instability, increased the frequency of divisions, caused multinucleation, and formation of aberrant chromosomes. These changes were associated with downregulation of p53 levels in a dose dependent manner [89]. In human umbilical vein endothelium cells, LANA-1 was found to prolong the life span in primary cultures, though alone itself it did not induce their transformation [201].

Monoclonal antibody against LANA-1 showed that this protein is expressed in a great majority of KS cells as a typical latency-associated protein. This is in accord with the observation that LANA promoter does not require tetradecanoyl phorbol acetate (TPA) for the stimulation of transcription. The pattern of episomal KSHV DNA latency (LANA-1 spontaneously expressed) found in KS was also demonstrated in primary effusion lymphoma, (PEL), which is a rare spontaneous body cavity based non-Hodgkin lymphoma, consisting of large neoplastic B cells. In both KSHV-associated diseases only very few tumor cells synthesize additional non-structural latency-associated proteins such as K2 (vIL-6 analog), K10/K11 (vIRF, viral interferon regulating factors), and K8 (the b-ZIP transactivator) (Table 4)[208]. Nevertheless, the expression of ORF73/LANA-1 in the KS cells may be closely associated with transcription of the neighbour gene ORF72, encoding viral cyclin (vCyclin) and ORF71, encoding the anti-apoptotic protein vFLIP [35].

The KSHV encoded vCyclin resembles to cellular D cyclin, which activates *cdk6* [186]. In this way, the Rb protein is indirectly phosphorylated to achieve the release and nuclear translocation of cellular transcription factors, such as NFκB or *c-jun* [126]. The vCyclin is the source of autonomic signaling, since it cannot be efficiently controlled by inhibitory kinases such as p21 [136]. In addition, the KSHV-coded vCyclin may cause degradation of another inhibitor kinase, the p27 protein [62]. Thus, vCyclin acts as in similar manner as deregulated cellular cyclin D when present in human tumors [147].

The ORF71 gene, located next to ORF72 (and in close vicinity of ORF73) encodes the viral FLIP (Fas-associated DD like ICE inhibitor protein). The vFLIP is a hybrid molecule inhibiting the activity of ICE, the interleukin-lβ convertase (caspase 1) acting as an apoptosis inducer. The KSHV coded inhibitor, vFLIP, has a death domain (DD), which otherwise would induce apoptotic signaling connected with its *Fas*-like ectomain, homologous to cellular FLICE (Fas-ligand ICE or caspase 8). However, the virus coded hybrid vFLIP reacts upon apoptotic stimuli in an opposite manner, by inhibiting the apoptotic pathway and blocking ICE. In this way, vFLIP can increase the probability of transformation [187]. The ORF71 sequence is present in tricistronic transcripts governed by the ORF73/LANA promoter (encoding LANA-1, vCyclin and vFLIP) as well as in spliced bicistronic transcripts presumed to encode vCyclin and vFLIP [53, 19]. Both mRNAs are transcribed in downstream (reversed) direction from the LANA promoter and were detected in KS cells [48]. The LANA promoter was analysed in detail, to determine the minimal sequence region needed for transcription in B cells as well as in endothelium cells [93]. The potential mechanism of independent initiation of vFLIP translation alone was related to an IRES site within the

ORF72 sequence [78]. The potential role of vFLIP in KSHV pathogenesis is reflected in its ability to promote transformation *in vitro* as well as *in vivo* [40]. In PEL cells, naturally expressing vFLIP, constitutive NF*k*B activation is associated with apoptosis inhibition; *vice versa,* inhibition of NF*k*B via the IKK complex induces apoptosis [103]. More precisely, TRAF2 and TRAF3 are required for vFLIP signaling, but mostly TRAF2 recruits the IKK complex [80].

The gene next of ORF73 is ORF74, which encodes a KSHV-associated cytokine receptor (IL-8R), also designated viral GPCR (G-protein Coupled Receptor) (vGPCR). In the presence of IL-8 the viral IL-8R activates the secretion of VEGF (vascular endothelium growth factor); this represents an important step in the pathogenesis of KS, especially in his malignant invasive form, so well documented in AIDS patients. Induction of VEGF synthesis was demonstrated *in vitro* using PEL derived cells, where vGPCR promiscuously binds CC as well as CXC chemokines [171]. Only a few KS cells express vGPCR, which – according to its transcription kinetics – belongs to the category of early proteins inducible by TPA. Under natural conditions, transcription of ORF74 and synthesis of vGPCR are induced by the transactivation protein *Rta*. Following IL-8 stimulation, the vGPCR molecule undergoes dimerization and activation of tyrosine kinase within its cytoplasmic tail. Next, the adaptor proteins *Grb2* and *Sos* interact with each other forming a complex, which, in turn, activates the oncogenic *Ras* protein. Recently, Montaner et al. [141] described activation of the nuclear factor of T cells (NFAT) via a small G protein called *Rac*. In contrast, the *Ras*/GTP complex generates a phosphorylation signal, which spreads via the MAKK (mitogen activated kinase) cascade to translocate transcription factors *c-jun* or AP-1 into the nucleus. Thus, in latent KSHV DNA carrier cells, the expression of the KSHV vGPCR causes constitutive activation of the ERK/p38/MAPK pathway [136] as well as of related mitogenic pathways. Furthermore, vGPCR may down-regulate the lytic switch to productive KSHV replication (via p21-mediated inhibition of *Cdk2*) and exert paracrine effects in neighbour cells [32]. Constitutive false signaling caused by the vGPCR dimer may come from a mutation within the second intracellular loop of the 7-transmembrane domain. As result of this, transgenic mice expressing KSHV vGPCR developed tumors with histological characteristics of Kaposi's sarcoma [201].

KSHV encodes an important interleukin homolog, vIL-6, which appears to be responsible for proliferation of non-infected B lymphocytes, at least in the pathogenesis of PEL. In KS, vIL-6 enhances VEGF production [65]. It seems that vIL-6 encoded by the K2 gene, is secreted from KSHV infected lymphocytes, fibroblasts and endothelium cells [151, 153]. The IL-6 receptor of lymphocytes consists of two subunits (gp80 and gp130), which are needed for the specific IL-6 binding (gp80) and signal transduction (gp130). However, vIL-6 has no requirement for gp80 binding, suggesting that a broader variety of receptors may get stimulated [36]. Direct gp130 signal transduction more easily activates the corresponding transcription factors (STAT1, STAT3 and/or STAT5), which are then translocated into nucleus [146]. Neither vIL-6 nor the viral inflammatory proteins (vMIP1/K4, vMIP3/K6) are expressed in carrier cells containing latent KSHV DNA. Thus, they cannot act at early stages of KS formation in LANA-1 positive cells [31]. In AIDS-associated KS, which shows quick progression, fibroblast proliferation occurs due to production of the basic fibroblast growth factor (b-FGF) induced by HIV-1 transactivator protein, *Tat*. It has been postulated that *Tat*, released from HIV-1 infected T lymphocytes would more widely activate the KSHV early transcription [63]. As a result, several signaling pathways may be activated in parallel, promote cellular DNA synthesis and drive infected cells into repeated division cycles, a prerequisite of blastic proliferation.

As described above, the KSHV coded early non-structural proteins expressed under special conditions, include the viral anti-apoptotic proteins vCyclin and vFLIP, virus coded interleukins and chemokines as well as their receptor(s) such as vGPCR. In addition, KSHV encodes several interferon-regulating factors (vIRFs), which are homologous to the family of cellular IRFs [143]. The vIRFs have an N-terminal DNA binding motif and a C-terminal repressor/transactivator region. IRFs bind to the interferon sequence responsive element (ISRE) within the promoters of IFN-responsive genes, but also to their positive regulatory domains [106]. Interestingly enough, vIRFs may also inhibit the IFN-γ associated cytokine response [195]. The viral IRF-1/K9 and IRF-3/K10.5-K10.6 prevent transcription from the IFN-α/β responsive promoter [123]. Furthermore, vIRF-l reduces the level of *cdk1* inhibitor p21 and can inhibit the activity of p53 by facilitating its degradation [179]. The vIRF-2 binds to NF-κB binding sites [28], inhibits p53 and may suppress the effect of dsRNA induced protein kinase R (PKR). The latter IFN regulator has been also named LANA-2, since it was found in nuclei of PEL derived cells but not in KS cells [168]. Taken together, KSHV encodes several proteins capable to modulate or mimic the action of cytokines, their receptors and/or to regulate IFN production. Understanding of their function may be helpful in exploiting the derivatives of immune modulators for therapeutic purposes, especially in AIDS patients [165].

The KSHV-specific K12 gene encodes an oncoprotein called kaposin [148]. The abundant latency-associated 0.7 kb transcript corresponding to K12 gene (T0.7) was found in all forms of KS as well as in PEL [34, 207]. Complex regulation and splicing of the K12 transcripts result into translation of three polypeptides, termed kaposin A, B and C [174]. The similarity of the hydrophobic N-terminus sequences between bovine papilomavirus 5 protein E5 and kaposin theoretically suggested a common mechanism of action. Namely, E5 and probably also kaposin was expected to bind to a component of vacuolar ATPase, which is important for processing of activated growth factor receptors [43]. Kaposin prolongs the activated state of the growth factor receptor upon external stimulation. As shown on the example PDGFR (platelet derived growth factor receptor), kaposin may also activate the cytoplasmic domain of this receptor in a constitutive manner. More recently, it was found that kaposin B stabilizes the cytokine mRNAs (i.e. the vIL-6 mRNA), which are rich in AU-elements at their 3'-ends. It also activates MK2 (mitogen kinase 2) a target of the p38/MAK (mitogen activated kinase) signaling pathway [130]. Kaposin A might be involved in activating of the extracellular signal regulated kinase (ERK-1, 2/MAPK) pathway [107].

The KSHV coded analog of EBV LMP-l is a product of the K1 gene (Table 4). This transmembrane glycoprotein has a conservative cytoplamic tail with an immunoreceptor tyrosine based activation motif, called ITAM [198, 100]. Under physiological condition, ITAM is involved in BCR (B cell receptor) and TCR (T cell receptor) signaling via phosphorylation of tyrosine residues [113]. Unlike to physiological conditions, the KSHV LMP-l surface domain does not require ligand cross-linking for initiation of the signaling cascade [117]. Due to the unic property of self-multimerization, the Kl protein was shown to induce host cell proliferation when expressed in fibroblasts similarly as the saimiri transformation protein (STP). The false stimulated ITAM domain induces expression of a transactivator protein NFAT. By a similar mechanism, the K1 homolog STP immortalizes HVS-infected T cells and induces lymphomas in HVS-infected marmoset monkeys (see below).

The K15 gene encodes an EBV LMP-2 analog termed LAMP (latency-associated membrane protein), which is located at the rightmost end of the KSHV genome (in opposite to the K1 gene) [38]. The cytoplasmic tail of LAMP (similarly to LMP-2) contains *src*-homology (SH2 or SH3) domains, which interact with *src*-tyrosine kinase family proteins. Under physiological conditions, *src*-kinases participate in signal transduction responding to various growth factors, which bind to external surface receptors on T cells, B cells, endothelium cells, bone marrow cells and/or fibroblasts [27]. The cytoplasmic region of K15/LAMP can be constitutively tyrosine phosphorylated, but elicits no signaling activity. It rather blocks B cell receptor signaling and intracellular calcium mobilization [39]. Because LAMP associates with HAX-1, a protein affecting cell contact and actin polymerization, it was assumed that this transmembrane protein would influence endothelium cell mobility [178]. In contrast to LAMP/LMP-2, the HVS subtype C encoded tyrosine kinase interacting protein (Tip), which is an LAMP homolog, more efficiently contributes to STP/ORF1 action (see below).

5. Mammalian Gammaherpesviruses and Cell Transformation

Murid herpesvirus 4 (MuHV-4) infection of mice is probably the most amenable animal model for studying the pathogenesis of human lymphoproliferative disorders caused by gammaherpesviruses [164]. MuHV-4, is a natural pathogen for free-living rodents [22]. It infects B lymphocytes and macrophages [184, 138]. Following intranasal inoculation of laboratory mice, the virus spreads to lungs, where it replicates in alveolar cells as well as vascular endothelial cells [163]. Similarly to other gammaherpesviruses, MuHV-4 establishes long-term latency in B lymphocytes (spleen, lymph nodes), macrophages but also in lung endothelial cells [183]. At acute stage, an infectious mononucleosis-like syndrome develops, during which the proliferating large atypical T/CD8 lymphocytes eliminate those B cells, which express non-structural early proteins [21]. Lymphoproliferative disease and solid tumors (lymphomas) were described in Balb/c mice infected with MHV-68 and MHV-72 strains of MuHV-4 [185, 139]. A chronic leukaemia-like syndrome associated with spleen enlargement and extremely high number of peripheral blood leukocytes was also noted, especially in MuHV-4 strain Šum-infected animals [140].

During non-productive latency, the MuHV-4 carrier B lymphocytes and mononuclear cells express a KSHV LANA homolog, encoded by the ORF73 gene [70]. Alike to EBNA-1, MuHV-4 ORF73 is involved in the replication and maintenance of the latent viral DNA. Its binding to host cell chromosome ensures an efficient partitioning of viral genomes to daughter cells during the mitosis of latently infected viral DNA carrier cell. Similarly to KSHV LANA, the MuHV-4 ORF73 may promote host cell proliferation, namely by decreasing the level of *cdk* inhibitor protein and/or kinase inhibitor protein (CIP/KIP) expression [58] and by p53 binding. By analogy to KSHV LANA that binds to the viral DNA terminal repeats [75], the ORF73/LANA is capable transcriptional autoregulation. The strain MHV-68 ORF73 was found transcribed during latency both *in vitro* and *in vivo* [129]. Its ORF73.STOP mutant grew well *in vitro* and induced acute phase infection *in vivo*. In lungs of immunocompetent mice the stop mutant exhibited a delayed replication and showed a severe defect in the establishment of latency. A similar latency deficit was also observed in splenocytes of animals infected with the ORF73 deletion mutants [144]. The latency deficient ORF73del virus was a potential live vaccine, since it did not persist in the immunized host [71].

In addition to ORF73/LANA, the MuHV-4 has additional powerful tools how to promote cellular DNA synthesis. It encodes the M11/*vBcl-2* anti-apoptotic protein and a vCyclin (ORF72), which is independent from cellular anti-*onc* inhibitors (Table 3). The gammaherpesvirus cyclins exhibit 25 to 31% of sequence identity with mammalian D-type cyclins; the highest level of sequence conservation is in the so-called cyclin box, a domain essential for the binding of the cellular cyclin-dependent kinase (*Cdk*). When complexed with cellular *Cdks*, the herpesvirus saimiri (HVS-2) and/or the KSHV vCyclin were found resistant to regulation by the cellular cyclin/*cdk* inhibitors (CIP/KIP) and the INK4 (inhibitor kinase 4) cell division regulator protein [186]. As mentioned above, vCyclins not only substitute for cellular cyclins, but they keep functioning despite of the presence of sufficient amounts of anti-*onc*-proteins (such as p53) and/or despite of the expression cyclin inhibitors such as CIP/KIP proteins [136]. To investigate the function of the strain MHV-68 vCyclin homolog, recombinant vCyclin.Lac.Z deletion/insertion constructs were prepared. The ORF72del/Lac.Z mutant was significantly compromised in the capacity to reactivate from latency. Independent studies using the MuHV-4 vCyclin deficient virus, confirmed that ORF72/vCyclin expression was rather critical for virus reactivation [59, 60]

The ORF74 situated next at the 3'-end of MuHV-4 encodes the IL-8 receptor (IL-8R), which is homologous with the G-protein coupled receptor protein (vGPCR) [197]. The splenocytes of mice infected with the ORF74del MuHV-4 mutant showed significantly reduced reactivation from latency [118]. The *in vitro* growth of the w.t. virus, but not of the ORF74del mutant, could be potentiated in the presence of a CXC chemokine and/or in the presence of the MIP-2 chemoattractant polypeptide. Furthermore, the MHV-68 ORF74/vGPCR was reported to induce the transformed phenotype in transfected 3T3 cells. The transformation frequency was comparable to that of LMP-1, the known EBV oncogene. To examine the role of MHV-68 v-GPCR *in vivo,* a mutant virus was generated, in which 440 bp of the gene ORF74 has been deleted (MHV68/v-GPCR440). The ability of the MHV68/v-GPCR440 deletion mutant to establish latency and to reactivate from latency was quantified on days 16 and 42 p.i. As compared to wild-type MHV-68 and to marker rescued viruses, there was a significant decrease in the efficiency of the vGPCR mutant to reactivate by day 42 p. i. [145].

The MuHV-4 viral *bcl-2* gene homolog was termed M11, since earlier it had been regarded for MuHV-4 specific (Table 5). The M11 gene is located in a close vicinity of γ-common genes, such as ORF72/vCyclin and ORF73/LANA. The v*Bcl-2* protein analog shows a single domain (BH1) homologous to the mammalian *Bcl-2* protein. MuHV-4/v*Bcl*-2 was found to protect cells from TNF induced apoptosis [199]. Possibly, it may reverse the processing of caspase-8 induced by *Fas* activation. The *Bcl-2* family proteins block the activation of caspase 8, occurring in response to cell death-induced signaling induced by *FasL* and mediated by cytoplasmic FADD/MORT1 adaptor proteins [101]. To terminate the *Bcl-2* action in *Fas*-stimulated cells, the *Bcl-2* itself is cleaved by caspases and converted into a potent pro-apoptotic factor [15]. The MHV-68 v*Bcl-2* was found susceptible to caspase digestion, but its cleavage product lacked pro-apoptotic activity. Thus, the γ-herpesvirus *Bcl-2* homologs escape negative down regulation by retaining anti-apoptotic activity and/or by the failure of getting converted into pro-apoptotic proteins in the course of the programmed cell death. During early infection of mice, M11 transcripts can be found in the spleen and lungs along with other lytic cycle mRNAs. In the course of latency, the M11 mRNA was still present in these organs, though no typical lytic transcripts (M7/gp150, ORF50/*Rta)* could be detected. This suggests that the MuHV-4 v*Bcl-2* protein promotes virus survival by protecting productively as well as persistently infected cells from apoptotic destruction.

Another latency associated protein M2 was found in the spleen of infected mice during the first month post-infection. The nuclear M2 protein down regulates the expression of STAT1 and STAT2 (signal transduction and transactivation) proteins, which moderate the transcription of IFN type I-reactive cellular enzymes. In MuHV-4 infected fibroblasts, the M2 acts as an IFN antagonist, favouring immune evasion and latency maintenance. Liang et al. [120] showed a cell type dependent localization pattern for M2 expression: in lymphocytes it was seen in the cytoplasm and cell membranes, while in epithelium cells and fibroblasts it was found solely in the nucleus. Mutational analysis indicated that M2 protein has positively charged internal amino acids. The mutation within the M2 gene did not affect the ability of the virus to replicate in tissue culture, nor did they affect MuHV-4 virulence. M2 expression was differentially required for acute replication *in vivo* being inevitable for virus production in the spleen but not in lungs [92]. The expression of the M2 gene was examined in B lymphocytes during acute infection and latency using mice inoculated by intranasal route. The induction of specific T/CD8+ cell response as followed from day 14 p.i., but became undetectable during long-term latency. Adoptive-transfer studies demonstrated that cytotoxic T cells specific to M2, reduced the initial, but not the long-term load of that protein [193]. In addition, it has been shown that vaccination with M2 reduces the load of latently infected B cells in the spleen at early, but not at late intervals p.i. [194]. While following intranasal inoculation, the cells positive for the M2 mutant genome inefficiently reactivated from latency, no significant defect was observed after intraperitoneal inoculation. The significance of the latter finding remains unclear.

The MuHV-4 specific M3 gene encodes a soluble 46kDa protein, which potentially interferes with the natural chemokines and their interactions to corresponding receptors [17]. Recently, the M3 protein has been shown capable of binding a broad variety of chemokines and to neutralize cellular responses to chemokines *in vitro* [157]. *In vivo* M3 probably attenuates the immune response to virus infection and assists at regulating leukocyte recruitment that could lead to an enhanced viral replication [177]. As recently shown, M3 protein when secreted from producer cells, generates a conformation pocket interacting with many residues of CCL2 chemokines (such as monocyte chemotactic proteins, MCPs, and/or macrophage inflammatory proteins, MIPs). Any interacting chemokine is recognized by the cellular receptor CCR2, which provides a structural basis for the ability of M3 to prevent the binding of CCL2 chemokines to the corresponding receptor. M3 binds to many inflammatory and chemotactic proteins (eotaxin, fractalkine, lymphotactine, RANTES etc.) and also interacts with some CXC chemokines (such as IL-8) as an immune evasion tool [3]. DNA vaccination of mice with an M3 expression plasmid yielded a partial protection lowering the infectious virus titer in the lungs of challenged animals [156]. The latter authors showed that M3 elicited a cytotoxic T cell mediated immune response starting during acute infection and persisting during latency.

A 9538 bp left-end sequence of strain MHV-68 encoding M2/M3 polypeptides is not present in certain MuHV-4 strains as demonstrated with the strain MHV-74 [124]. The left hand region starts with four virus specific ORFs (ORF1/M1/serpin, ORF2/M2, ORF3/M3, M4 and ORF4). From these, the ORF1/M1 displays similarity to *crmA* genes encoding the poxvirus SP1-2 proteins. The members of the serpin protein family are caspase-1 inhibitors [108]. The function of Ml was investigated by inserting a LacZ cassette into the M1 ORF to create a recombinant M1.LacZ virus. Despite of decreased splenic virus titers during acute infection (at 4-9 days p.i.) in immunocompetent as well as immunodeficient mice, the M1.LacZ recombinant had established latent infection comparable to that of w.t. virus, it exhibited in comparison with w.t. virus an approximately fivefold increase in the efficiency of reactivation. These results indicated that the establishment of latency was not determined by the extent of acute virus replication. Because the inactive precursors of IL-18 and IL-lβ are converted into active chemokines by caspase 1, the impairment of caspase 1 activity by MuHV-4 coded serpin protected against apoptosis. The Ml protein was also shown hampering the development of cytotoxic and NK cell responses via decreased IFNγ formation.

Herpesvirus saimiri 2 (HVS/SaHV-2) is a rhadinovirus, which infects squirrel monkeys without apparent disease [66], but in other monkey species (i.e. in marmosets) it may cause acute lymphomas and/or lymphoproliferative disease. It should not be confused with herpesvirus saimiri 1 (HVS-1/SaHV-1), which is an alphaherpesvirus enzootic in squirrel monkeys and related to the B herpesvirus, enzootic in rhesus monkeys [61]. The neural spread of HVS-1 caused myelitis as demonstrated in Balb/c mice [23]. To avoid any confusion, in this review we use the abbreviation HVS-2 for the gamma-2 rhadinovirus commonly referred to as HVS. There are three different subgroups of the lymphotropic HVS-2 rhadinovirus, entitled A, B and C [51]. Subgroup B strains do not cause disease in heterogenous species, such as adult marmosets; only type A and C subgroups transform the marmoset T lymphocytes in vitro [131]. The most oncogenic type C HVS-2 strains cause acute lymphoma in marmoset and tamarin monkeys as well as in rhesus and cynomolgus species. The T cell lymphomas developing in cynomolgus monkeys are widespread and pleomorphic, but all stain positively for the CD3 marker [68]. A good example of an oncogenic HVS-C is the isolate C-488, which may produce fulminant lymphoma in rhesus monkeys [20, 25]. The variations in question correlate with differences in the up most left hand region of the HVS genome, which contains the ORFs encoding proteins critical for oncogenicity [52]. Deletion of this region can abolish the transformation capacity of HVS-C for T cells [109], even when the oncogenic HVS-2 remains capable of productive replication [149]. The critical ORF1 gene, encodes a protein, originally termed saimiri transformation protein, STP [55], which is analogous to the KHSV Kl gene product LMP-1 of KSHV and/or to EBV LMP-1 (Table 4). All the three HVS-2 subtypes encode an STP, but only STPs type A and C activate the intracellular signaling pathway resulting in activation of NFκB or AP-1 transcription factors. Their transforming ability for rodent fibroblasts is related to a polypeptide region within the cytoplasmic domain of STP-C and/or STP-A, referred to as collagen-like [95]. While STP-C has a relative long compact collagen-like domain, the STP-A polypeptide shows short scattered stretches of collagen-like repeats located even in the N-terminal AD domain [191, 39]. Thus, the molecular structure of STPs points at the diverse nature of genes, which encode variably functioning oncogenes among different gammaherpesviruses [48]. While EBV LMP-1 cytoplasmic domain interacts with the TRAF adapter protein, which activates the JNK pathway or the Pi3K pathway, the K1 encoded LMP-l analog interacts with the ITAM adapter protein by means of the SH2 domain (see above). The STP-C collagen repeats associate with *Ras* protein, providing an interaction critical for transformation [96], while the STP-A activates other *src*-kinases [115]. Definitely, the former interaction is considerably more potent than the latter. In addition to this difference, in HVS-C genome, the ORF nearby to ORF1 encodes a protein called TIP (tyrosine kinase interacting protein)[206]. TIP interacts with the *src*-related kinases Lck [97] and Zap [88, 155], and with a novel cellular protein called TIP-associated protein (Tap) [205]. The co-expression of STP and TIP dramatically up-regulates NFκB mediated transcription. Retroviral plasmid constructs carrying STP-C and TIP genes were used for transfection of human lymphoblastic cell lines such as MOLT4, Jurkat and JCaM1, which otherwise would be refractory to DNA transfection [135]. Using this system a versatile expression of both essential HVS-2 oncogens could be achieved. It was confirmed that STP-C does not transform the cytotoxic T cells alone as previously suggested [18]. Both STP-C and TIP potently activate the tyrosine kinase signaling pathway via the Lck and/or Zap adaptor proteins. According to this model, the adaptors phosphorylate and activate the GDP/GTP exchanger (mainly the *Ras*-protein), which has a key position in the activation of NFκB transcription factor. As result of signaling, NFκB is released from the IKK blockade and translocated to nucleus either directly or via the activated MAKK pathway. The adaptor protein Lck can also phosphorylate Pi3K, which modulates the Ca^{2+}/calcitonin pathway activating transcription mediated by the nuclear factor of activated T cells, NFAT [191]. Neither STP-C nor TIP is required for HVS-2 persistence, but both are essential for transformation and lymphoma induction [55].

In the meantime there was shown that for the maintenance of latent infection in helper T cells and for their proliferation, a secreted glycoprotein specified by the HVS-2 ORF14 gene is at least as important as STP-C and TIP [202]. The 50 kDa glycoprotein in question binds to MHC class II molecules and stimulates T lymphocytes by a superantigen presentation mechanism, when interacting with the HLA-DR molecules on the surface of marmoset T cells. This binding was demonstrated using the strain C488 mutant deleted at ORF14 [57]. In similar manner acts the mouse mammary tumor virus (MMTV) superantigen, which stimulates T-cells via the class Vβ TCRs [82]. In the above-mentioned HVS deletion mutant the missing ORF14 gene was replaced with the MMTV superantigen gene. This insertion restored the previously abolished transformation capacity of the deletion mutant for marmoset T lymphocytes. In both, HVS-2 and KSHV, ORF71 and ORF72 encode a vFLICE [187] and a vCyclin [35], respectively (Table 3). In various cell types vFLICE inhibited DD-dependent apoptosis as mediated by *Fas*-ligand and/or TNFR.

Furthermore, the HVS-2 ORF73 encodes a LANA-1 homolog a vGPCR (IL-8R) homolog. The sequence homology of HVS-2 ORF73 and its KSHV counterpart is relatively limited, being confined to the AD, a short region of the N-terminus, the two nuclear signal localization domains and the C-terminus [81]. This suggests that HVS-2 LANA may have a similar role in latency maintenance as KSHV LANA has. The HVS-2 ORF73 gene product forms multimers and interacts with host cell mitotic chromosomes by its C-terminus [29]. In contrast, EBNA-1 binds to metaphase chromosomes via a human EBNA binding protein, EPB-2 [99]. The HVS-2 coded anti-apoptotic *vBcl-2* was shown to act at the level of mitochondrial stabilization and to inhibit apoptosis following Sendai virus infection, *Fas*-ligand activation or chemical induction [150, 50].

The best defined virokine encoded by HVS-2 is the IL-17 homolog, encoded by ORF13 [69]. Initially designated *ctla8,* it is specifically produced by HVS-infected T lymphocytes. The virus coded IL-17 was found to promote proliferation of T cells. It induces secretion of IL-6, IL-8, G-GSF (granulocyte colony stimulating factor) and prostaglandin E in fibroblasts, endothelium and stromal cells. The most striking alteration in this respect is CD2 hyper-reactivity, triggered by co-expression of the ligand CD58 [137]. The transformed T lymphocytes over-express great many markers such as CD2/LFA2 (leukocyte function antigen 2), CD3, CD4 or CD8, CD7, CD11a/LFA-1, CD45 (tyrosine phosphatase), CD54/ICAM-l (intercellular adhesion molecule) and CD58/LFA-3, a CD2 ligand [133]. Since HVS transformed T cells express at their surface a great number copies of the adhesion receptor (LFA-2) as well as of its ligand (LFA-3), their interaction with each other enhances autonomous growth [68]. A novel cellular gene, akt55 was identified when over expressed in transformed T cells (but not in B cells), encoding a secreted protein Akt155. This protein was classified as a new lymphokine, homologous to IL-10, which contributes to the transformed phenotype.

Summing up, similarly as in the case of MuHV-4, the HVS genome has two sets of genes involved in host cell transformation and/or promoting proliferation. The left 5'-end of the genome encodes STP and TIP and a complement (C3) inhibitor (CCP/ORF4). In addition, ORF2 encodes a dihydrofolate reductase (DHFR) and a formyl glycinamide ribotide amino transferase (FGARAT), both important for nucleotide metabolism. The right 3'-end encodes the set of genes involved in host cell proliferation, such as vFLIP/ORF71, vCyclin/ORF72 and vGPCR/ORF74. It also encodes the above-mentioned LANA-1/ORF73 homolog. Also the middle of HVS genome encodes proteins, which enhance T cell proliferation, such as vIL-17/ORF13, the superantigen (*vSag*/ORF14) and the apoptosis inhibitor *vBcl-2* [98]. Their products are cellular signaling pathway homologs and immune response modulators, which contribute to host cell transformation by different mechanisms but in a manner achieving synergic effect activating proliferation and deregulation of growth control.

Using serological techniques, antibodies to EBV capsid antigen (VCA) were found in many Old World non-human primates, but not in the New World primates. Later on, cell lines expressing VCA were established from lymphomas occurring in a baboon colony [55] similar EBNA positive lines were established from lymphocytes of chimpanzees (Gerber et al., 1976; [76], gorillas [152], orangutans [162] and macaque species [24]. As soon as the

EBV genome was cloned, about 40% homology was found between this genome and that of the rhesus EBV-like lymphocryptovirus (LCV), also called herpesvirus papio 1 or Cercopithecine herpesvirus 12. The EBV-like LCV should not be confused with the monkey alphaherpesvirus, the Cercopithecine herpesvirus 16, also called *Herpesvirus papio 2* [173]. The most variable EBV-like LCV regions encode the EBNA-3 proteins, LMP-1 and LMP-2, respectively [200]. The rhesus and baboon LCV LMP-1 can activate NFκB and induce ICAM-1 synthesis [72]. It has a preserved domain for interaction with TNFR associated factor 3 (TRAF3) and the C-terminal cytoplasmic domain for interaction with the TNFR associated death domain (TRADD) adaptor molecule [91]. Finally the LCV LMP-1 can activate the transcription factor AP-1 suggesting that the c-jun N-terminal kinase (JNK) pathway becomes activated in its presence [37]. The baboon and rhesus LCV LMP-2A homolog was also identified according to a conserved immunoreceptor tyrosine activated motif (ITAM) and careful analysis demonstrated the presence of LMP-2B transcripts [167]. The LCV EBNA-1 is one of most conserved ORFs within the latent LCV sequence found in LCV-infected cell lines [204], while the EBNA-2 much less conserved [158]. The interaction with transcription factor RBP-Jκ – important for B cell immortalization – has remained conserved. Recently, Ramer et al. [161] noted that the high incidence of B cell lymphomas in common marmosets (*Callitrix jacchus*) might be associated an EBV-like lymphocryptovirus. The new virus was isolated from tumor tissue [37] and designated *Callitrichine herpesvirus* 3 (CalHV-3). At least three CalHV-3-specific genes, C1 – C3 were detected. From these, C1 is homologous to K1/LMP-l of KSHV, C2 encodes a putative glycoprotein and C3 is a positional analog of EBNA-3 gene family [200]. An EBNA-1 homolog was also identified within the CalHV-3 genome. It comes from these findings, that also the New World non-human primates may be infected with a lymphocryptovirus, which might induce lymphoproliferation.

To make the list of non-human primate rhadinoviruses complete – in addition to the New World monkey rhadinoviruses such as HVS-2 and *Herpesvirus ateles* – rhadinoviruses infecting Old World monkeys should be mentioned. The unic long segment of RRV has at least 84 ORFs organized in an order similar to KSHV with exception of the dihydrofolate reductase gene [4]. All the KSHV genes have RRV homologs except of K3, K5, K7 and K12 (see Table 4). The RRV26-95 genome contains one MIP-1 and eight vIRF genes as compared to three MIP and four vIRF genes within the KSHV genome. With on exception, the ORFs of the isolate 29-95 are homologous to the genome of isolate 17577; they differed in a single ORF not found in the RRV17577 genome. The rhesus rhadinovirus RRV/CeHV-17 and the novel recently isolated homologous rhadinoviruses from macaques were in general termed RV2mac. Their wide sequence homology confirms that RV2/RRV is the main gammaherpevirus naturally infecting macaques. Furthermore, RRV-related, but still more distinct sequences (RVlmac) were amplified by PCR from rhesus monkeys suffering of retroperitoneal fibromatosis. In addition, PCR amplifications revealing highly related but still distinct DNA sequences were found in African green monkeys (RVlagm as well as RV2agm) and in hominoid apes (RV1pan as well as Rv2pan). Phylogenetic analyses showed at least two rhadinovirus linages in primates, namely HHV-8 and the newly discovered RV1 sequences on one hand and the related RV2/RRV/CeHV-17 classical isolates and the novel

RV-2 sequences on other hand. Summing up, however, the current evidence still suggests that both primate rhadinovirus linages are related to HHV-8 [47].

6. Conclusion

The development of lymphoproliferative disease and/or sarcoma-like malignancies associated with gammaherpesvirus infections was found related to unusual genes believed to represent cellular gene homologs. The proteins specified by these genes fall into three categories. One can recognize pirated and modified cellular gene products, which mimick the function of cyclins regulating cell division. Other viral oncogenes, such as LMP-1/STP activate the NFκB responsive synthesis of enzymes needed for cellular DNA synthesis. Alternative signaling pathways become activated, which generate additional transcription factors (*c-jun*/AP1). Further powerful tools for the immortalization of host cells are anti-apoptotic proteins. The gammaherpesvirus coded *Bcl-2* is a good example. In case of rhadinoviruses the effect of v*Bcl-2* may be combined with that of vFLIP (Fas-associated death domain-like inhibitory protein), which is a caspase 1 antagonist. The third group of gammaherpesvirus genes of cellular origin encodes immunomodulator proteins such as vMIP, vIRF, viral interleukins and/or viral interleukin receptors (for example vGPCR). Despite of the rich oncogenic potential of gammaherpesviruses, they cause tumors relatively rarely. One reason for this is the immune surveillance by cytotoxic T cells, which may be eliminated or at least hampered during immunosuppression. In AIDS patients, the HIV specific transactivator proteins (such as *Tat*) actively promote the transcription of early regulatory genes within the KSHV genome. An important condition promoting the action of gammaherpesvirus oncogenic proteins is the continuous growth stimulation through physiological receptors, such as BCR (in infected B cells) and/or TCR (especially in infected helper T cells). Under the influence of cytokines, chemokines and/or due to co-infection with other viruses, especially with lentiviruses such as HIV-1, the latent gammaherpesvirus genome becomes activated to express a full set of latency-associated proteins. These oncogenic proteins, when abundantly expressed in non-productively infected B cells, epithelial or endothelial cells, accelerate the transformation escaping anti-oncoprotein control.

Acknowledgments

This work was supported by the Slovak Research and Development Agency under the contract No. APVV-51-005005 and the joint grant agency of Slovak Ministry of Education and Slovak Academy of Sciences VEGA (#2/7096/27 and #2/7095/27)

References

[1] Albrecht, JC; Nicholas; Biller, D; Cameron, KR; Biesinger, B; Newman, C; Wittmann, S; Craxton, MA; Coleman, H; Fleckenstein, B; Honess, RW. Primary structure of the *herpesvirus saimiri* genome. *J. Virol.,* 1992, 66, 5047-5058.

[2] Albrecht, JC. Primary structure of the *herpesvirus ateles* genome. *J. Virol.,* 2000, 74, 1033-1037.

[3] Alcami, A. Structural basis of the herpesvirus M3-chemokine interaction. *Trends in Microbiol,* 2003, 11, 191-192.

[4] Alexander, AL; Danekamp, L; Knapp, A; Auerbach, MR; Damania, B; Desrosiers, RC. The primary sequence of rhesus monkey rhadinovirus isolate RRV26-95: sequence similarities to Kaposi's sarcoma-associated herpesvirus and rhesus monkey rhadinovirus isolate 17477. *J. Virol.*, 1999, 75, 3040-3053.

[5] Allday, MJ; Farrel, PJ. Epstein-Barr virus nuclear antigen EBNA3C -6 expression maintains the level of latent membrane protein 1 in G1-arrested cells. *J. Virol.,* 1994, 68, 3491-3498.

[6] Altmann, M. and Hammerschmidt, W. Epstein-Barr virus provides a new paradigm: a requirement for the immediate inhibition of apoptosis. *PLoS Biology*, 2005, 12, 2148-2157.

[7] Ambinder, RF; Shah, WA; Rawlings, DR; Hayward, GS; Hayward, SD. Definition of the sequence requirements for binding of the EBNA1 protein to its palindromic target sites in Epstein-Barr virus DNA. *Cell,* 1990, 58, 527-535.

[8] Ambinder, RF; Mullen, MA; Chang, YN; Hayward, GS; Hayward, SD. Functional domains of Epstein Barr virus nuclear antigen EBNA1. *J. Virol.,* 1991, 65, 1466-1478.

[9] An, FQ; Compitello, N; Horwitz, M; Sramkoski, M; Knudsen, ES; Renner, R. The latency-associated nuclear antigen of Kaposi's sarcoma associated herpesvirus modulates cellular gene expression and protects lymphoid cells from p16INK4A-induced cell arrest. *J. Biol. Chem.* 2005, 280, 3862-3874.

[10] Baer, R; Bankier, AT; Biggin, MD; Deininger, PL; Farrell, PJ; Gibson, TJ; Hatfull, G; Hudson, GS; Satchwell, SC; Seguin, C; Tufnell, PS; Barrell, BG. DNA sequence and expression the B95-8 Epstein-Barr virus genome. *Nature*, 1984, 310, 207-211.

[11] Baichwal, V. R. and Sugden, B. Transformation of Balb/c 3T3 cells by the BNLF-1 gene of Epstein-Barr virus. *Oncogene*, 1988, 2, 461-467.

[12] Ballestas, ME; Chatis, PA; Kaye. KM. Efficient persistence of extrachromosomal KSHV DNA mediated by latency-associated nuclear antigen. *Science*, 1999, 284, 641-644.

[13] Barbera, AJ; Chodaparambil, JV; Kelley'Clarke, B; Joukov, V; Walter, JC; Luger, K; Kaye, KM. The nucleosomal surface as docking station for Kaposi's sarcoma herpesvirus LANA. *Science*, 2006, 311, 856-860.

[14] Beaulieu, B.L., and Sullivan, J.L. (2002). Epstein-Barr virus. In Fichman, D.D, Whitley, R.J., and Hayden, F.G. (eds.): *Clinical Virology*, (2nd edition pp 479-494), Washington, ASM Press.

[15] Bellows, DS; Chau, BN; Lee, P; Lazebnik, Y; Burns, WH; Hardwick, JM. Antiapoptotic herpesvirus Bcl-2 homologs escape caspase-mediated conversion to proapoptotic proteins. *J. Virol.*, 2000, 74, 5024-5031.

[16] Bellows, DS; Howel, M; Pearson, G; Hazlewood, SA; Handwick, JM. Epstein-Barr virus BALF1 is a Bcl-2 like antagonist of the herpesvirus antiapoptotic Bcl-2 proteins. *J. Virol.*, 2002, 76, 2469-2479.

[17] vanBerkel, V; Preiter, K; Virgin IV, HW; Speck, SH. Identification and initial characterization of the murine gammaherpesvirus 68 gene M3, encoding an abundantly secreted protein. *J. Virol.*, 1999, 73, 5110-5122.

[18] Berend, KR; Jung JU' Boyle, TJ; DiMayo, JM; Mungal, SA; Desrosiers, RC; Lyerly, HK. Phenotypic and functional consequences of *Herpesvirus saimiri* infection of human CD8 cytototoxic lymphocytes. *J. Virol.*, 1993, 67, 6317-6321.

[19] Bieleski, L. and Talbot, S. Kaposi's sarcoma-associated herpesvirus vCyclin Open reading frame contains an internal ribosomal entry site. *J. Virol.*, 2001, 75, 1864-1869.

[20] Biesinger, B; Muller-Fleckenstein, I; Simmer, G; Lang, S; Whittmann, E; Desrosiers, RC; Fleckenstein, B. Stable growth transformation of human T lymphocytes by herpesvirus saimiri. *Proc. Natn. Acad. Sci. USA*, 1992, 89, 3116-3119.

[21] Blackman, MA; Flano, E; Usherwood, E; Woodland, DL. Murine gamma-herpesvirus-68: a mouse model for infectious mononucleosis? *Mol. Med. Today,* 2000, 6, 488-490.

[22] Blaškovič, D; Stančeková, M; Svobodová, J; Mistríková, J. Isolation of five strains of herpes viruses from two species of free living small rodents. *Acta virol*, 1980, 24, 468-473.

[23] Breshears, MA; Eberle, R; Ritchie, JW. Characterization of gross and histological lesions in Balb/c mice experimentally infected with herpesvirus saimiri 1 (HVS 1). *J. comp Pathol.*, 2001, 125, 25-33.

[24] Broker, JE; Tiederman, KH; Bornkamm, GW; zurHausen, H. Characterization of an EBV-like virus from African green monkey lymphoblasts. *Virology*, 1980, 101, 291-295.

[25] Broker, BM; Tsygankov, AY; Muller-Fleckenstein, I; Guse, AH; Chitaev, NA; Biesinger, B; Fleckenstein, B; Emmrich, F. Immortalization of human T cell clones by *Herpesvirus saimiri*. *J. Immunol.*, 1993, 151, 1184-1192.

[26] Bublot, M; Lomonte, P; Lequarre, AS; Albrecht, JC; Nicholas, J; Fleckenstein; B; Pastoret, PP.; Thiry, E. Genetic relationships between bovine herpesvirus 4 and the gammaherpesviruses Epstein-Barr virus and *herpesvirus saimiri*. *Virology*, 1992, 190, 654-665.

[27] Burkhardt, AL; Bolem, JB; Kieff, E; Longnecker, R. An Epstein-Barr virus transformation-associated membrane protein interacts with *src* family tyrosine kinases. *J. Virol.*, 1992, 66, 5161-5167.

[28] Burysek, L, Yeow, WS, Lubyova, B, Kellum, M, Schafer, SL, Huang, IQ, Pitha, PM: Functional analysis of human herpesvirus 8-encoded viral interferon regulatory factor I and its association with cellular regulatory factors and p300. *J. Virol,* 1999, 73, 7334-7342.

[29] Calderwood, MA, Hall, KT, Matthews, DA, Whitehouse, A: The herpesvirus saimiri ORF73 gene interacts with host cell mitotic chromosomes and self-associates via C-terminus. *J. Gen. Virol.,* 2004, 85, 147-153.

[30] Caldwell, RG; Wilson, JB; Anderson, SJ; Longnecker, R. Epstein-Barr virus LMP2A drives B cell development and survival on in vitro infection in the absence of normal B cell receptor signals. *Immunity*, 1998, 9, 405-411.

[31] Cannon, JS; Nicholas, J; Orenstein, JM; Mann RB; Murray, PG; Browning, PJ; diGuiseppe, JA; Cesarman, E; Hayward, GS; Ambinder, RF. Heterogeneity of viral IL-6 expression in HHV-8 associated disease. *J. Infect. Dis.*, 1999, 180, 824-828.

[32] Cannon, M, Cesarman, E, Boshoff, C. KSHV G-protein-coupled receptor inhibits lytic gene transcription in primary-effusion lymphoma cells via p21-mediated inhibition of Cdk2. *Blood*, 2006, 107, 277-284.

[33] Chabot-Fletcher, M. Cellular signaling to NFκB: role in inflammation and therapeutic promise, pp. In: Letts, G.L., and Morgan, D.W. (eds.): *Inflammatory process: Molecular mechanisms and therapeutic opportunities*, Birkhauser; Basel, 2000, pp 23-38.

[34] Chang, Y; Cesarman, E; Pessin, MS; Lee, F; Culpepper, J; Knowles, DM; Moore, PS. Identification of herpesvirus-like DNA sequences in AIDS-associated Kaposi's sarcoma. *Science*, 1994, 266, 1865-1869.

[35] Chang, Y; Moore, PS; Talbot, SJ. Cyclin encoded by KS herpesvirus. *Nature*, 1996, 382, 410-11.

[36] Chatterjee, M; Osborne, J; Bestetti G; Chang, Y; Moore, PS. Viral IL-6-induced cell proliferation and immune evasion of interferon activity. *Science*, 2002, 298, 1432-1435.

[37] Cho, Y; Ramer, J; Rivailler, P; Quink, C; Garber, RI,; Beier, D; Wang, F. Epstein Barr related herpesvirus from marmoset lymphomas. *Proc. Natn. Acad Sci. USA*, 2001, 98, 1224-1229.

[38] Choi, JK; Lee, BS; Shim, SN; Li, M; Jung, JU. Identification of the novel K15 gene at the rightmost end of the Kaposi's sarcoma associated herpesvirus genome. *J. Virol.,* 1999, 74, 436-446.

[39] Choi, JK; Lee, BS; Shim, SN; Li M; Jung JU. Identification of the novel K15 gene at the rightmost end of the Kaposi´s sarcoma genome. *J. Virol.*, 2000, 74, 436-446.

[40] Chugh, P; Matta, H; Schaumus, S; Zachariac, S; Kumar, A; Richardson, JA; Smith, AL; Chaudhary, PM. Constitutive NFκB activation, normal Fas-induced apoptosis and increased incidence of lymphoma in human herpesvirus 8 K13 transgenic mice. *Proc. Natn. Acad. Sci. USA,* 2005, 102, 12885-12890.

[41] Cohen, JI; Wang, F; Manninck, J; Kieff, E. Epstein-Barr virus nuclear protein 2 is a key determinant of lymphocyte transformation. *Proc. Natn. Acad. Sci. USA* 1989, 86, 9558-9562.

[42] Cohen, J.I. A region of herpes simplex virus VP16 can substitute for a transforming domain of Epstein-Barr virus nuclear protein 2. *Proc. Natn. Acad. Sci. USA*, 1992, 9, 8030-8034.

[43] Cohen, BD; Goldstein, DJ; Rutlege, L. Wass, WC; Lowy, DR; Schlegel, R; Schiller, JT.Transformation specific interaction of the bovine papillomavirus E5 oncoprotein

with the platelet derived growth factor receptor domain and the epidermal growth factor receptor cytoplasmic domain. *J. Virol.*, 1993, 67, 5303-5311.

[44] Craighead, J. E. Epstein-Barr virus (EBV). In: *Pathology and Pathogenesis of Human Viral Disease*. San Diego, Academic Press, 2000, pp.117-146.

[45] Craighead, J. E. Kaposi sarcoma-associated herpesvirus (KSHV, HHV-8). In: *Pathology and Pathogenesis of Human Viral Disease*. San Diego, Academic Press, 2000, pp. 171-186.

[46] Damania, B; Cho Joong-Kook; Jung, JU. Signaling activities of gammaherpesvirus membrane proteins. *J. Virol.*, 2000, 74, 1593-1601.

[47] Damania, B; Desrosiers, RC. *Simian homologues of human herpesvirus* 8. Phil Trans R Soc London B, 2001, 356, 535-543.

[48] Damania, B. Oncogenic gammaherpesviruses: comparison of viral proteins involved in tumorigenesis. *Nature* (Reviews), 2004, 2, 656-668.

[49] Davis, MA; Sturzl, MA; Blasig, C; Schreier, A; Gui, HG; Reitz, M; Opalenik, SR; Browning PJ. Expression of human herpesvirus 8-encoded cyclin D in Kaposi´s sarcoma spindle cells. *J. Natn. Cancer Inst.* 1997, 89, 1868-1874.

[50] Derfuss, T; Fickenscher, H; Kraft, MS; Henning, G; Lengenfelder, D; Fleckenstein, B; Meinl, E. Antiapoptotic activity of the *Herpesvirus saimiri*-encoded Bcl-2 homolog: stabilization of mitochondria and inhibition of caspase-3-like activity. *J. Virol.,* 1998, 72, 5897-5904.

[51] Desrosiers, R.C and Falk, L.A. *Herpesvirus saimiri* strain variability. *J. Virol.*, 1982, 43, 352-356.

[52] Desrosiers, RC; Baker, A; Kamine, J; Falk, LA; Hunt, RD; King, NW. A region of the *Herpesvirus saimiri* genome required for oncogenicity. *Science*, 1985, 228, 184-187.

[53] Desrosiers, RC; Sasseville, VG; Czajak, SC; Zhang, X; Mansfield, KG; Kaur, A; Johnson, RP; Lackner, AA; Jung, JU. A herpesvirus of rhesus monkeys related to the human Kaposi´s sarcoma-associated herpesvirus. *J. Virol.*, 1997, 71, 9764-9769.

[54] Dittmer, D; Lagunoff, M; Renne, R; Staskus, K; Haase, A; Ganem, D. A cluster of latently expressed genes in Kaposi's sarcoma –associated herpesvirus. *J. Virol.,* 1998 72, 8309-8315.

[55] Djatchenko, AG; Kakubava, VV; Lapin, BA; Agrba, VZ; Yakovleva, LA; Samolchuk, EI. Continuous lymphoblastoid suspension cultures from cells of haemopoetic organs of baboons with malignant lymphoma – biological characterization and properties of the herpes virus associated with culture cells. *Exp. Pathol.,* 1976, 12, 163-168.

[56] Duboise, SM; Guo, J; Czajak, S; Desrosiers RC; JUng, J. STP and TIP are essential for *Herpesvirus saimiri* oncogenicity. *J. Virol.,* 1998, 72, 1808-1813.

[57] Duboise, M; Guo, H; Czajak, S; Lee, H; Veazey, R; Desroisiers, RC; Jung, JU. A role for herpesvirus saimiri orf14 in transformation and persistent infection. *J. Virol.,* 1998 72, 6770-6776.

[58] Dutia, BM; Clarke, CJ; Allen, DJ; Nash, AA. Pathological changes in the spleens of gamma interferon receptor-deficient mice infected with murine gammaherpesvirus: a role for CD8 T cells. *J. Virol.,* 1997, 71, 4278-4283.

[59] vanDyk, LF; Hess, JL; Katz, JD; Jacoby, M; Speck, SH; Virgin IV, HI. The murine gammaherpesvirus 68 v-cyclin is a oncogene that promotes cell cycle progression in primary lymphocytes. *J. Virol.* 1999, 73, 5119-5122.

[60] vanDyk, LF; Virgin IV, HW; Speck, SH. The murine gammaherpesvirus 68 v-Cyclin is a critical regulator of reactivation from latency. *J. Virol.*, 2000, 74, 7451-7461.

[61] Eberle, R, Hilliard, J. Review: the simian herpesviruses. *Infect Agents and Disease* 1995, 4, 55-70.

[62] Ellis, M; Chew, YP; Fallis, L. Degradation of p27KIP *cdk* inhibitor triggered by Kaposi's sarcoma virus cyclin/cdk6 complex. *EMBO J.,* 1999, 18, 644-653.

[63] Ensser, A; Pflanz, R; Fleckenstein, B. Primary structure of the alcephaline herpesvirus 1 genome. *J. Virol.,* 1997, 71, 6517-6525.

[64] Ensoli, B; Buonaguro, L; Barrilari, G; Fiorelli, V; Gendelman, R; Morgan, RA; Wingfield, P; Gallo, RC. Release, uptake and effects of extracellular HIV-Tat protein in induction of Kaposi's sarcoma. *J. Virol,* 1993, 67, 277-287.

[65] Ensoli, B; Sturzl, M; Monini, P. Cytokine-mediated growth promotion of Kaposi's sarcoma and primary effusion lymphoma. *Cancer Biol.,* 2000, 10, 367-381.

[66] Falk, L; Wolfe, L; Deinhardt, F. Isolation of *herpesvirus saimiri* from blood of squirrel monkeys (*Saimiri sciurcius*). *J. Natn. Cancer Inst.,* 1972, 48, 1499-1505.

[67] Falk, L; Deinhardt, F; Nonoyama, M; Wolfe, LG; Bergholz, C. Properties of a baboon lymphotropic herpesvirus related to Epstein-Barr virus. *Int. J. Cancer*, 1976, 18, 798-807.

[68] Fickenscher, H; Bokel, C; Knappe, A; Biesinger, B; Meinl, E; Fleischer, B; Fleckenstein, B; Broker, BM. Functional phenotype of transformed human alphabeta and gammadelta T cells determined by different subgroup C strains of *Herpesvirus saimiri*. *J. Virol.,* 1997, 71, 2252-2263.

[69] Fickenscher, H. and Fleckenstein, B. Herpesvirus saimiri. *Phil. Trans R Soc.* (Lond) B 2001, 356, 545-576.

[70] Fowler, P; Marques, S; Simas, JP; Efstathiou, S. ORF73 of murine herpesvirus-68 is critical for the establishment and maintenance of latency. *J. Gen. Virol.*, 2003, 84, 3405-3416.

[71] Fowler, P. and Efstathiou, S. Vaccine potential of a murine gammaherpesvirus-68 mutant deficient for ORF73. *J. Gen. Virol.*, 2004, 85, 609-613.

[72] Franken, M; Annis, B; Ali, AN; Wang, F. 5'-coding and regulatory region sequence divergence with conserved function of the Epstein-Barr, virus LMP-2A homolog in Herpesvirus papio. *J. Virol.,* 1995, 69, 8011-8019.

[73] Friborg, Jr; Kong, W; Hottiger, MO; Nabel, GJ. p53 inhibition of by the LANA protein of KSHV protects against cell death. *Nature*, 1999, 402, 889-894.

[74] Gahn, T.A. and Schildkraut, C.L. The Epstein-Barr virus origin of replication, oriP, contains both the initiation and termination sites of DNA replication. *Cell*, 1989, 58, 527-535.

[75] Garber, AC; Hu, J; Renne, R. Latency-associated nuclear antigen (LANA) cooperatively binds to two sites within the terminal repeat, and both sites contribute to the ability of LANA to suppress transcription and to facilitate DNA replication. *J. Biol. Chem.,* 2002, 277, 27401-27411.

[76] Gerber, P; Pritchett, RF; Kieff, ED. Antigens and DNA of a chimpanzee agent related to Epstein-Barr virus. *J. Virol.,* 1976, 19, 1090-1099.

[77] Gompels UA; Nicholas, J; Lawrence, G. The DNA sequence of human heroesvirus 6: structure, coding content and genome evolution. *Virology*, 1995, 209, 29-51.

[78] Grundhoff, A. and Ganem, D. Mechanisms governing expression of the v-FLIP gene of Kaposi´s sarcoma-associated herpesvirus. *J. Virol.,* 2001, 75, 1857-1863.

[79] Gires, O; Zimber-Strobl, U; Gonnella, R; Ueffing, M; Marschall, G; Zridler, R; Pich, D; Hammerschmidt, W. Latent membrane protein of Epstein-Barr virus mimics a constitutively active receptor molecule. *EMBO J.*, 1997. 16, 6131-6140.

[80] Guasparri, I; Keller, SA; Cesarman, E. KSHV vFLIP is essential for the survival of infected lymphoma cells. *J. Exp. Med.,* 2004, 199, 993-1003.

[81] Hall, K; Giles, T; Goodwin, MS; Calderwood, MA; Markham, AF; Whitehouse, A. Characterization of the herpesvirus saimiri ORF73 gene product. *J. Gen. Virol.*, 2000, 81, 2653-2658.

[82] Held, W; Wanders, GA; Shakhov, A; Scarpellino, L; Acha-Obea, H; MacDonald, HR. Superantigen-induced immunone stimulation amplifies mouse mammary tumor virus infection and allows virus transmission. *Cell,* 1993, 74, 529-540.

[83] Henkel, T; Link PD; Hayward, SD; Peterson, MG. Mediation of Epstein Barr virus EBNA-2 transactivation by recombination signal binding protein J kappa. *Science*, 1994, 265, 92-95.

[84] Henessy, K; Fennewald, SW; Hummel, M. A membrane protein encoded by Epstein-Barr virus. *Proc. Natn. Acad. Sci. USA,* 1985, 985, 5944-5948.

[85] Heskett, R. Bcl-2. In: *The Oncogene Facts Book*, Academic Press, Harcourt Brace and Company Publ., London, 1995, pp. 52-56.

[86] Hoge, AT; Hendrickson, SB; Burns, WH. Murine gammaherpesvirus 68 cyclin D homologue is required for efficient reactivation from latency. *J. Virol.,* 2000, 74, 7016-7023.

[87] Horner, D; Lewis, M; Farell, PJ. Novel hypothesis for the roles of EBNA-1 and BHFR1 in EBV-related cancers. *Intervirology*, 1995, 38, 195-205.

[88] Howe, LR. and Weiss, A. Multiple kinases mediate T cell receptor signaling. *Trends Biochem Sci.,* 1995, 20, 59-64.

[89] Huaxin, S. and Robertson, E. Kaposi's sarcoma-associated herpesvirus encoded latency-associated nuclear antigen induces chromosomal instability through inhibition of p53 function. *J. Virol.,* 2006, 80, 697-709.

[90] Irusta, PM; Chen, YB; Hardwick, JM. Viral modulators of cell death provide new links to old pathways. *Curr. Opinion Cell Biol.,* 2003, 15, 700-7005.

[91] Izumi, KM and. Kief, ED. The Epstein-Barr virus oncogenic product latent membrane protein engages the tumor necrosis factor death domain protein to mediate B lymphocyte growth transformation and activate NFκB. *Proc. Natn. Acad. Sci. USA*, 1997, 94, 12592-12597.

[92] Jacoby, MA; Virgin IV, HW; Speck, SH. Disruption of the M2 gene of murine gammaherpesvirus 68 alters splenic latency following intranasal, but not intraperitoneal inoculation. *J. Virol.*, 2002, 76, 1790-1801.

[93] Jeong, J; Papin, J; Dittmer, D. Differential regulation of the overlapping Kaposi's sarcoma-associated herpesvirus vGCR (orf74) and LANA (orf73) promoters. *J. Virol.* 2001, 75, 1798-1807.

[94] Johanessen, I. and Crawford, DH. In vivo models for Epstein-Barr virus (EBV-associated) B cell lymphoproliferative disease (BLPD). *Rev. Med. Virol.,* 1999, 9, 263-277.

[95] Jung, JU; Trimble, UJ; King, NW; Biesinger, B; Fleckenstein, BW; Desrosiers, RE. Identification of transforming genes of subgroup A and C strains of *herpesvirus saimiri*. *Proc. Natn. Acad. Sci. USA*, 1991, 88, 7051-7055.

[96] Jung, J.U. and Desrosiers, R.C. Distinct functional domains of STP-C488 of *herpesvirus saimiri*. *Virology*, 1994, 204, 751-758.

[97] Jung, JU; Lang, SM; Jun, T; Roberts, TM; Veilette, A; Desrosiers, RC. Downregulation of Lck-mediated signal transduction by *Tip* of *herpesvirus saimiri*. J Virol, 1995, 69, 7814-7822.

[98] Jung, JU; Choi, J-K; Ensser, A; Biesinger, B. Herpesvirus saimiri as a model for gammaherpesvirus oncogenesis. *Cancer Biology*, 1999, 9, 231-239.

[99] Kapoor, P. and Frappier, L. EBNA-1 partitions of Epstein-Barr virus plasmids in yeast cells by attaching to human EBNA-1 binding protein 2 on mitotic chromosomes. *J. Virol.*, 2003, 77, 6946-6956.

[100] Kasolo, FC; Monze, M; Obel, N; Anderson, RA; French, C; Gompels, UA. Sequence analyses of human herpesvirus 8 strains from both African human immunodeficiency virus-negative and -positive childhood endemic Kaposi's sarcoma show a close relationship with strains identified in febrile children and variation in the K1 glycoprotein. *J. Gen. Virol.,* 1998, 79, 3055-3065.

[101] Kawahara, A; Kobayashi, T; Nagata, S. Inhibition of Fas-induced apoptosis by *Bcl-2*. *Oncogene*, 1998, 19, 2549-2554.

[102] Kedes, DH; Lagunoff, M; Renne, R; Ganem, D. Identification of the gene encoding the major latency-associated nuclear antigen of the Kaposi's sarcoma-associated herpesvirus. J Clin Invest, 1997, 100, 2602-2610.

[103] Keller, SA; Schattner, EJ; Cesarman, E. Inhibition of NFkB induces apoptosis of KSHV-infected primary effusion lymphoma cells. *Blood*, 2000, 96, 2537-2542.

[104] Kieff, E., and Rickinson, A. (2001). Epstein-Barr virus and its replication In: Knipe, D.M., and Howley, P.M. (eds.): *Field's Virology*, (4th edition, pp. 2511-2574) Philadelphia, Lippincott Williams and Wilkins.

[105] Kim, AL; Maher, MA; Hayman, JB. An imperfect correlation between DNA replication activity of Epstein Bar virus nuclear antigen and binding to the nuclear import receptor, Rcb/importin alpha. *Virology*, 1997, 39, 340-351.

[106] King, P. and Goodbourn, S. The β-interferon promoter responds to priming through multiple independent regulatory elements. *J. Biol. Chem.* 1994, 269, 30609-30615.

[107] Kliche, S; Nagel, W; Kremmer, E; Atyler, C; Ege, A; Knorr, T; Koszinovsky, U; Kolanus, W; Haas, J. Signaling by human herpesvirus 8 kapopsin A through direct membrane recruitment of cytohesin-I. *Mol. Cell*, 2001, 7, 833-843.

[108] Komiyama, T; Ray, CA; Pickup, DJ. Inhibition of interleukin-1 beta converting enzyme by the cowpox virus serpin *crmA*: an example of cross-class inhibition. *J. Biol. Chem.,* 1994, 269, 19331-19337.

[109] Koomy, JM; Mulder, C; Burghoff, RL; Fleckenstein, B; Desrosiers, RC. Deletion of DNA sequences in a immunogenic variant of herpesvirus saimiri. *J. Virol.,* 1984, 50, 662-665.

[110] Krithivas, A; Fujimuro, M; Weidner, M; Young, DB; Hayward, SD. Human herpesvirus 8 LANA interacts with proteins of the mSin3 correpressor complex and negatively regulates Epstein-Barr virus gene expression in dually infected PEL cells. *J. Virol.* 2000, 74, 9637-9645.

[111] Krithivas, A; Fujimoro, M; Weidner, M; Young, DB; Hayward, SD. Protein interactions targeting the latency-associated herpesvirus to cell chromosomes. *J. Virol.,* 2002, 76, 11596-11604.

[112] Kuppers, R. Mechanisms of B cell lymphoma pathogenesis. *Nature Reviews,* 2005, 5, 251-262.

[113] Lagunoff, MR; Majett, R; Weiss, A; Ganem, D. Deregulated signal transduction by the K1 gene product of Kaposi's sarcoma-associated herpesvirus. *Proc. Natn. Acad. Sci. USA,* 1999, 96, 5704-5709.

[114] Lan, K; Kuppers, DA; Verma, SC; Robertson, ES. Kaposi's sarcoma-associated herpesvirus-encoded latency-associated nuclear antigen inhibits lytic replication by targeting Rta: a potential mechanism for virus-associated control of latency. *J. Virol.,* 2004, 78, 6585-6594.

[115] Lee, H; Trimble, JJ; Yoon, DW; Regier, D; Desrosiers, RC; Jung, JU. Genetic variation of *herpesvirus saimiri* subgroup A transforming protein and its association with cellular *src*. *J. Virol.* 1997, 71, 3817-3825.

[116] Lee, H; Gun, J; Li, M; Choi, JK; DeMaria, M; Rosenyweig, M; Jung, JU. Identification of an immunoreceptor tyrosine-based activation motif of K1 transforming protein of Kaposi's sarcoma –associated herpesvirus. *Mol. Cell Biol.,* 1998, 18, 5219-5228.

[117] Lee, H; Veazey, R; Williams, K; Li, M; Guo, J; Neipel, F; Fleckensteinm, B; Lackner, A; Desrosiers, RC; Jung, JU. Deregulation of cell growth by the K1 gene of Kaposi's sarcoma-associated herpesvirus. *Nat. Med.,* 1998, 4, 435-440.

[118] Lee, BJ; Koszinowski, UH; Sarawar, SR; Adler, H. A gammaherpesvirus G-protein receptor homolog is required for increased viral replication in response to chemokines and efficient reactivation from latency. *J. Immunol.*, 2003b, 170, 243-251.

[119] Leight, E.R. and Sugden, B. EBNA1: a protein pivotal to latent infection by Epstein-Barr virus. *Rev. Med. Viro*l., 2000, 10, 83-100.

[120] Liang, X; Shin, YC; Means, RE; Jung, JU. Inhibition of interferon-mediated activity by murine gammaherpesvirus 68 latency-associated M2 protein. *J. Virol.*, 2004, 78, 12416-12427.

[121] Liebowitz, D; Wang, D; Kieff E. Orientation and patching of the latent infection membrane protein encoded by Epstein-Barr virus. *J. Virol.,* 1986, 58, 233-237.

[122] Lim, C; Gwack, Y; Hwang, S; Kim, S; Choe, J. The transcriptional activity of cAMP response element-binding protein is modulated by the latency-associated nuclear antigen of Kaposi's sarcoma herpesvirus. *J. Biol. Chem.,* 2001, 276, 31016-31022.

[123] Lubyova, B. and Pitha, PM. Characterization of a novel human herpesvirus 8-encoded protein, vIRF3 that shows homology to viral and cellular interferon regulatory factors. *J. Virol.,* 2000, 74, 8194-8201.

[124] Macrae, AI; Dutia, BM; Milligan, S; Brownstein, DG; Allen, DJ; Mistríková, J; Davison, A; Nash, AA; Stewart, JP. Analysis of a novel strain of murine gammaherpesvirus reveals a genomic locus important for acute pathogenesis. *J. Virol.*, 2001, 75, 5315-5327.

[125] Magrath, L. The pathogenesis of Burkitt´s lymphoma. Adv. Cancer Res. 1990, 55, 133-269.

[126] Manning, A.M. Small molecule regulators of AP-1 and NFκB, In: Letts, G.L., and Morgan, D.W. (eds.): *Inflammatory process: Molecular mechanisms and therapeutic opportunities*, Birkhauser; Basel, 2000, pp 39-52.

[127] Marshall, W.I. and Sample, D.C. Epstein-Barr virus nuclear antigen 3C is a transcriptional regulator. *J. Virol.,* 1995, 69, 3624-3630.

[128] Marshall, WI; Yim, C; Gustafson, E; Graf, T; Sage DR et al. Epstein-Barr virus encodes a novel homolog of the bcl-2 oncogene that inhibits apoptosis and associates with Bax and Bak. *J. Virol.,* 1999, 73, 5181-5185.

[129] Martinez-Guzman, DA; Rickabough, T; Wu, TT; Brown, H; Cole, S; Song MJ; Tong, L; Sun, R. Transcription program of murine gammaherpesvirus. *J. Virol.,* 2003, 77, 10488-10503.

[130] McCormick, C. and Ganem, D. The kaposin B protein of KSHV activates the p38/MK2 pathway and stabilizes cytokine mRNAs *Science*, 2005, 307, 739-741.

[131] Medveczky, P; Szomolayi, E; Desrosiers, RC; Mulder, C. Classification of *herpesvirus saimiri* into three subgroups based on extensive variation in a DNA region required for oncogenicity. *J. Virol.* 1984, 52, 935-944.

[132] Medveczky, MM; Geck, P; Clarke, C; Byrnes, J; Sullivan, JL. Medveczky, PG. Arrangement of repetitive sequences in the genome of *herpesvirus sylvilagus. J. Virol,* 1989, 63, 1010-1014.

[133] Meinl, E; Hohlfeld, R; Wekerle, H; Fleckenstein, B. Immortalization of human T cells by *Herpesvirus saimiri*. *Immunol Today*, 1995, 16, 55-58.

[134] Melendez, LV; Hunt, RD; King, J; Daniel, MD; Garcia, FG; Fraser, CE. *Herpesvirus saimiri* II. Experimentally induced malignant lymphoma in primates. *Lab. Anim. Care,* 1969, 19, 378-386.

[135] Merlo, KJ; Romano, G; Gordon, SS; Feschchenko, EA; Peng, G; Henderson, EE; Tsygankov, A. Human T cells transduced by a retroviral vector to express herpesvirus saimiri proteins TIP and STPC. *Anticancer Research*, 1998, 18, 2389-2396.

[136] Mittnacht, S. and Boshoff, Ch. Viral cyclins. *Rev. Med. Virol.,* 2000, 10, 175-184.

[137] Mittrucker, HW; Muller-Fleckenstein, I; Fleckenstein, B; Fleischer, B. CD2-mediated autocrine growth of *Herpesvirus saimiri*-transformed human T lymphocytes. *J. Exp. Med.,* 1992, 176, 909-913.

[138] Mistríková, J; Remeňová, A; Leššo, J; Stančeková, M. Replication and persistence of murine herpesvirus 72 in lymphatic system and peritoneal blood mononuclear cells of Balb/c mice. *Acta Virol.,* 1994, 38, 151-156.

[139] Mistríková, J; Rajčáni, J; Mrmusová, M; Oravcová, I. Chronic infection of Balb/c mice with murine herpesvirus 72 is associated with neoplasm development. *Acta Virol.*, 1996, 40, 297-301.

[140] Mistríková, J; Mrmusová-Šupolíková, M; Rajčáni, J. Leukemia like syndrome in Balb/c mice infected with the lymphotropic gammaherpesvirus MHV-Šumava: an analogy to EBV infection. *Neoplasma*, 2004, 51, 71-74.

[141] Montaner, S; Sodhi, A; Servitja, J.-M; Ramsdell, AK; Barac, A; Sawai, ET; Gutkind, JS. The small GTPase Rac1 links the Kaposi sarcoma-associated herpesvirus vGPCR to cytokine secretion and paracrine neoplasia. *Blood,* 2004, 104, 2903-2911.

[142] Moore, P.S., and Chang, Y. (2001). Kaposi´s sarcoma-associated herpesvirus. In: Knipe, D.M., and Howley, P.M. (eds.): *Field´s Virology*, (4th edition, pp. 2803-2833) Philadelphia, Lippincott Williams and Wilkins.

[143] Moore, PS. and Chang, Y. Molecular virology of Kaposi´s sarcoma-associated herpesvirus. *Phil. Trans R Soc.* London B, 2001, 356, 499-516.

[144] Moorman, NJ; Willer, DO; Speck, SH. The gamma herpesvirus 68 latency: associated nuclear antigen homolog is critical for the establishment of splenic latency. *J. Virol.,* 2003, 77, 10295-10303.

[145] Moorman, NJ; Virgin, IV HW; Speck, SH. Disruption of the gene encoding the HV68 v-GPCR leads to decreased efficiency of reactivation from latency. *Virology,* 2003, 307, 179-190.

[146] Molden, J; Chang, Y; You, Y; Moore, PS; Goldsmith, MA. A Kaposi's sarcoma-associated herpesvirus-encoded cytokine homolog (vIL-6) activates signaling through the shared gp130 receptor subunit. *J. Biol. Chem.,* 1997, 272, 19 625-19 631.

[147] Motokura, T; Bloom, T; Kim, HG; Juppner, H; Ruderman, JV; Kronenberg, HM; Arnold, A. A novel cyclin encoded by a *bcl-1* linked candidate oncogene. *Nature*, 1991, 350, 512-525.

[148] Muralidhar, S; Pumpery, AM; Hassani, M; Sadaie, MR; Azumi, N; Kishishita, M; Brady JN; Doniger, J; Medveczky, P; Rosenthal, LJ. Identification of kaposin (open reading frame K12, as a human herpesvirus 8 (Kaposi's sarcoma-associated herpesvirus) transforming gene. *J. Virol.,* 1998, 72, 4980-4988.

[149] Murthy, SC; Trimble, JC; Desrosiers, RC. Deletion mutants of herpesvirus saimiri define and open reading frame necessary for transformation. *J. Virol.,* 1989, 63, 3307-3314.

[150] Nava, VEl Cheng, EH; Veliuona, M; Zou, S; Clem, RJ; Mayer, MI; Hardwick, JM. *Herpesvirus saimiri* encodes a functional homolog of the human bcl-2 oncogene. *J. Virol.,* 1997, 71, 4118-4122.

[151] Neipel, F; Albrecht, JC; Ensser, A; Huang, YQ; Li, JJ; Friedman, KA; Fleckenstein, B. Human herpesvirus 8 encodes a homologues of macrophage inhibitory protein-1 and interleukin-6. *J. Virol.,* 1997, 71, 839-842.

[152] Neubauer, RH; Rabin, RH; Strnad, BC; Nonoyama, M; Nelson, RW. Establishment of a lymphoblastoid cell line and isolation of an Epstein-Barr related virus of gorilla origin. *J. Virol.,* 1979, 31, 845-848.

[153] Nicholas, J; Ruvolo, VR; Burns, WH; Sandford, G; Wan, X; Giufo, D; Hendrickson, SB; Guo, HG; Hayward, GS; Reitz, MS. Kaposi's sarcoma –associated human

herpesvirus-8 encodes homologues of macrophage inflammatory protein 1 and interleukin-6. *Nature* (Med), 1997, 3, 287-292.

[154] Nicholas, J. Evolutionary aspects of oncogenic herpesviruses. *J. Clin. Molec. Pathol.*, 2000, 53, 222-237.

[155] Noraz, N; Saha, K; Ottones, F; Smith, S; Taylor, N. Constitutive activation of TCR signaling molecules in IL-2 independent Herpesvirus saimiri-transformed T cells. *J. Immunol.*, 1998, 160, 2042-2045.

[156] Obar, JJ; Donovan, DC; Crist, SG; Silvia, O; Stewart, JP; Usherwood, EJ. T cell responses to the M3 immune evasion protein of murid gammaherpesvirus 68 are partially protective and induced with lytic antigen kinetics. *J. Virol.*, 2004, 78, 10839-10832.

[157] Parry, CM; Simas, JP; Smith CA; Stewart, AC; Minson, CA; Efstathiou, S; Alcami, A. A broad spectrum secreted chemokine-binding protein encoded by a herpesvirus. *J. Exp. Med.*, 2000, 191, 573-578.

[158] Peng, R; Gordadze, AV; Fuentes Panana, EM; Wang, F; Zong, J; Hayward. GS; Tan, J; Ling, PD. Seuqnce and functional analysis of EBNA-LP and EBNA-2 proteins from nonhuman primate lymphocryptoviruses. *J. Virol.*, 74, 379-389, 2000.

[159] Phelan, A, Clements, JB: Posttranscriptional regulation in herpes simplex virus. *Semin. Virol.*, 1998, 8, 309-318.

[160] Radkov, SA; Kellam, P; Boshoff, C. The latent nuclear antigen of Kaposi's sarcoma-associated targets the retinoblastoma-E2F pathway and with the oncogene H-ras transforms primary rat cells. *Nat. Med.*, 2000, 6, 1121-1127.

[161] Ramer, JC; Garber, RL; Steeler, KE; Boyson, JF; O'Rourke, C; Thomspn, J. Fatal lymphoproliferative disease associated with a novel gammaherpesvirus in captive population of common marmosets. *Comp. Med.*, 2000, 50, 59-68.

[162] Rasheed, S; Rongey, RW; Bruszweski, J; Nelson-Rees, WA; Rabin, H; Neubauer, RH; Esra, G; Gardner, MB. Establishment of a cell line with associated Epstein-Barr like virus from a leukemic orangutan. *Science*, 1977, 198, 407-409.

[163] Rajčáni, J; Blaškovič, D; Svobodová, J; Čiampor, F; Hučková, D; Staneková, D. Pathogenesis of acute and persistent murine herpesvirus infection in mice. *Acta virol.*, 1985, 29, 51-60.

[164] Rajčáni, J. and Kúdelová, M. Murine herpesvirus pathogenesis: a model for the analysis of molecular mechanisms of gamma herpesvirus infections. *Acta Microbiol. Immunol. Hung*, 2005, 52, 41-71.

[165] Rezaee, SA; Cunningham, Ch; Davison, AJ; Blackbourn, DJ. Kaposi's sarcoma-associated herpesvirus immune modulation: an overview. *J. Gen. Virol.*, 2006, 87, 1781-1804.

[166] Rickinson, A. B., and Kieff, E. (2001). Epstein-Barr virus. In: Knipe, D.M., and Howley, P.M. (eds.): *Field's Virology*, (4th edition, pp. 2575-2627) Philadelphia, Lippincott Williams and Wilkins.

[167] Rivailler, P; Quink, C; Wang, F. Strong selective pressure for evolution of an Epstein-Barr virus. *J. Virol.*, 1999, 73, 8867-8872.

[168] Rivas, C; Thlick,A-E; Parravicini, C; Moore, PS; Chang, Y. Kaposi's sarcoma-associated herpesvirus LANA2 is a B cell specific viral protein that inhivits p53. *J. Virol.,* 2001, 75, 429-438.

[169] Roizman, B. (1990). Herpesviridae: a brief introduction. In: Fields, B.N, and Knipe, DM (eds.) *Field's Virology* (2nd edition, pp. 1787-1794) New York, Raven Press.

[170] Roizman, B. and Pellet, P. (2001). The family Herpesviridae. A brief introduction. In: Knipe, D.M., and Howley, P.M. (eds.): *Field's Virology*, (4th edition, pp. 2381-2398) Philadelphia, Lippincott Williams and Wilkins.

[171] Rosenkilde, MM; Kledal, TN; Brauner-Osborne, H; Schwartz, TW. Agonists and inverse agonists for the herpesvirus 8-encoded constitutively active seven-transmembrane oncogene product, ORF74. *J. Biol. Chem.*, 1999, 274, 956-961.

[172] Russo, JJ; Bohenzky, RA; Chien, MC; Chen, J; Yan M; Maddalena, D; Parry, JP; Peruzzi, D; Edelman, IS; Chang, Y; Moore, PS. Nucleotide sequence of the Kaposi's sarcoma-associated herpesvirus (HHV8). *Proc. Natn. Acad. Sci. USA*, 1996, 93, 14862-14867.

[173] vanRegenmortel, M.H.V., Fauquet, C,M., and Bishop. D.H.L. (2000). Herpesvirus family. In *Virus Taxonomy: Classification and Nomenclature of Viruses* (7th ICTV Report, pp. 220-226). San Diego, Academic Press.

[174] Sadler, R; Wu, L; Forghani, B; Renne, R; Zhong, W; Herndler, B; Ganem, D. A complex translational program generates multiple proteins from the latently expressed kaposin (K12) locus of Kaposi's sarcoma herpesvirus. *J. Virol.,* 1999, 73, 5722-5730.

[175] Sample, J; Liebowitz, D; Kieff, E. Two related Epstein-Barr membrane proteins are encoded by separate genes. *J. Virol.,* 1989, 63, 933-937.

[176] Van Santen, VL: Characterization of the bovine herpesvirus 4 major immediate early transcript. *J. Virol.,* 1991, 65, 5211-5224.

[177] Sarawar, SR; Lee, BJ; Anderson, M; Teng, Ych; Zuberi, R; vonGejsen, S. Chemokine induction and leukocyte trafficking to the lungs during murine gammaherpesvirus 68 (MHV-68) infection. *Virology*, 2002, 293, 54-62.

[178] Sharp, TV; Wang, HW; Kuomi, A; Hollyman, D; Endo, Y; Ye, H; Du, MQ; Boshoff, Ch. K15 protein of Kaposi's sarcoma-associated herpesvirus is latently expressed and binds to HAX-1, a protein with anti-apoptotic function. *J. Virol.,* 2002, 76, 802-806.

[179] Shin, YC; Nakamura, H; Liang X; Feng, P; Chang, H; Kowalik, TF; Jung, JU. Inhibition of the ATM/p53 signal transduction pathway by Kaposi's sarcoma-associated herpesvirus interferon regulatory factor. *J. Virol.,* 2006, 80, 2257-2266.

[180] Skare, J; Farley, J; Strominger, JL; Fresen, K; Fresen, O; Cho MS; zurHausen, H. Transformation by Epstein Barr virus requires DNA sequences in the region of BamHI fragments Y and H., *J. Virol.,* 1985, 55, 286-297.

[181] Song HY; Regnier, CH; Kisching CJ; Goeddel, DV; Rothe, M. Tumor necrosis factor (TNF) mediated cascades: bifurcation of nuclear factor κB and c-jun N-terminal kinase (JNK/SAPK) pathways at the TNF receptor associated factor 2. *Proc. Natn. Acad. Sci. USA*, 1997, 94, 9792-9796.

[182] Staskus, KA; Zhong, W; Gebhard, K; Herndier, B; Wang, H; Renne, R; Beneke, J; Pudney, J; Anderson, DJ; Ganem, D; Haase, AT. Kaposi's sarcoma-associated

herpesvirus gene expression in endothelial (spindle) tumor cells. *J. Virol.*, 1997, 71, 715-719.

[183] Stewart, J.P; Usherwood, E.J; Ross, A; Dyson, H; Nash, A.A. Lung epithelial cells are a major site of murine gammaherpesvirus persistence. *J. Exp. Med.,* 1998, 187, 1941-1951.

[184] Sunil-Chandra, NP; Efsthathiou, S; Nash, AA. Interaction of murine gammaherpesvirus 68 with B and T cell lines. *Virology*, 1993, 193, 825-833.

[185] Sunil-Chandra, N.P; Fazakerley, A.J; Nash, A.A. Lymphoproliferative disease in mice infected with murine gammaherpesvirus 68. *Am. J. Pathol.,* 1994, 145, 818-826.

[186] Swanton, C; Mann, DJ; Fleckenstein, B; Neipel, F; Peters, O; Jones, N. Herpes viral /cdk6 complexes evade inhibition by CDK inhibition proteins. *Nature*, 1997, 390, 187-189.

[187] Thome, P; Schneider, R; Hofmann, K; Fickenscher, K; Meinl, E; Neipel, F; Mattman, C; Burns, K; Bodmer, JL; Schroter, M; Scaffidi, C; Krammer, PH; Peter, ME; Tschopp, J. Viral FLICE inhibitory proteins prevent apoptosis induced by death receptors. *Nature*, 1997, 386, 517-521.

[188] Telford, EAR; Watson, MS; Aird, HC; Perry, J; Davison, AJ. The DNA sequence of Equine herpesvirus 2. *J. Mol. Biol.,* 1995, 249, 520-528.

[189] Tokai, N; Fujimoto, NA; Toyoshima Y. Kid, a novel kinesin-like DNA-binding protein, is localized to chromosomes and the mitotic spindle. *EMBO J.*, 1996, 15, 457-467.

[190] Tong, XR; Drapkin, D; Reinberg, D; Kieff, E. The 62- and 80-kDa subunits of transcription factor mediate the interaction with Epstein-Barr virus nuclear protein 2. *Proc. Natn. Acad. Sci. USA*, 1993, 92, 3259-32636.

[191] Tsigankov, AY, Romano, G: Mechanisms of cell transformation by *Herpesvirus saimiri. Anticancer Research*, 19, 973-984, 1999.

[192] Tsui, S. and Schubach, W H. Epstein-Barr virus nuclear protein 2A form oligomers *in vitro* and *in vivo* through a region required of B-cell transformation. *J. Virol.,* 1994, 68, 4287-4294.

[193] Usherwood, EJ; Roy, D J; Ward, SL; Surman, BM; Dutia, MA; Blackman, J; Stewart, P; Woodland, DL. Control of gammaherpesvirus latency by latent antigen-specific CD8+ T cells. *J. Exp. Med.*, 2000, 192, 943-952.

[194] Usherwood, E J; Ward, K; Blackman, MA; Stewart, J P; Woodland, DL. Latent antigen vaccination in a model gammaherpesvirus infection. *J. Virol.*, 2001, 75, 8283-8288.

[195] Vilcek, J., and Sen, G.C. (1996). Interferons and other cytokins, In B.N. Fields, D.M. Knipe, and P.M. Howley, (Eds.), *Fields Virology* (3rd ed, pp. 375-399). Philadelphia, Lippincott-Raven Publishers.

[196] Virgin IV, HW; Latreille, P; Wamsley, P; Hallsworth, K; Weck, KE; Dal Canto, AJ; Speck, HS. Complete sequence and genomic analysis of murine gammaherpesvirus 68. *J. Virol.,* 1997, 71, 5894-5904.

[197] Wakeling, MN; Roy, DJ; Nash, AA; Stewart, JP. Characterization of the murine gammaherpesvirus ORF74 product: A novel oncogenic G protein-coupled receptor. *J. Gen. Virol.*, 2001, 82, 1187-1197.

[198] Wang, F; Gregory, C; Sample, C; Rowe, M; Liebowitz, R; Rickinson, A; Kieff, E. Epstein-Barr virus latent membrane protein (LMP1) and nuclear proteins 2 and 3C are

effectors of phenotypic changes in B lymphocytes: EBNA-2 and LMP1 cooperatively induce CD23. *J. Virol.*, 1990, 64, 2309-2318.

[199] Wang, GH; Garvey, TL; Cohen, JI. The murine gammaherpesvirus 68 M11 inhibits *Fas*- and TNF-induced apoptosis. *J. Gen. Virol.,* 1999, 80, 2737-2740.

[200] Wang, F; Rivailler, P; Rao, P; Cho, Y-G. Simian homologues of Epstein-Barr virus. *Phil. Trans R Soc.* London B, 2001, 356, 489-497.

[201] Watanabe, T; Sugaya, M; Atkins, M; Aquilino, EA; Yang, A; Barris, DLl Brady, J; Blauvelt, A. Kaposi's sarcoma-associated herpesvirus latency nuclear antigen prolongs the life span of primary human umbilical vein endothelial cells. *J. Virol.,* 2003, 77, 6188-6196.

[202] Yang, T.Y; Chen, S.C; Leach, M.W; Manfra, D; Homey B; Wiekowksi, M; Sullivan, L; Jenh, CH; Narula, SK; Chensue, SW; Lira, S.A. Transgenic expression of the chemokine receptor encoded by human herpesvirus 8 induces an angioproliferative disease resembling Kaposi's sarcoma. *J. Exp. Med.,* 2000, 191, 445-454.

[203] Yao, Z; Maraskowsky, E; Spriggs, MK; Cohen, JI; Armitage, RJ; Alderson, MR. Herpesvirus saimiri open reading frame 14, a protein encoded by a T lymphotropic herpesvirus, binds in MHC class II molecules and stimulates T cell proliferation. *J. Immunol.*, 1996, 156, 3260-3266.

[204] Yates, JL; Warren, N; Sugden, B. Stable replication of plasmids derived from Epstein-Barr virus in various mammalian cells. *Nature,* 1985, 313, 812-815.

[205] Yates, JL; Camiolo, SM; Ali, S; Ying, A. Comparison of EBNA-1 like proteins of Epstein-Barr virus and *Herpesvirus papio* in sequence function. *Virology*, 1996, 222, 1-13.

[206] Yoon, DW; Lee, H; Scol, W; DeMaria, M; Rosenzweig, M; Jung, JU. Tap, a novel cellular protein that interacts with Tip. *Immunity,* 1997, 6, 571-582.

[207] Zhang, S. and Nonoyama, M. The cellular proteins that bind specifically to the Epstein-Barr virus belong to the family of plasmid DNA replication origin. *Proc. Natn. Acad. Sci. USA,* 1994, 91, 2843-2847.

[208] Zhong, W; Wang, H; Herndier, B; Ganem, D. Restricted expression of Kaposi sarcoma associated herpesvirus (human herpesvirus 8) genes in Kaposi sarcoma. *Proc. Natn. Acad. Sci. USA*, 1996, 93, 6641-6646.

[209] Zimmermann, W; Broll, H; Ehlers, B; Buhk, H-J; Rosenthal, A; Goltz, M. Genome sequence of bovine herpesvirus 4, a bovine rhadinovirus, and identification of an origin of DNA replication. *J. Virol.,* 2001, 75, 1186-1194.

In: Herpesviridae Viral Structure, Life Cycle and Infections
Editor: Toma R. Gluckman
ISBN 978-1-60692-947-6

Chapter 9

Present Focus on HPV-Virus-Induced Carcinoma

Viroj Wiwanitkit
Wiwanitkit House, Bangkhae, Bangkok 10160, Thailand

Abstract

The human papilloma virus (HPV) is a DNA virus that can be the cause of many carcinomas. This DNA virus has been proven as a DNA tumor virus. Cervical carcinoma is the main carcinoma that relates to HPV infection. Screening for HPV DNA is a new laboratory analysis in gynecology, and a vaccine for HPV is presently available. In this work, current knowledge on HPV laboratory diagnosis, therapy and prevention are reviewed and discussed. In addition, the author also performs a meta-analysis of the previous reports on cervical carcinoma, the most common female carcinoma in Thailand, and HPV virus infection in Thailand.

Introduction: HPV Virus and Carcinoma

Human papillomavirus (HPV) is an important double-stranded DNA virus associated with a broad spectrum of clinical states. The virus is transmitted by direct contact with site-subtype specificity. It is accepted as a tumor virus [1]. Previous biochemical and serological studies have demonstrated the existence of at least four distinct types of HPVs causing benign skin pathological lesions [2]. These virions show no strong antigenic relationships; their DNAs differ by their sensitivity to restriction endonucleases, and present little, if any, sequence homology, as detected by molecular hybridization using complementary RNAs transcribed in vitro [2]. The recognition of the virion is important owing to the different morphology of the pathological lesions generated and their various oncogenic potentials [3]. There are many types of HPV, but four main well-realized classical types. HPV1 is mostly responsible for plantar warts; HPV2 for common (hand) warts; and HPV3 has been detected both in flat warts and in the variety of epidermodysplasia verruciformis (EV) in which pathological skin lesions are of the flat wart type, the course is relatively more benign, and commonly malignant transformation is not to be imagined [3]. HPV4 was up to now found exclusively in the scenarios of EV with prevalent red and red-brownish plaques and hyper- and depigmentations similar to those of pityriasis versicolor. In all scenarios of this variety of EV, cancers invariably occured [3]. For HPV1-related diseases, plantar warts are thick, endophytic, hyperkeratotic pathological lesions caused by human papilloma virus [4]. Because they are frequently mistaken for other conditions, they are often misdiagnosed in athletes [4]. The diagnosis of a plantar wart is made by paring down the hypertrophic epithelium until multiple seeds are detected in the dermis representing the thrombosed vessels supplying the wart [4]. Concerning HPV2-related diseases, most people get warts on their hands at some time in their lives [5]. They are most common in childhood, with 4–20% of schoolchildren getting warts at any one time [5]. For HPV3- and HPV4-related disorders, EV is a rare genodermatosis characterized by persistent human papilloma virus infection with a possible autosomal recessive inheritance pattern [6]. Clinically, it is characterized by flat wart-like pathological lesions, scaly hypo- and hyperpigmented macules and/or patches, which resemble pityriasis versicolor, and development of early nonmelanoma cutaneous carcinomas [6]. In addition to simple hyperplasia, HPV is also related to many malignant disorders. The association of HPV-16 and HPV-18 with anogenital malignancy has been recently reported.

In oncology, HPV is strongly correlated with cervical carcinoma. HPV infection has been implicated in the intraepithelial cervical changes that cause most abnormal Pap smears [7]. To date, more than 10 types of HPVs have been identified [7]. Summarized are icosahedral DNA viruses that share a common internal antigen. In scenarios of cervical HPV infection, the koilocytes and dyskeratocytes are the most frequently seen cell types. Most infections are flat aceto-white pathological lesions [7]. Virologically, HPVs are double-stranded DNA viral particles that infect the cutaneous and mucosal epithelium. Infection by specific HPV types has been related to the development of cervical carcinoma [8]. HPV infects epithelial cells that undergo terminal differentiation and so encode multiple mechanisms to override the normal regulation of differentiation to generate progeny virions [8]. HPVs play an essential function in the pathogenesis of cervical carcinoma. Although infections by these viruses are very common in the general population, only a few result in clinically relevant pathological lesions [9,10]. A strong association between cervical and oral carcinoma with high-risk human papillomavirus (HPV) 16 and 18 infections underlines the importance of the virus in the pathogenesis of these squamous cell carcinomas [9]. Functionally high-risk HPV infection leads to carcinogenesis and tumor progression predominantly through the actions of viral oncogenes [9].

HPV is a contributing factor, but probably not the sole cause of cervical precarcinoma and carcinoma [11]. Secondary exogenous and endogenous factors, HPV cofactors, may lead to the probability of a carcinoma-associated (oncogenic) HPV infection progressing to cervical precarcinoma and carcinoma [11]. For these cofactors to influence the natural history of HPV infection, they must act on cervical tissue to promote viral persistence, progression to precarcinoma or carcinoma given viral persistence, or both [11]. However, HPV alone may not be sufficient to induce carcinomas, because even the E6 and E7 oncogenes ORFs of HPV-16 could not transform rat primary cells immediately after infection, but could do so after a long latency. Cervical carcinoma is preventable and it should be a high priority in national carcinoma control programmes. In order to be highly effective, various methods warrant joint usage [12]. Tristen and Bergstrom noted that the screening of the entire population in the 35–64 year age groups every 10 years could reduce the incidence of invasive cervical carcinoma by about 55% [13]. Screening for CIN, the curable pathological lesion, is a good preventive method for the control of cervical carcinoma. Several alternatives are available for screening for CIN in present medical practice. According to the study of De Vuyst et al. [14], sensitivity for HPV DNA-PCR is significantly higher than other alternatives. For the use of screening in the developing world with limited resources, the concept of laboratory economics should also be examined.

For skin carcinoma, HPV is also documented as an important etiological factor. The skin is an organ in which direct contact with viruses, solar ultraviolet (UV) irradiation and increased susceptibility to immune suppression gather to support viral tumorigenesis [15]. Viruses transform keratinocytes by activation of carcinoma-promoting genes [5]. Viral proteins may directly act as oncogenes that cause cells to proliferate or generate inflammatory responses and cause regeneration of injured cells that eventually lead to malignant transformation [15]. Pathophysiologically, HPV infects cutaneous and mucosal epithelia and induces benign and malignant pathological lesions [16]. Non-melanoma skin carcinoma, encompassing basal cell carcinoma and squamous cell carcinoma, is the most common carcinoma among the Caucasian population, and the incidence has increased dramatically worldwide [16]. The relationship between HPV and non-melanoma skin carcinoma is clinically significant, since non-melanoma skin carcinoma is the most common form of malignancy among fair-skinned populations [17]. It is well established that solar UV irradiation is the main risk factor for developing non-melanoma skin carcinoma, but a pathogenic expression for HPV in the development of non-melanoma skin carcinoma has also been proposed [17]. Molecularly, high-risk mucosal HPV types encode two major oncoproteins, E6 and E7, which inactivate two suppressor proteins, p53 and pRb, respectively, and are sufficient for host-cell immortalization. A polymorphism resulting in either a proline or an arginine at codon 72 might be a relevant risk factor for mucosal HPV-type-associated non-melanoma skin carcinoma [18]. By contrast, E6 of skin HPV types fails to interact with p53, but prevents infected cells from UV-generated apoptosis, thus leading to the propagation of deleterious UV-generated mutations [18]. The antiapoptotic activities of E6 proteins of cutaneous HPV could be relevant to oncogenesis in the interplay with UV exposure [19]. For EV scenarios, EV results from an abnormal susceptibility to infection by specific HPV genotypes (beta-papillomaviruses) which include the potentially oncogenic HPV5 [20]. Of interest, EV-specific HPVs are considered harmless for the general population [20]. Jenson et al. concluded that in normal people most of the HPV has been shown to establish a latent infection of the skin, most likely as normal flora residing in hair follicles; however, in patients with various systemic and localized depressions of cell-mediated immunity, some HPV infections have been shown to be involved in the development of nonmelanotic skin carcinoma and its precursor pathological lesions in skin, usually in sunlight-exposed settings [21]. They also report that that all HPVs might have a function in promoting proliferative pathological lesions of the skin, although the sites of active infection are unknown [21].

While much is realized about the natural history of cervical human HPV infection and its consequences, including cervical intraepithelial neoplasia and cervical carcinoma, relatively little is realized about the natural history of anogenital HPV infection and diseases in men [22]. Concerning carcinoma of the penis, HPV is an important etiological factor similar to the case of cervical carcinoma. Infection with high-risk HPV has been associated with intraepithelial neoplasia and carcinomas at various sites of the anogenital tract, including the cervix, vulva, vagina, penis and anus [23]. HPV, specifically types 16, 18, 31, 33, 35, 39, 45 and 52, have been related to the etiology of anogenital carcinoma [24]. For the penis, herpes genitalis and infections caused by HPV are increasing, particularly in young sexually active people [25]. Squamous cell carcinoma is the most common malignancy of the penis, and the function of oncogenic HPV-types has been also been established in squamous cell carcinoma of the penis [25]. The relationship between carcinomas of the penis and cervix uteri is very important in married couples [26]. Genital HPV infections manifest themselves as condylomas [26]. Malek et al. said that the combination of the host of carcinogenic factors and currently rampant immunologic disorders will likely lead to an increase in the historically low incidence of squamous cell carcinoma of the penis [27]. Therefore, any men who carry the virus must be identified and treated [26]. Prevention of squamous cell carcinoma of the penis presupposes an identification of risk factors, early determination of pre-carcinomaous pathological lesions and treatment of phimosis [25].

Laboratory Diagnosis and Screening for HPV DNA as a Preventive Measure

A variety of new tests for detecting the presence of oncogenic HPV types in biological specimens are available at present [28]. These rely on the various stages of infection and viral life cycle [28]. There are three basic classes of detectable markers for HPVs: molecular markers rely on determination of nucleic acid sequences, serological markers rely on determination of antibodies against viral proteins, and cellular markers rely on determination of proteins expressed intracellularly, upon either infection or carcinogenesis [28]. Also, there is a classical marker for determination of HPV-related carcinoma, the Papanicolaou (Pap) smear. Since HPVs now comprise many different HPV types, the polymerase chain reaction (PCR) has been the preferred methodology for virus identification and typing on isolated DNA. At present, HPV infection is mainly diagnosed by molecular methods, since reliable serological tools are not available and culture of the virus is not possible [29]. Methods are divided according to three groups: hybridization based, PCR based and a combination of both. The accurate determination and diagnosis of cervical carcinoma and its malignant precursors (collectively referred to as high-grade cervical disease) represents one of the current challenges in clinical medicine and cytopathology [30]. HPV DNA testing is a sensitive test for the presence of squamous intraepithelial pathological lesions, with excellent negative predictive value for the absence of squamous intraepithelial pathological lesions [31]. Also, HPV DNA testing might be an effective screening test in the initial evaluation and management of cytological atypical glandular cells [31]. The advent of molecular diagnostics and the use of whole-genome profiling using DNA microarrays promises to yield improved understanding of the disease process with the subsequent development of more accurate diagnostic procedures based upon these discoveries [30]. It is accepted that PCR primers that target the L1 or E1 region can be unreliable and may miss more advanced disease, whereas those directed at the E6 or E7 regions, which encode oncogenic products, are preferable because 1) the LI/E1 regions, but never the E6/E7 regions, are lost during integration of viral DNA into host genomic DNA, a process that can represent an integral component of progression from infection to tumorigenesis; and 2) the E6/E7 nucleotide sequence exhibits less nucleotide variation [32]. The determination sets the stage for a prospective follow-up study currently being undertaken to evaluate the prognostic relevance of the determination of high-risk HPV E6/E7 oncogene transcripts for the persistence of a high-risk HPV infection, and the possible evolution and further development of a CIN. Future applications of the assay described may include the monitoring of women in studies investigating antiviral treatment or vaccination.

There are some interesting previous reports on the clinical use of HPV oncogene screening in cervical carcinoma. In 2002, Wang-Johanning et al. performed a study to determine the potential clinical applications of real-time PCR and reverse transcription-PCR methods for evaluating HPV-16 E6 and E7 oncogene expression [33]. In this work, ThinPrep cervical samples were tested for expression of oncogenes of HPV-16 by real-time PCR or RT-PCR analysis and were compared with determination of expression by conventional PCR and RT-PCR analysis [33]. According to this study, the determination of HPV-16 E6 and E7 expression by real-time RT-PCR or PCR analysis in ThinPrep cervical cytologic specimens may serve as a quick, reliable, and sensitive tool to identify a subset of patients who express HPV-16 oncoproteins [33]. Sasagawa et al. established a new assay to detect the E6-E7 DNA of mucosal HPV by a PCR-based method using four pairs of degenerate LCR and E7 primers (LCR-E7 PCR) and compared this assay with the first generation hybrid captured assay (HCA-I) and the MY09/11-PCR method [34]. According to this study, the discordant results were mostly observed in samples with a low-copy number of the HPV genome or with multiple HPV infection [34]. Naucler et al. performed an interesting study to compare HPV DNA test and Papanicolaou tests to screen for cervical carcinoma [35]. They said that the addition of an HPV test to the Papanicolaou test to screen women in their mid-30s for cervical carcinoma effectively reduced the incidence of grade 2 or 3 cervical intraepithelial neoplasia or carcinoma detected by subsequent screening examinations [35]. Mayrand et al. performed a similar report and found that as compared with Pap testing, HPV testing had greater sensitivity for the determination of cervical intraepithelial neoplasia [36]. Kulasingam et al. reported that testing for HPV had a higher sensitivity but lower specificity than thin-layer Pap screening [37]. They also reported that in some settings, particularly where screening intervals are long or haphazard, screening for HPV DNA might be a reasonable alternative to cytology-based screening of reproductive-age women [37]. Costa et al. found that the potential combinations of Pap with cervicography and with a hybrid capture test were more sensitive in detecting cervical intraepithelial neoplasia 2 and 3 compared with Pap alone and retained a positive predictive value similar to that of Pap [38]. Kuhn et al. reported that HPV DNA testing had a sensitivity equivalent to, or better than, that of cytology [39]. Since

HPV DNA testing programs might be easier to implement than cytologic screening, and that HPV testing should be considered for primary cervical carcinoma screening in low-resource settings [39]. In addition, Manos et al. proposed that for women with atypical squamous cells of undetermined significance in Pap tests, HPV DNA testing of residual specimens collected for routine cervical cytology could help identify those who have underlying high-grade squamous intraepithelial pathological lesions [40]. Bistoletti et al. also studied the cost-effectiveness of primary cytology and HPV DNA cervical screening in Sweden [41]. They found that population-based, organized cervical cytology screening between the ages of 32 to 60 was highly cost-efficient for cervical carcinoma prevention [40]. They also noted that if screening intervals were increased to at least nine years, combined cytology and HPV DNA screening were shown to be even more effective and less expensive [41].

HPV Therapy at Present

In the few previous years, extensive research has led to the documentation of the molecular mechanisms of HPV virus persistence and malignant transformation, confirming a direct function of viral proteins in these processes [42]. Previously, major breakthroughs emerged from immunological studies [42]. Indeed, these studies paved the way for the medical treatment of HPV infections [42]. There are many new immunomodulation drugs for the treatment of HPV infection. Imiquimod is a new synthetic molecule with potent immune-modifying activities [43]. Formulated in a 5% vanishing cream as Aldara, this self-applied therapy has shown good efficacy and safety in the treatment of external genital and perianal warts caused by human papillomavirus (HPV) infection (Condyloma acuminata) [43]. The molecule does not demonstrate direct antiviral activity, but through induction of cytokines results in immune-based resolution of wart tissue and reduction of viral burden [43]. Imiquimod increases in interferon and tumor necrosis factor in cultures of cells isolated from animal skin, and increases interleukin-8 concentrations in human keratinocyte and fibroblast cultures [44]. Although in vitro studies have shown that imiquimod has no direct antiviral effects, the drug does exhibit antiviral and antitumor effects in vivo through induction of human cytokines [44]. Although imiquimod cream previously became available for the treatment of genital and perianal warts, the topical mechanism of action of imiquimod is not yet fully understood [44]. It is believed that stimulation of local cytokines by imiquimod leads to a reduction in HPV load, to wart regression and to the normalization of keratinocyte proliferation without evidence of scarring [44]. Treatment with topical 5% imiquimod cream has shown promising results in the treatment of genital warts in immunocompetent individuals [44]. In addition to new antiviral immunomodulation drugs, it remains to be investigated whether HPV-specific therapeutic vaccines can be developed [45].

HPV Vaccine: A New Way to Prevent Infection

Cervical carcinoma is the second leading cause of carcinoma-related death in women worldwide. Approximately 70% of cervical carcinoma is caused by infection with HPV types

16 and 18 and approximately 90% of genital warts are caused by HPV types 6 and 11 [46]. Vaccine for the prevention of the HPV infection is the hope for success in control of cervical carcinoma [46]. The challenges of the journey from target identification through development of a prophylactic quadrivalent HPV vaccine have been met in Gardasil [46,47]. Gardasil (Merck, Whitehouse Station, NJ) is a non-infectious recombinant, quadrivalent vaccine set from the highly purified virus-like particles (VLPs) of the major capsid proteins of HPV types 6, 11, 16, and 18. Gardasil is the first vaccine confirmed for use in women aged 9–26 years for the prevention of cervical carcinoma and genital warts, and vulvar and vaginal precarcinomaous pathological lesions [47]. Prophylactic HPV vaccination has demonstrated 100% efficacy in preventing type-specific persistent infections and associated genital dysplasias [48,49]. The Food and Drug Administration has confirmed Gardasil as the first vaccine developed to prevent cervical carcinoma and precarcinomaous genital pathological lesions and genital warts owing to certain types of HPV [50]. The vaccine is approved for use in females aged 9 to 26 years [50]. Several issues, such as the duration of protection, the need for the development of post-exposure vaccination strategies and the availability of such a vaccine in low-income countries, are open and need further discussion [51,52].

Cervical Carcinoma and HPV Infection: Experience in Thailand

Women in Thailand have a relatively high risk of getting cervical carcinoma [53]. Vatanasapt et al. noted that an appropriate cervical carcinoma carcinoma screening program can lower the previous prevalence rate and lead to better results of treatment [54]. Swaddiwudhipong et al. reported that greater efforts should be made to encourage the use of screening among older women [55]. Promotion of cervical carcinoma screening among Thai adult women, particularly in the rural area, is recommended [55]. There was a previous report on cervical carcinoma screening among Thai women immigrants in Australia (not the local population in Thailand) [56]. A similar low rate among the rural female populations in Thailand can be expected. The medical workers should work harder to increase the coverage rate of cervical carcinoma screening for Thai females. Wiwanitkit summarized and meta-analysed the previous reported results from cervical screening programs established by several settings in Thailand [57]. According to the meta-analysis, 101,107 scenarios were studied [57,63]. The overall prevalence of cervical carcinoma is 0.38% (383/101,107) [57]. The overall prevalence of pre-carcinomaous scenarios and other pathological lesions (infection and inflammation) are 2.39% (2,405/101,107) and 5.30%, respectively (5,358/101,107) [57]. There is no significant association between the prevalence rate and the setting of the study (region) [57]. These results demonstrate the significance of cervical carcinoma in Thailand [57]. Indeed, the high determination rate of pre-carcinomaous pathological lesions also implies the usefulness of a screening program for secondary prevention of cervical carcinoma in Thailand [57]. Health education seems to play an important function in the success of a cervical carcinoma screening program for the Thai female population [57].

Table 1. Some reports on HPV infection and cervical carcinoma in Thailand

Authors	Details
Sukvirach et al. [64]	This study was performed to determine the prevalence and HPV type in normal and cervical carcinoma tissues of Thai females. Biopsy samples from 105 invasive cervical carcinoma patients (histologically confirmed) and cervical smears from 298 normal subjects were collected. Carcinoma patients and normal subjects were those who attended the Out-patient Division of the National Carcinoma Institute. HPV-DNA was assayed by PCR-based method using general and specific probes. HPV-DNA was found in 95 scenarios (90.48 percent) of cervical carcinoma with eight "high risk" types of HPV (HPV 16, 18, 31, 33, 35, 39, 52 and 58) being observed in 88 scenarios (83.81 per cent) and HPV X (unrealized HPV) in seven scenarios (6.67 percent). In normal cervical smears, HPV-DNA was found in only 28 scenarios (9.4 percent); 14 scenarios (4.7 percent) were found positive for "high risk" type HPV (HPV 16, 33, 52 and 58) and the other 14 scenarios (4.7 percent) were found to be HPV X.
Poonnaniti and Bhattarakosol [65]	In this study, purified plasmid HPV-16 DNA and HeLa-NA, containing HPV-18 DNA, were amplified by PCR using Ll consensus primers specific for HPV. The amplified product was then analysed by gel electrophoresis (GE) and dot hybridization (DH). The generic oligonucleotide probes (GPs) labelled with Enhanced Chemiluminescence 3' labelling kit (ECL) were used in DH. The sensitivity of PCR reaction after determination by GE was one copy per cell for purified plasmid HPV-16 DNA and 20–80 copies per cell for HeLa-DNA, while determining by DH was only 0.1 and 2–8 copies per cell, respectively. Thus, the determination of amplified product by DH using an enhanced chemiluminescence system improved not only the specificity but also the sensitivity of HPV determination at least 10-fold.

References

[1] Schulz H. Virus tumors. *Dtsch Med Wochenschr*. 1970 Jun 19;95(25):1367-70.

[2] Orth G, Jablonska S, Breitburd F, Favre M, Croissant O. The human papillomaviruses. *Bull Carcinoma*. 1978;65(2):151-64.

[3] Jablonska S, Orth G, Jarzabek-Chorzelska M, Obalek S, Rzesa G, Croissant O, Favre M. New developments relating to papillomaviruses. *Hautarzt*. 1979 Aug;30(8):411-7.
[4] Esterowitz D, Greer KE, Cooper PH, Edlich RF. Plantar warts in the athlete. *Am J Emerg Med.* 1995 Jul;13(4):441-3.
[5] Tackling warts on the hands and feet. *Drug Ther Bull.* 1998 Mar;36(3):22-4.
[6] Gül U, Kiliç A, Gönül M, Cakmak SK, Bayis SS. Clinical aspects of epidermodysplasia verruciformis and review of the literature. *Int J Dermatol.* 2007 Oct;46(10):1069-72.
[7] Roy M, Morin C, Casas-Cordero M, Meisels A. Human papillomavirus and cervical pathological lesions. *Clin Obstet Gynecol.* 1983 Dec;26(4):949-67.
[8] Hebner CM, Laimins LA. Human papillomaviruses: basic mechanisms of pathogenesis and oncogenicity. *Rev Med* Virol. 2006 Mar-Apr;16(2):83-97.
[9] Nair S, Pillai MR. Human papillomavirus and disease mechanisms: relevance to oral and cervical carcinomas. *Oral Dis*. 2005 Nov;11(6):350-9.
[10] Trunk MJ, Wentzensen N, von Knebel Doeberitz M. Molecular pathogenesis of cervical carcinoma and its first steps. *Pathologe*. 2005 Jul;26(4):283-90.
[11] Castle PE. Beyond human papillomavirus: the cervix, exogenous secondary factors, and the development of cervical precarcinoma and carcinoma. *J Low Genit Tract Dis.* 2004 Jul;8(3):224-30.
[12] Singer A. Cervical carcinoma screening: state of the art. *Baillieres Clin Obstet Gynaecol.* 1995 ;9:39-64.
[13] Tristen C, Bergstrom S. Cervical carcinoma in geting countries. A threat to reproductive health. *Lakartidningen*. 1996;93:3374-6.
[14] De Vuyst H, Calaeys P, Njiru S, Muchiri L, Steyaert S, De Sutter P, Van Marck E, Bwayo J, Temmerman M. Comparison of pap smear, visual inspection with acetic acid, human papilloma virus DNA-PCR testing a cervicography. *Int J Gynaecol Obstet* 2005; 89: 120-26.
[15] Molho-Pessach V, Lotem M. Viral carcinogenesis in skin carcinoma. *Curr Probl Dermatol.* 2007;35:39-51.
[16] Nindl I, Gottschling M, Stockfleth E. Human papillomaviruses and non-melanoma skin carcinoma: basic virology and clinical manifestations. *Dis Markers*. 2007;23(4):247-59.
[17] Akgül B, Cooke JC, Storey A. HPV-associated skin disease. *J Pathol.* 2006 Jan;208(2):165-75.
[18] Aubin F, Humbey O, Guérrini JS, Mougin C, Laurent R. Non-melanoma skin carcinomas and human papillomavirus. *Ann Dermatol Venereol.* 2003 Dec;130(12 Pt 1):1131-8.
[19] Pfister H. Chapter 8: Human papillomavirus and skin carcinoma. *J Natl Carcinoma Inst Mo*nogr. 2003;(31):52-6.
[20] Orth G. Genetics of epidermodysplasia verruciformis: Insights into host defense against papillomaviruses. *Semin Immunol.* 2006 Dec;18(6):362-74.
[21] Jenson AB, Geyer S, Sundberg JP, Ghim S. Human papillomavirus and skin carcinoma. *J Investig Dermatol Symp Proc.* 2001 Dec;6(3):203-6.
[22] Palefsky JM. HPV infection in men. *Dis Markers*. 2007;23(4):261-72.

[23] Steenbergen RD, de Wilde J, Wilting SM, Brink AA, Snijders PJ, Meijer CJ. HPV-mediated transformation of the anogenital tract. *J Clin Virol.* 2005 Mar;32 Suppl 1:S25-33.

[24] zur Hausen H. The function of papillomaviruses in anogenital carcinoma. *Scand J Infect Dis Suppl.* 1990;69:107-11.

[25] Buechner SA. Common skin disorders of the penis. *BJU Int.* 2002 Sep;90(5):498-506.

[26] Dutkiewicz S, Witeska A. Human papillomavirus (HPV) infection in premalignancy and carcinoma of the penis. Clinical relevance. *Mater Med Pol.* 1994 Oct-Dec;26(4):139-41

[27] Malek RS, Goellner JR, Smith TF, Espy MJ, Cupp MR. Human papillomavirus infection and intraepithelial, in situ, and invasive carcinoma of penis. *Urology.* 1993 Aug;42(2):159-70.

[28] Pagliusi SR, Garland SM. International standard reagents for HPV determination. *Dis Markers.* 2007;23(4):283-96.

[29] Molijn A, Kleter B, Quint W, van Doorn LJ. Molecular diagnosis of human papillomavirus (HPV) infections. *J Clin Virol.* 2005 Mar;32 Suppl 1:S43-51.

[30] Malinowski DP. Molecular diagnostic assays for cervical neoplasia: emerging markers for the determination of high-grade cervical disease. *Biotechniques.* 2005 Apr;Suppl:17-23.

[31] Irvin W, Evans SR, Andersen W, Jazaeri A, Taylor P, Stoler M, Pastore L, Rice L. The utility of HPV DNA triage in the management of cytological AGC. *Am J Obstet Gynecol.* 2005 Aug;193(2):559-65

[32] Morris BJ. Cervical human papillomavirus screening by PCR: advantages of targeting the E6/E7 region. *Clin Chem Lab Med.* 2005;43(11):1171-7.

[33] Wang-Johanning F, Lu DW, Wang Y, Johnson MR, Johanning GL. Quantitation of human papillomavirus 16 E6 and E7 DNA and RNA in residual material from ThinPrep Papanicolaou tests using real-time polymerase chain reaction analysis. *Carcinoma.* 2002 Apr 15;94(8):2199-210.

[34] Sasagawa T, Minemoto Y, Basha W, Yamazaki H, Nakamura M, Yoshimoto H, Sakaike J, Inoue M. A new PCR-based assay amplifies the E6-E7 genes of most mucosal human papillomaviruses (HPV). *Virus Res.* 2000 Apr;67(2):127-39.

[35] Naucler P, Ryd W, Törnberg S, Strand A, Wadell G, Elfgren K, Rådberg T, Strander B, Forslund O, Hansson BG, Rylander E, Dillner J. Human papillomavirus and Papanicolaou tests to screen for cervical carcinoma. *N Engl J Med.* 2007 Oct 18;357(16):1589-97.

[36] Mayrand MH, Duarte-Franco E, Rodrigues I, Walter SD, Hanley J, Ferenczy A, Ratnam S, Coutlée F, Franco EL; Canadian Cervical Carcinoma Screening Trial Study Group. Human papillomavirus DNA versus Papanicolaou screening tests for cervical carcinoma. *N Engl J Med.* 2007 Oct 18;357(16):1579-88.

[37] Kulasingam SL, Hughes JP, Kiviat NB, Mao C, Weiss NS, Kuypers JM, Koutsky LA. Evaluation of human papillomavirus testing in primary screening for cervical abnormalities: comparison of sensitivity, specificity, and frequency of referral. *JAMA.* 2002 Oct 9;288(14):1749-57.

[38] Costa S, Sideri M, Syrjänen K, Terzano P, De Nuzzo M, De Simone P, Cristiani P, Finarelli AC, Bovicelli A, Zamparelli A, Bovicelli L. Combined Pap smear, cervicography and HPV DNA testing in the determination of cervical intraepithelial neoplasia and carcinoma. *Acta Cytol.* 2000 May-Jun;44(3):310-8.

[39] Manos MM, Kinney WK, Hurley LB, Sherman ME, Shieh-Ngai J, Kurman RJ, Ransley JE, Fetterman BJ, Hartinger JS, McIntosh KM, Pawlick GF, Hiatt RA. Identifying women with cervical neoplasia: using human papillomavirus DNA testing for equivocal Papanicolaou results. *JAMA.* 1999 May 5;281(17):1605-10.

[40] Kuhn L, Denny L, Pollack A, Lorincz A, Richart RM, Wright TC. Human papillomavirus DNA testing for cervical carcinoma screening in low-resource settings. *J Natl Carcinoma Inst.* 2000 May 17;92(10):818-25.

[41] Bistoletti P, Sennfält K, Dillner J. Cost-effectiveness of primary cytology and HPV DNA cervical screening. *Int J Carcinoma.* 2008 Jan 15;122(2):372-6.

[42] Menzo S, Marinelli K, Bagnarelli P, Rolla S, Clementi M. Human papillomavirus infections: new perspectives for prevention and treatment. *New Microbiol.* 2007 Jul;30(3):189-212.

[43] Slade HB, Owens ML, Tomai MA, Miller RL. Imiquimod 5% cream (Aldara). *Expert Opin Investig Drugs.* 1998 Mar;7(3):437-49.

[44] Wiwanitkit V. Imiquimod: a new immunomodulatory drug. *Chula Med J* 2004 May; 48(5): 325 – 38.

[45] Müller M, Gissmann L. Prophylactic and therapeutic HPV immunization. *Hautarzt.* 2007 Jun;58(6):483-4, 486-8.

[46] Bryan JT. Geting an HPV vaccine to prevent cervical carcinoma and genital warts. *Vaccine.* 2007 Apr 20;25(16):3001-6.

[47] Shi L, Sings HL, Bryan JT, Wang B, Wang Y, Mach H, Kosinski M, Washabaugh MW, Sitrin R, Barr E. GARDASIL: prophylactic human papillomavirus vaccine development--from bench top to bed-side. *Clin Pharmacol Ther.* 2007 Feb;81(2):259-64.

[48] New vaccine prevents cervical carcinoma. *FDA Consum.* 2006 Sep-Oct;40(5):37.

[49] Glastetter E, Kaufmann AM. Humoral and cellular immune response in HPV vaccination. *Hautarzt.* 2007 Jun;58(6):493-4, 496-500.

[50] Gissmann L, Müller M. Development of prophylactic HPV vaccines. *Coll Antropol.* 2007 Apr;31 Suppl 2:113-5.

[51] Kirnbauer R. HPV vaccines. Prophylactic vaccines from virus-like particles. *Hautarzt.* 2007 Jun;58(6):489-92.

[52] Gariglio P, Benitez-Bribiesca L, Berumen J, Alcocer JM, Tamez R, Madrid V. Therapeutic uterine-cervix carcinoma vaccines in humans. *Arch Med Res.* 1998 Winter;29(4):279-84.

[53] Punyaratabandhu P, Supanvanich S, Tirapat C, Podhipak A. Epidemiologic study of risk factors in carcinoma of the cervix uteri in Thai women. *J Med Assoc Thai* 1982;65:231-9

[54] Vatanasapt V, Sriamporn S, Vatanasapt P. Carcinoma control in Thailand. *Jpn J Clin Oncol* 2002 ;32 Suppl:S82-91

[55] Swaddiwudhipong W, Chaovakiratipong C, Nguntra P, Mahasakpan P, Lerdlukanavonge P, Koonchote S. Effect of a mobile unit on changes in knowledge and use of cervical carcinoma screening among rural Thai women. *Int J Epidemiol* 1995;24:493-8

[56] Jirojwong S, Maclennan R, Manderson L. Health beliefs and Pap smears among Thai women in Brisbane, Australia. *Asia Pac J Public Health* 2001;13:20-3

[57] Wiwanitkit V. Screening for cervical carcinoma, results from Thailand. *Asian Pac J Carcinoma Prev*. 2006 Apr-Jun;7(2):329-30.

[58] Nopdonrattakoon L. Results of the cervical carcinoma screening programme at Maesot General Hospital. *Bull Dept Med Serv* 1993; 18: 586-591

[59] Veskijkul S, Kanchanaporn K, Chicharoen S, Wattanakitkrailert S, Srivongpanish S, Wacharapiyanan S, Arrerak K. Cervical carcinoma screening in Ratapum District: cost benefit analysis. *Songklanagarind Med J* 1991; 6: 406-412

[60] Kanwatanasirikul T. Cytologic screening for cervical carcinoma in Northern Thailand. *Bull Chiang Mai Assoc Med Sci* 1980; 14: 23-33

[61] Kanjanavirojkul N, Sripa C. Cervical carcinoma screening in Srinagarind Hospital. *Bull Dept Med Serv* 1995; 20: 349-354

[62] Pongnikorn S. Cervical carcinoma screening in Lampang Regional Carcinoma Centre. *Thai Carcinoma J* 1995 ; 21: 116-122

[63] Khunchairuk T. The results of cervical carcinoma screening in Charoenkrung Pracharak Hospital. *J Charoenkrung Pracharak Hosp* 2003 ; 19: 13-17.

[64] Sukvirach S, Pitakpraiwan P, Kosiyatrakul T, Hankittipongpaisarn P. Determination of human papillomavirus DNA in normal and cervical carcinoma tissues of Thai females. *Thai Carcinoma J.* 1994; 20(3-4): 85-91.

[65] Poonnaniti A, Bhattarakosol P. Improvement of PCR determination of HPV-DNA using enhanced chemiluminescence system and dot hybridization. *J Med Assoc Thai.* 1996 Dec;79 Suppl 1:S96-103.

In: Herpesviridae Viral Structure, Life Cycle and Infections
Editor: Toma R. Gluckman
ISBN 978-1-60692-947-6

Short Commentary 1

Human Herpesvirus-6 and Acute Liver Failure

Irmeli Lautenschlager [1,2*]***, Maiju Härmä*** [1,2] ***and Krister Höckerstedt*** [2]
Departments of [1]Virology and [2]Surgery, Transplantation and Liver Surgery Clinic and Transplant Unit Research Laboratory, Helsinki University Central Hospital and University of Helsinki, Helsinki, Finland

Abstract

Human herpesvirus-6 (HHV-6) is a lymphotropic virus, which was first isolated from immunocompromised patients. Two variants of HHV-6 have been categorized: HHV-6A and HHV-6B, of which the variant B is the most common. HHV-6B causes *exanthema subitum,* febrile seizures and other infectious syndromes of early childhood. The clinical symptoms are usually mild and self-limitted, but complications such as encephalitis and hepatitis have been described. Infection with HHV-6A appears to be much less frequent, but is suggested to be more neurotropic than HHV-6B. In the adult population, there is a high HHV-6 seroprevalence of 90-95%. Like other herpesviruses, after primary infection, HHV-6 persists in latency for life time and may reactivate later.

Acute liver failure (ALF) is a significant cause of liver transplantation. Common causes of ALF are hepatitis B, drug toxicity and vascular disorders. The etiology of ALF remains often unknown, but viral infections are thought to be involved. HHV-6 has been demonstrated to cause acute hepatitis as a complication of primary infection. HHV-6 DNA is also frequently detected in hepatocytes of liver of children with various liver diseases. Also cases of HHV-6-related acute liver failure in immunocompetent adults have been reported. In our study, HHV-6 was found in most explanted livers of adult patients with ALF of unknown origin ending-up with liver transplantation. HHV-6 antigens were demonstrated in the explants with numerous positive inflammatory cells

* Correspondence to: Irmeli Lautenschlager, MD, PhD, Transplant Unit Research Laboratory, Helsinki University Hospital, Meilahti, P-Floor, PL 340, FIN-00029 HUS, Helsinki, Finland; Tel. +358-9-47175867, Fax +358-9-47175866; E-mail Irmeli.Lautenschlager@hus.fi

and even in a few hepatocytes. No other viruses but HHV-6 were found in these explanted livers. This indicates, that ALF and hepatocyte necrosis may be caused by HHV-6. On the other hand, it is also possible, that the hepatocyte necrosis seen in this and other studies, is not caused by HHV-6 directly, but the immunoresponse triggered by the virus leads to destruction of hepatocytes. On the other hand, the impact of HHV-6 infection on the immunological events of the liver and triggering inflammation could be one of the mechanisms of HHV-6 to enhance acute liver failure. Despite the lack of definitive evidence of the direct causality of HHV-6 in liver failure, these observations strongly support its involvement in some cases, and probably a systematic research in cases of unexplained ALF could be recommended.

Human Herpesvirus-6

Human herpesvirus (HHV-6) is a lymphotropic virus, which was first isolated from peripheral blood of immunocompromised patients (1). HHV-6 belongs to the betaherpesviruses, together with its close relatives cytomegalovirus (CMV) and human herpesvirus-7 (HHV-7). Two variants of HHV-6 have been categorized: HHV-6A and HHV-6B (2, 3), of which the variant B is the most common (4). HHV-6B causes *exanthema subitum* (5), febrile seizures and other infectious syndromes of early childhood (6). In immunocompetent children, the clinical symptoms are usually mild and self-limitted, but complications such as encephalitis or hepatitis have been described (6-8). Infection with HHV-6A appears to be much less frequent, but is suggested to be more neurotropic than HHV-6B (9). Seroconversion mostly occurs by the age of two years in 90% of children (10). In the adult population, there is a high HHV-6 seroprevalence of approximately 95% (11) and primary infections are rare.

After primary infection, HHV-6 persists in latency for life time and may reactivate later. HHV-6 is a lymphotropic virus replicating in CD4+ T-lymphocytes (12) but by using CD46 molecule as its cellular receptor (13), may also infect other cell types, such as monocytes and macrophages, astrocytes, fibroblasts, and cells of endothelial or epithelial origin (14-18). HHV-6 infects various tissues, icluding brain (19), salivary glands (20), tonsils (21), lungs (22), kidneys (23) and liver (24). In addition to the direct virological patogenicity of HHV-6, it induces various immunological alterations (25, 26), which may lead to indirect reactions and tissue damage.

HHV-6 and the Liver

HHV-6 has been demonstrated to cause acute fulminant hepatitis as a complication of primary infection (7, 27-30). Also chronic hepatitis associated with HHV-6 has been described (31). HHV-6 DNA has been frequently detected in hepatocytes of liver of children with various liver diseases by in situ hybridization (24). The histopathology of acute HHV-6 infection of the liver has been described together with the detection of HHV-6 DNA expression in portal vein endothelial cells (32). There is also evidence that HHV-6 can infect hepatocytes (24, 33). However, HHV-6 DNA could by found in the liver tissue of asymptomatic healthy individuals, as well, when a sensitive PCR-method was used (34).

In transplant patients, the virus reactivates frequently, and HHV-6 infection of the liver has been described to cause graft dysfunction or hepatitis and be associated with allograft rejection (35-40). We have demonstrated that intrahepatic HHV-6 infection induces immunological events in the liver allografts, such as inflammatory infiltrate, lymphocyte activation and increased expression of vascular adhesion molecules (41).

HHV-6 and Acute Liver Failure

Acute liver failure (ALF) is a significant cause of liver transplantation (42). Common causes of ALF are hepatitis B, drug toxicity and vascular disorders (43-45). The etiology of ALF remains often unknown, but viral infections are thought to be involved. Herpesviruses are thought to be possible causative agents of ALF of unknown origin, but only in some cases Herpes simplex virus (HSV) or Epstein-Barr virus (EBV) have been found in the explanted livers (45, 46).

Recently, HHV-6 DNA has been detected also in retrospective analysis of explanted livers of acute liver failure patients (33). HHV-6 was detected by DNA hybridization in the liver tissues in 9 of 22 patients with acute fulminant hepatitis (33). In this study, viral DNA and RNA were localized in hepatocytes, and viral antigens were also demonstrated in the hepatocytes by immonohistochemistry. Also cases of HHV-6-related acute liver failure in immunocompetent adults have been reported (47). High amounts of HHV-6 DNA was detected in liver tissue by PCR, and the decrease of intrahepatic viral load was also recorded after antiviral treatment with ganciclovir (47). In a prospective study on pediatric patients HHV-6 was demonstrated to cause fulminant hepatic failure and acute decompensation of chronic liver disease in children (48).

In our study on adult patients with ALF of unknown origin ending-up with liver transplantation, HHV-6 was found in most explanted livers (49). All these hepatic infections were caused by the variant B. Most of these patients showed HHV-6 antigenemia and one patient had a serologial diagnosis of recent HHV-6 infection. HHV-6B antigens were demonstrated in the explants in numerous positive inflammatory cells and even in a few hepatocytes. No other viruses but HHV-6 were found in the explanted livers of ALF patients. After transplantation, half of the patients with pre-transplant HHV-6 infection, developed HHV-6 infection of liver allograft together with HHV-6 antigenemia during the first six months postoperatively (50). None of the ALF patients without pre-transplant HHV-6 infection showed HHV-6 antigens in the post-transplant patients. HHV-6B antigens were located in the mononuclear cells of the portal areas and in a few hepatocytes. The results were confirmed by detecting of HHV-6 DNA by in situ hybridization in the same structures of the liver. In histological examination of intragraft HHV-6 relapse, the findings were suggestive for viral infection with mild to moderate portal lymphocytic infiltration and hepatocellular damage without endothelialitis or clear damage of the bile ducts. All patients with post-transplant HHV-6 infection of the liver had graft dysfunction. At the time of HHV-6 positive liver biopsy impaired liver function was seen by serum liver function tests in all patients. However, the patients did not develop acute HHV-6 hepatitis or liver failure. Post-transplant HHV-6 infection of the liver had no effect on patient or graft survivals, and during the follow-up of 4-8 years no significant long-time effects of HHV-6 infection were recorded (51).

The actual pathogenic role of HHV-6 in ALF remains still suggestive only, as a viral reactivation could alternatively be induced by an unknown factor, which leads to ALF and the occurring of HHV-6 that enters the scene after the onset of liver failure. The results of our series and other previous reports indicate, that ALF and hepatocyte necrosis may be caused by HHV-6. On the other hand, it is also possible, that the hepatocyte necrosis seen in these and other studies, is not caused by HHV-6 directly, or but the immunoresponse triggered by the virus leads to destruction of hepatocytes. On the other hand, the impact of HHV-6 infection on the immunological events of the liver and triggering inflammation could be one of the mechanisms of HHV-6 to enhance acute liver failure. However, this does not explain the fact that the post-transplant intragaft HHV-6 relapse did not lead to ALF. After all, the mechanisms of the causal involvement of HHV-6 in ALF are remain still suggestive. Despite the lack of definitive evidence of causality of HHV-6 in ALF, these observations strongly support its involvement in some cases, and probably a systematic research in cases of unexplained ALF could be recommended.

References

[1] Salahuddin SZ, Ablashi DV, Markham PD, Josephs SF, Sturzenegger S, Kaplan M, et al. Isolation of a new virus, HBLV, in patients with lymphoproliferative disorders. *Science*. 1986;234(4776):596-601.

[2] Ablashi DV, Balachandran N, Josephs SF, Hung CL, Krueger GR, Kramarsky B, et al. Genomic polymorphism, growth properties, and immunologic variations in human herpesvirus-6 isolates. *Virology*. 1991;184(2):545-52.

[3] Schirmer EC, Wyatt LS, Yamanishi K, Rodriguez WJ, Frenkel N. Differentiation between two distinct classes of viruses now classified as human herpesvirus 6. *Proc Natl Acad Sci U S A*. 1991;88(13):5922-6.

[4] Dewhurst S, McIntyre K, Schnabel K, Hall CB. Human herpesvirus 6 (HHV-6) variant B accounts for the majority of symptomatic primary HHV-6 infections in a population of U.S. infants. *J Clin Microbiol*. 1993;31(2):416-8.

[5] Yamanishi K, Okuno T, Shiraki K, Takahashi M, Kondo T, Asano Y, et al. Identification of human herpesvirus-6 as a causal agent for exanthem subitum. *Lancet*. 1988;1(8594):1065-7.

[6] Hall CB, Long CE, Schnabel KC, Caserta MT, McIntyre KM, Costanzo MA, et al. Human herpesvirus-6 infection in children. A prospective study of complications and reactivation. *N Engl J Med*. 1994;331(7):432-8.

[7] Asano Y, Yoshikawa T, Suga S, Yazaki T, Kondo K, Yamanishi K. Fatal fulminant hepatitis in an infant with human herpesvirus-6 infection. *Lancet*. 1990;335(8693):862-3.

[8] Asano Y, Yoshikawa T, Kajita Y, Ogura R, Suga S, Yazaki T, et al. Fatal encephalitis/encephalopathy in primary human herpesvirus-6 infection. *Arch Dis Child.* 1992;67(12):1484-5.

[9] Hall CB, Caserta MT, Schnabel KC, Long C, Epstein LG, Insel RA, et al. Persistence of human herpesvirus 6 according to site and variant: possible greater neurotropism of variant A. *Clin Infect Dis.* 1998;26(1):132-7.

[10] Okuno T, Takahashi K, Balachandra K, Shiraki K, Yamanishi K, Takahashi M, et al. Seroepidemiology of human herpesvirus 6 infection in normal children and adults. *J Clin Microbiol.* 1989;27(4):651-3.

[11] Clark DA. Human herpesvirus 6. *Rev Med Virol.* 2000;10(3):155-73.

[12] Takahashi K, Sonoda S, Higashi K, Kondo T, Takahashi H, Takahashi M, et al. Predominant CD4 T-lymphocyte tropism of human herpesvirus 6-related virus. *J Virol.* 1989;63(7):3161-3.

[13] Santoro F, Kennedy PE, Locatelli G, Malnati MS, Berger EA, Lusso P. CD46 is a cellular receptor for human herpesvirus 6. *Cell.* 1999;99(7):817-27.

[14] Kondo K, Kondo T, Okuno T, Takahashi M, Yamanishi K. Latent human herpesvirus 6 infection of human monocytes/macrophages. *J Gen Virol.* 1991;72 (Pt 6)(Pt 6):1401-8.

[15] He J, McCarthy M, Zhou Y, Chandran B, Wood C. Infection of primary human fetal astrocytes by human herpesvirus 6. *J Virol.* 1996;70(2):1296-300.

[16] Luka J, Okano M, Thiele G. Isolation of human herpesvirus-6 from clinical specimens using human fibroblast cultures. *J Clin Lab Anal.* 1990;4(6):483-6.

[17] Chen M, Popescu N, Woodworth C, Berneman Z, Corbellino M, Lusso P, et al. Human herpesvirus 6 infects cervical epithelial cells and transactivates human papillomavirus gene expression. *J Virol.* 1994;68(2):1173-8.

[18] Caruso A, Rotola A, Comar M, Favilli F, Galvan M, Tosetti M, et al. HHV-6 infects human aortic and heart microvascular endothelial cells, increasing their ability to secrete proinflammatory chemokines. *J Med Virol.* 2002;67(4):528-33.

[19] Luppi M, Barozzi P, Maiorana A, Marasca R, Torelli G. Human herpesvirus 6 infection in normal human brain tissue. *J Infect Dis.* 1994;169(4):943-4.

[20] Fox JD, Briggs M, Ward PA, Tedder RS. Human herpesvirus 6 in salivary glands. *Lancet.* 1990;336(8715):590-3.

[21] Roush KS, Domiati-Saad RK, Margraf LR, Krisher K, Scheuermann RH, Rogers BB, et al. Prevalence and cellular reservoir of latent human herpesvirus 6 in tonsillar lymphoid tissue. *Am J Clin Pathol.* 2001;116(5):648-54.

[22] Hammerling JA, Lambrecht RS, Kehl KS, Carrigan DR. Prevalence of human herpesvirus 6 in lung tissue from children with pneumonitis. *J Clin Pathol.* 1996;49(10):802-4.

[23] Gupta M, Diaz-Mitoma F, Feber J, Shaw L, Forget C, Filler G. Tissue HHV6 and 7 determination in pediatric solid organ recipients--a pilot study. *Pediatr Transplant.* 2003;7(6):458-63.

[24] Ozaki Y, Tajiri H, Tanaka-Taya K, Mushiake S, Kimoto A, Yamanishi K, et al. Frequent detection of the human herpesvirus 6-specific genomes in the livers of children with various liver diseases. *J Clin Microbiol.* 2001;39(6):2173-7.

[25] Flamand L, Gosselin J, D'Addario M, Hiscott J, Ablashi DV, Gallo RC, et al. Human herpesvirus 6 induces interleukin-1 beta and tumor necrosis factor alpha, but not interleukin-6, in peripheral blood mononuclear cell cultures. *J Virol.* 1991;65(9):5105-10.

[26] Krueger GR, Ablashi DV. Human herpesvirus-6: a short review of its biological behavior. *Intervirology.* 2003;46(5):257-69.

[27] Ward KN, Gray JJ, Efstathiou S. Brief report: primary human herpesvirus 6 infection in a patient following liver transplantation from a seropositive donor. *J Med Virol.* 1989;28(2):69-72.

[28] Dubedat S, Kappagoda N. Hepatitis due to human herpesvirus-6. *Lancet.* 1989;2(8677):1463-4.

[29] Mendel I, de Matteis M, Bertin C, Delaporte B, Maguer D, Collandre H, et al. Fulminant hepatitis in neonates with human herpesvirus 6 infection. *Pediatr Infect Dis J.* 1995;14(11):993-7.

[30] Sobue R, Miyazaki H, Okamoto M, Hirano M, Yoshikawa T, Suga S, et al. Fulminant hepatitis in primary human herpesvirus-6 infection. *N Engl J Med.* 1991;324(18):1290.

[31] Tajiri H, Tanaka-Taya K, Ozaki Y, Okada S, Mushiake S, Yamanishi K. Chronic hepatitis in an infant, in association with human herpesvirus-6 infection. *J Pediatr.* 1997;131(3):473-5.

[32] Aita K, Jin Y, Irie H, Takahashi I, Kobori K, Nakasato Y, et al. Are there histopathologic characteristics particular to fulminant hepatic failure caused by human herpesvirus-6 infection? A case report and discussion. *Hum Pathol.* 2001;32(8):887-9.

[33] Ishikawa K, Hasegawa K, Naritomi T, Kanai N, Ogawa M, Kato Y, et al. Prevalence of herpesviridae and hepatitis virus sequences in the livers of patients with fulminant hepatitis of unknown etiology in Japan. *J Gastroenterol.* 2002;37(7):523-30.

[34] Chen T, Hudnall SD. Anatomical mapping of human herpesvirus reservoirs of infection. *Mod Pathol.* 2006;19(5):726-37.

[35] Lautenschlager I, Hockerstedt K, Linnavuori K, Taskinen E. Human herpesvirus-6 infection after liver transplantation. *Clin Infect Dis.* 1998;26(3):702-7.

[36] Griffiths PD, Ait-Khaled M, Bearcroft CP, Clark DA, Quaglia A, Davies SE, et al. Human herpesviruses 6 and 7 as potential pathogens after liver transplant: prospective comparison with the effect of cytomegalovirus. *J Med Virol.* 1999;59(4):496-501.

[37] Humar A, Kumar D, Caliendo AM, Moussa G, Ashi-Sulaiman A, Levy G, et al. Clinical impact of human herpesvirus 6 infection after liver transplantation. *Transplantation.* 2002;73(4):599-604.

[38] Feldstein AE, Razonable RR, Boyce TG, Freese DK, El-Youssef M, Perrault J, et al. Prevalence and clinical significance of human herpesviruses 6 and 7 active infection in pediatric liver transplant patients. *Pediatr Transplant.* 2003;7(2):125-9.

[39] Yoshikawa T. Human herpesvirus 6 causes hepatitis in transplant recipients. *Intern Med.* 2006;45(7):417-8.

[40] Ljungman P, Singh N. Human herpesvirus-6 infection in solid organ and stem cell transplantation. *J Clin Virol.* 2006;3 (Suppl. 1):S87-91.

[41] Lautenschlager I, Harma M, Hockerstedt K, Linnavuori K, Loginov R, Taskinen E. Human herpesvirus-6 infection is associated with adhesion molecule induction and lymphocyte infiltration in liver allografts. *J Hepatol.* 2002;37(5):648-54.

[42] Polson J, Lee WM, American Association for the Study of Liver Disease. AASLD position paper: the management of acute liver failure. *Hepatology.* 2005;41(5):1179-97.

[43] Shakil AO, Kramer D, Mazariegos GV, Fung JJ, Rakela J. Acute liver failure: clinical features, outcome analysis, and applicability of prognostic criteria. *Liver Transpl.* 2000;6(2):163-9.

[44] Brandsaeter B, Hockerstedt K, Friman S, Ericzon BG, Kirkegaard P, Isoniemi H, et al. Fulminant hepatic failure: outcome after listing for highly urgent liver transplantation-12 years experience in the nordic countries. *Liver Transpl.* 2002;8(11):1055-62.

[45] Ostapowicz G, Fontana RJ, Schiodt FV, Larson A, Davern TJ, Han SH, et al. Results of a prospective study of acute liver failure at 17 tertiary care centers in the United States. *Ann Intern Med.* 2002;137(12):947-54.

[46] Schiodt FV, Davern TJ, Shakil AO, McGuire B, Samuel G, Lee WM. Viral hepatitis-related acute liver failure. *Am J Gastroenterol.* 2003;98(2):448-53.

[47] Cacheux W, Carbonell N, Rosmorduc O, Wendum D, Paye F, Poupon R, et al. HHV-6-related acute liver failure in two immunocompetent adults: favourable outcome after liver transplantation and/or ganciclovir therapy. *J Intern Med.* 2005;258(6):573-8.

[48] Chevret L, Boutolleau D, Halimi-Idri N, Branchereau S, Baujard C, Fabre M, et al. Human herpesvirus-6 infection: a prospective study evaluating HHV-6 DNA levels in liver from children with acute liver failure. *J Med Virol.* 2008;80(6):1051-7.

[49] Harma M, Hockerstedt K, Lautenschlager I. Human herpesvirus-6 and acute liver failure. *Transplantation.* 2003;76(3):536-9.

[50] Harma M, Hockerstedt K, Krogerus L, Lautenschlager I. Pretransplant human herpesvirus 6 infection of patients with acute liver failure is a risk factor for posttransplant human herpesvirus 6 infection of the liver. *Transplantation.* 2006;81(3):367-72.

[51] Harma M, Hockerstedt K, Lautenschlager I. Long-time survival of patients transplanted due to acute liver failure; with or without intrahepatic HHV-6 infection. *Transplant Int.* 2007; 20 (Suppl.2):280.

In: Herpesviridae Viral Structure, Life Cycle and Infections ISBN 978-1-60692-947-6
Editor: Toma R. Gluckman

Short Commentary 2

Herpesviruses Type 1 (HHV-1), 6 (HHV-6) and 7 (HHV-7) Role in Chronic Human Diseases

J.L. Leite, N.E. Bufalo, E.C. Morari, A.C.T. Guilhen, R.B. Santos and L.S. Ward

Laboratory of Molecular Genetics of Cancer Faculty of Medical Sciences
PO Box 6111 University of Campinas – UNICAMP
13083-970, Campinas, SP, Brazil

Abstract

We investigated the role of herpesviruses in human chronic pathologies such as cancedrf and autoimmune diseases. Our first focus was on HHV6 and HHV1 role in the susceptibility to sporadic skin cancers. HHV6 (31.7%) and HHV1 (23.8%) fragments were detected more frequently in 120 skin cancer patients cancer than in 41 normal control individuals (14.6% and 5%, respectively). The risk of presenting a Basal Cell Carcinomas (BCC) was more than 3 times higher for HHV6 infected patients (OR= 3.182; 95% CI: 1.125-8.997). The risk for HHV1 infected individuals of presenting BCC and SCC was increased 8 and 6 times, respectively (OR= 8.125; 95% CI: 1.735-38.043 and OR= 6.290; 95% CI: 1.283-30.856, respectively). Because a subset of immunocompromised patients appeared to be more susceptible to HHV-associated skin cancer, we further investigated the influence of the variants of codon 72 and codon 47 of exon 4 on the susceptibility to HHV6 and 1 HHV1 infection in immunosuppressed patients. We examined 78 renal transplant recipients and 151 controls. HHV6 infection was more frequent among the renal transplant patients (35.89%) than in the control population (11.25%). HHV1 infection rate was similar in renal transplant patients (7.28%) and controls (2.56%). HHV6 positive cases were more frequent among patients with codon 72 of *p53* variants (60.71%) than among wild-type *p53* patients (28.20%) despite the higher frequency of codon 72 of *p53* wild-type variant in renal transplant patients compared to controls (64.1% *versus* 36.4%; $p < 0.001$). The presence of a codon

72 of *p53* germ line variant genotype increased the risk for HHV6 infection more than 5 times (OR= 5.479; 95% CI= 1.992-15.069). More recently, we have aimed to study the relationship between HHV6 and HHV7 infection, p53 apoptotic ability as represented by 72p53 polymorphisms, and Graves Disease (GD) susceptibility. Sixty GD patients were paired to 60 controls. Both viruses infection demonstrated to increase the risk for GD, especially HHV7 that was more frequent among GD (64.64%) than in controls (38.73%). Patients presenting 72TP53 Pro/Pro variants had more chance to develop GD and to be infected by HHV7.

Introduction

HHV6 and HHV1 and the Non-Melanoma Skin Cancer

Human lymphotropic herpesviruses, including Human herpesvirus 6, variants A and B (HHV-6A, HHV6-B), Human herpesvirus 7 (HHV7), and others herpesviruses, are responsible for a wide variety of human diseases, caused either by primary infection or by reactivation in immunosuppressive conditions [1].

HHV6 has been detected in oral squamous carcinomas, cervical carcinomas, Hodgkin's and Non-Hodgkin's lymphomas, among other malignancies [2,3]. The mechanism involved in HHV6 associated malignancy may be related to the fact that, in both immunocompetent and immunosuppressed hosts, HHV6 produces an oncogenic protein called ORF-1 (open reading frame 1) that binds to wild-type p53 and inhibits regulation of the cell cycle [4,5].

HHV1 can infect both skin and nerves and develop latent infection within the dorsal root and trigeminal ganglia [6]. HHV1 was also associated with many types of cancer, including Squamous Cell Carcinomas (SCC), and there is evidence that the virus may determine genetic cellular modifications in vitro and in experimental in vivo models [4,7,8].

We investigated the role of HHV6 and HHV1 in the susceptibility to sporadic skin cancers in a case-control prospective study [9]. Comparing HHV6 and HHV1 fragments detected in DNA samples extracted from 120 lesions and 41 normal skin tissues, we demonstrated that HHV6 (31.7%) and HHV1 (23.8%) were found more frequently in patients with skin cancer than in control individuals (14.6% and 5%, respectively) (p= 0.0391 and p= 0.00094, respectively). The risk of presenting a Basal Cell Carcinomas (BCC) was more than 3 times higher for HHV6 infected patients (OR= 3.182; 95% CI: 1.125-8.997), but we did not find a significant increase in the risk for SCC. The risk for HHV1 infected individuals of presenting BCC and SCC was increased 8 and 6 times, respectively (OR= 8.125; 95% CI: 1.735-38.043 and OR= 6.290; 95% CI: 1.283-30.856, respectively) [9]. Also, we demonstrated the presence of both HHV6 and HHV1 in autologous normal tissue from patients with skin lesions and in normal control skin, indicating that the skin is one of the reservoirs for persistent infection in the adult.

A control group of healthy skin donors from the general population of our region with no skin conditions was very hard to obtain and the comparison with the 41 healthy skin donors obtained increased the strength of these data [9]. Also, it was very hard to pair patients and controls not only for gender, age and color, but also for environmental specific exposures, medical history and current medical conditions, especially immunosuppressive therapy and other malignancies. Therefore, the power of calculation of the cohort obtained is relatively low. Another limitation of these findings includes the non description of HHV1 patients with frequent recrudescence.

HHV6 and HHV1 and the Immunosuppressed Patient with Cancer

Herpesviruses, like every infectious agent that requires the replication of its own genome in the host nucleus, have to overcome the barrier presented by *p53* tumor suppressor gene. Normal (wild-type) *p53* maintains the integrity of the genome by causing a pause in the cell cycle until damage has been repaired or by inducing apoptosis in cells constituting a risk for the organism [10]. Both herpesvirus type 6 (HHV6) and herpesvirus type 1 (HHV1) have been demonstrated to induce programmed cell death [11-13]. The immunosuppressive post-transplant state favors viral reactivation. In addition, patients that have escaped infection up to the time of transplant face the risk of acquiring cytomegalovirus or other herpesvirus from the donor organ or from blood products when receiving immunosuppressive agents to prevent or treat rejection [14].

A critical region of *p53* for signaling apoptosis lies between codons 64 and 92, encoding a proline-rich region of the gene in which there is a common polymorphism resulting in either an arginine or a proline at codon 72 of exon 4. Proline polymorphic alleles (P72) have a markedly poorer ability to induce apoptosis than arginine variants [10]. More recently, another polymorphism site, at codon 47 of the same exon 4 of *p53*, was also demonstrated to significantly decrease p53 ability to induce apoptosis [15]. Codon 47 encodes proline in wild type *p53*, but in a small subset of individuals it can encode serine (CCG-TCG) [15]. S47 was described to occur in *cis* with P72, suggesting both polymorphisms are linked [15].

Because our previous findings in skin cancer indicated that a group of immunosuppressed patients could be more susceptible to develop herpesviruses-associated malignancies, we decided to investigate the influence of the variants of codon 72 and codon 47 of exon 4 on the susceptibility to HHV6 and 1 HHV1 infection in immunosuppressed patients [16]. We examined 78 renal transplant recipients and 151 controls. HHV6 infection was more frequent among the renal transplant patients (35.89%) than in the control population (11.25%) ($p < 0.001$). HHV1 infection rate was similar in renal transplant patients (7.28%) and controls (2.56%). HHV6 positive cases were more frequent among patients with codon 72 of *p53* variants (60.71%) than among wild-type *p53* patients (28.20%) ($p= 0.001$) despite the higher frequency of codon 72 of *p53* wild-type variant in renal transplant patients compared to controls (64.1% *versus* 36.4%; $p< 0.001$). The presence of a codon 72 of *p53* germ line variant genotype increased the risk for HHV-6 infection more than 5 times (OR= 5.479; 95% CI= 1.992-15.069) [16]. Our data suggests that codon 72 of *p53* polymorphism genotyping may be useful to screen for patients at higher risk for post-transplant infections hence identifying individuals that could benefit from preventive treatment [16].

A major drawback from our findings is, once again, the relatively small number of patients investigated and the consequent low power of calculation of these data. Especially regarding S47 polymorphism, which is quite rare in the population, we were not able to establish any conclusive relationship with herpesviruses infection [16].

HHV-7 and Graves´ Disease

Graves´ Disease (GD) is a multifactorial condition presumably provoked by environmental factors, including viruses, whose interactions with the immune system have been proposed to trigger the disease [17].

More recently, we have aimed to study the relationship between HHV6 and HHV7 infection, p53 apoptotic ability as represented by 72p53 polymorphisms, and GD susceptibility. Sixty GD patients were paired to 60 controls with respect to gender, age, color and environmental exposure. Through of nested-primers we identify HHV6 and HHV7 and Polimerase Chain Reaction-Restriction Fragment Length Polymorphisms (PCR-RFLP) to sort out 72p53 polymorphisms. Patients were treated according to a same protocol, followed-up for Mo= 36 months and considered cured when they did not need antithyroid drugs to maintain euthyroidism one year after radioiodine therapy. Both viruses infection demonstrated to increase the risk for GD, especially HHV7 that was more frequent among GD (64.64%) than in controls (38.73%). Patients presenting 72TP53 Pro/Pro variants had more chance to develop GD and to be infected by HHV7 (data not published). We were not able to find any relationship between viral infection and patients' clinical features, including ophthalmopathy, or their outcome. These preliminary data suggest that both HHV infections, especially HHV7, increase the susceptibility to GD and this may be related to a deficient *TP53* apoptotic activity.

Conclusion

The HHV6 presence and, mainly, HHV1 considerably increased the risk for skin cancer in infected individuals, suggesting that these viruses may play a role in susceptibility to skin malignancies, perhaps through reactivation of a latent infection [9]. Although this observational study needs confirmation in biological models, it is tempting to suggest that HHV presence in the epithelial cells might contribute to the genomic instability, driving these cells to a cumulative multistep mutagenic process towards certain types of skin cancers [9].

The ability of *p53* inducing apoptosis is significantly reduced by 2 polymorphisms, at codons 47 and 72 of exon 4 of *p53* [16]. We found a higher prevalence of HHV6 infection among individuals with the less effective P72 alleles, suggesting that HHV6 infection is facilitated by the presence of the polymorphism of codon 72. Arresting cells, rather than destroying them, may be an evolutionary developed advantage for HHV6. Indeed, hiding from the immune system and keeping infected cells alive may prevent the immune reactions initiated by the liberation of viral proteins from apoptotic cells. Hence, infection of cells that are less able to undergo apoptosis may favor HHV6 survival [16].

References

[1] Pozo, F; Tenorio, A. Detection and typing of lymphotropic herpesviruses by multiplex polymerase chain reaction. *J Virol Methods,* 1999 79, 9-19.

[2] Levy, J. Three new herpesvirus (HHV6,7,8). *Lancet*, 1997 349, 558–562.

[3] Kosuge, H. HHV-6, 7 and their related diseases. *Can.Commun. Dis. Rep.* 2000 26, 1–27.

[4] Flaitz, CM; Hicks, MJ. Molecular piracy: the viral link to carcinogenesis. *Oral Oncol.* 1998 34, 448–453.

[5] Lusso, P; Secchiero, P; Crowley, RW; Garzino-Demo, A; Berneman, ZN; Gallo, RC. CD4 is a critical component of the receptor for human herpesvirus 7: interference with human immunodeficiency virus. *Proc Natl Acad Sci U S A*. 1994 26, 3872-3876.

[6] Dwyer, DE; Cunningham, AL. Herpes simplex and varicellazoster virus infections, *Med. J. Aust.* 2002 177, 267–273.

[7] Rotola, A; Gerna, G; Di Lica, D; Virgili, AR; Manservigi, R; Cassai, E. Herpes simplex virus and human cancer. III. Search for relationship of herpes simplex antibodies and cervical dysplasia and labial neoplasia, *Tumori*, 1983 69, 83–87.

[8] Abrahams, PJ; Van der Keij, AA; Schouten, R; Van der Eb, AJ. Absence of induction of enhanced reactivation of Herpes Simplex Virus in cells from Xeroderma Pigmentosum patients without cancer, *Cancer Res.* 1998 48, 6054–6057.

[9] Leite, JL; Stolf, HO; Reis, NA; Ward, LS. Human herpesvirus type 6 and type 1 infection increases susceptibility to nonmelanoma skin tumors. *Cancer Lett.* 2005 224, 213.

[10] Lane, DP. p53, guardian of the genome. *Nature,* 2002 358,15.

[11] Yasukawa, M; Inoue, Y; Ohminami, H; Teradam K; Fujitam, S. Apoptosis of CD4+ T lymphocytes in human herpesvirus- 6 infection. *J Gen Virol.* 1998 79, 143.

[12] Secchiero, P; Flamand, L; Gibellini, D; et al. Human herpesvirus 7 induces CD4(+) T-cell death by two distinct mechanisms: necrotic lysis in productively infected cells and apoptosis in uninfected or nonproductively infected cells. *Blood,* 1997 90, 4502.

[13] Winkler, MT; Dosterm A; Jonesm C. Bovine herpesvirus 1 can infect CD4(+) T lymphocytes and induce programmed cell death during acute infection of cattle. *J Virol.* 1999 73, 8657.

[14] Pass, R. Editorial: Herpesvirus Infections in Transplant Recipients. *Herpes*, 2000 7, 3.

[15] Li, X; Dumont, P; Della Pietram A; Shetlerm C; Murphy, ME. The codon 47 polymorphism in p53 is functionally signifi- cant. *Biol Chem.* 2005 280, 242-245.

[16] Leite, JL; Manfrinatto, JA; Mazzali, M; Ward, LS. Polymorphisms at exon 4 of p53 and the susceptibility to herpesvirus types 6 and 1 infection in renal transplant recipients.*Transpl Int.* 2006 19,732-737.

[17] Weetman, A.P. Autoimmune thyroid disease: propagation and progression. *European Journal of Endocrinology*, 2003 148, 1–9.

In: Herpesviridae Viral Structure, Life Cycle and Infections ISBN 978-1-60692-947-6
Editor: Toma R. Gluckman

Short Commentary 3

Induction of Anticardiolipin Antibodies Associated with Human Herpesvirus-6 Infection

***Mitsuo Toyoshima*[1*] *and Yoshihiro Maegaki*[2]**

[1]Department of Pediatrics, Graduate School of Medical and Dental Sciences, Kagoshima University, Kagoshima City, Kagoshima,

[2]Division of Child Neurology, Institute of Neurological Science, Tottori University Faculty of Medicine, Yonago City, Tottori, Japan

Human herpesvirus-6 (HHV-6) is a causative virus of exanthema subitum which is characterized by high fever followed by rash in young children. HHV-6 infection is associated with variety of acute and chronic neurologic diseases, including febrile seizure, encephalitis, meningitis, facial palsy, Guillain-Barré syndrome and multiple sclerosis, possibly through immune-mediated reactions [1, 2]. Although cerebral infarctions have been also reported following HHV-6 infection on rare occasions, the underlying mechanism has not yet been elucidated [4, 5].

Antiphospholipid syndrome (APS) is an autoimmune disease characterized by thrombosis, repeated abortions, or thrombocytopenia associated with elevated antiphospholipid antibodies (aPL) [6]. APS often appears in association with autoimmune diseases or infections, while the cause of aPL induction is obscure in many patients with APS. Anticardiolipin antibodies (aCL) are the most common aPL and are one of the risk factors for cerebral vascular disease or myocardial infarctions in both adults and children [7-13]. Recent epidemiologic studies suggested that the infectious environment in infancy influence the likelihood producing aCL [14].

* Correspondence to: Mitsuo Toyoshima, Department of Pediatrics, Graduate School of Medical and Dental Sciences, Kagoshima University, 8-35-1 Sakuragaoka, Kagoshima City, Kagoshima, 890-8520, Japan; Phone: 81-99-275-5354; Fax: 81-99-265-7196; Email: toyoshim@m2.kufm.kagoshima-u.ac.jp

We recently reported a child with cerebral infarction associated with transient elevation of aCL following primary human herpesvirus-6 infection (HHV-6) [15].

The patient was the fourth child of nonconsanguineous healthy parents. There was no family history of stroke, recurrent intrauterine fetal death, or autoimmune disease. At the age of 10 months, he had a high fever for three days. He had no convulsions and no consciousness disturbance. On the third day of illness, while the fever abated, he suffered from left arm and leg weakness. On the fourth day the typical skin rash appeared on the trunk. The serum titer of the IgG antibody against HHV-6 using the fluorescent antibody method was less than 1:10 on the sixth day and increased to 1:320 on the 15th day. The IgM titer was 1:10 on the sixth day and less than 1:10 on the 15th day. The serum IgM and IgG against human herpesvirus-7 were negative. Therefore, a definite diagnosis of primary HHV-6 infection was made. His physical examination was unremarkable. Neurological examinations demonstrated left hemiplegia with hypertonus and brisk tendon reflex on the left upper and lower extremities. He did not show any other abnormal findings such as meningeal sign, consciousness disturbance, involuntary movements or an impairment of the cranial nerves.

Brain MRI performed on the 24th day showed abnormal intensity areas in the right caudate nucleus, putamen and globus pallidus. Brain MRA demonstrated the constriction of the right middle cerebral artery and the obstruction of the A1 segment of the right anterior cerebral artery without enlargement of the collateral vessels. A serological analysis studied on the 28th day revealed an elevated IgG aCL antibody of 37.4 U/ml (reference range; <10). Both the IgM aCL antibody and anti-beta-2-glycoprotein-I (β_2-GPI) antibody were negative. The following laboratory tests were normal: complete blood cell count, blood chemistry, urinalysis, plasma and urine amino acids, blood glucose, blood lactate and pyruvate, CRP, urinary organic acids and serum acylcarnitine by gas chromatography-mass spectrometry. There were no abnormal findings on coagulation, fibrinolysis tests and lupus anticoagulant. All autoantibodies, except for the aCL antibody, were negative. The IgM and IgG antibodies against varicella zoster virus (VZV) were also negative. The HHV-6 and VZV genomes were not detectable from the CSF by polymerase chain reaction. His clinical and laboratory findings ruled out the known causes of stroke, including moyamoya syndrome, fibromuscular dysplasia, congenital heart disease, trauma, congenital coagulopathy, VZV infection, and metabolic disorders such as homocystinuria and mitochondrial cytopathy.

The aCL IgG level had transiently increased to 52.4 U/mL on the 71st day and gradually decreased thereafter, but was still above the normal upper limit. The patient is now three years old, and although his left hemiplegia has persisted, he is able to walk independently and his mental development is normal. Oral aspirin therapy had continued and he showed no further infarction or no signs of autoimmune disease during the follow-up periods.

According to the international classification criteria for APS proposed by International Congress on aPL [6], he was definitely diagnosed as having antiphospholipid antibody syndrome. APS often appears as secondary autoimmune diseases, particularly in association with systemic lupus erythematosus, but some patients without any overt symptoms of autoimmune disease show APS [16]. Because our patient did not have any other symptoms of autoimmune diseases except for cerebral infarction and also demonstrated no other autoimmune antibodies except for the aCL antibody, underlying autoimmune diseases in this case were thus ruled out.

Cerebral infarction associated with HHV-6 infection is an uncommon but serious neurological complication. Our patient showed cerebral infarction and transient elevation of the aCL IgG antibody. This observation suggests that HHV-6 infection can induce APS, thus resulting in cerebral infarction.

Syphilis, leprosy, hepatitis C virus, human immunodeficiency virus, cytomegalovirus, Epstein-Barr virus, VZV, human T lymphotrophic virus, adenovirus, and parvovirus B19 have been reported to induce aPL [16-18]. However, there have been no previous reports dealing with the association between HHV-6 and aPL except for our recent report. Although cerebral infarction following HHV-6 infection has been reported in a few patients [4, 5, 15], the patient was the first case in which cerebral infarction was diagnosed as APS.

Although the clinical significance of infection-associated aPL remains unclear, the presence of these antibodies was closely associated with thrombosis in many instances [16-18]. We suspect that the prevalence of aCL production associated with HHV-6 infection is much higher than expected. Further studies with a large number of cases regarding the induction of aPL by HHV-6 infection may lead to one of the risk factors of vascular events and thus facilitate preventive treatment.

Manco-Johnson et al. described that pediatric post-infectious APS may be severe, but normally tends to be transient [19]. However, the aCL antibody persisted at a low level in the present patient. Differently from other infectious agents such as syphilis, hepatitis C virus, human immunodeficiency virus and so on, HHV-6 is ubiquitous in the human population, with approximately 90% of children seropositive at 12 months of age; by three years of age nearly all children are infected. After primary infection the virus persists in a latent form, the virus DNA can be detected in peripheral blood mononuclear cells, in saliva, and in cerebrospinal fluid [2]. Therefore, HHV-6 infection may be the most important etiological cause of the persistent presence of aCL not only in children but also in adults.

In conclusion, induction of aCL should be considered one of the possible causes of HHV-6 infection-associated neurologic complications. The transient elevation in the antiphospholipid antibody level suggests that the HHV-6 infection can induce APS, thus resulting in a cerebral infarction.

References

[1] Yoshikawa T, Asano Y. Central nervous system complications in human herpesvirus-6 infection. *Brain Dev*. 2000;22:307-314.

[2] Dewhurst S. Human herpesvirus type 6 and human herpesvirus type 7 infections of the central nervous system. *Herpes*. 2004;11 Suppl 2:105A-111A.

[3] Mannonen L, Herrgård E, Valmari P, Rautiainen P, Uotila K, Aine MR, Karttunen-Lewandowski P, Sankala J, Wallden T, Koskiniemi M. Primary human herpesvirus-6 infection in the central nervous system can cause severe disease. *Pediatr Neurol*. 2007;37:186-191.

[4] Webb DW, Bjornson BH, Sargent MA, Hukin J, Thomas EE. Basal ganglia infarction associated with HHV-6 infection. *Arch Dis Child.* 1997;76:362-364.

[5] Tanaka M, Kimura S, Nezu A, Ohtsuki N, Takeshita S. Focal brain legion accompanied by exanthema subitum: report of two cases. *No To Hattatsu.* 1998; 30:65-68. (in Japanese)

[6] Miyakis S, Lockshin MD, Atsumi T, Branch DW, Brey RL, Cervera R, Derksen RH, DE Groot PG, Koike T, Meroni PL, Reber G, Shoenfeld Y, Tincani A, Vlachoyiannopoulos PG, Krilis SA. International consensus statement on an update of the classification criteria for definite antiphospholipid syndrome (APS). *J Thromb Haemost*. 2006;4:295-306.

[7] Vaarala O, Mänttäri M, Manninen V, Tenkanen L, Puurunen M, Aho K, Palosuo T. Anti-Cardiolipin Antibodies and Risk of Myocardial Infarction in a Prospective Cohort of Middle-Aged Men. *Circulation.* 1995;91:23-27.

[8] Baca V, Garcia-Ramirez R, Ramirez-Lacayo M, Marquez-Enriquez L, Martinez I, Lavalle C. Cerebral infarction and antiphospholipid syndrome in children. *J Rheumatol.* 1996;23:1428-1431.

[9] Liu C, Xia Y, Sun S, Yuan G, Tong E. Study on relationship between anticardiolipin antibody and cerebrovascular diseases. *J Tongji Med Univ*. 1999;19:59-62.

[10] Heinzlef O, Abuaf N, Cohen A, Amarenco P; French Study of Aortic Plaques in Stroke Group. Recurrent stroke and vascular events in elderly patients with anticardiolipin antibodies: a prospective study. *J Neurol.* 2001;248:373-379.

[11] Nojima J, Kuratsune H, Suehisa E, Kitani T, Iwatani Y, Kanakura Y. Strong correlation between the prevalence of cerebral infarction and the presence of anti-cardiolipin/beta2-glycoprotein I and anti-phosphatidylserine/prothrombin antibodies—Co-existence of these antibodies enhances ADP-induced platelet activation in vitro. *Thromb Haemost*. 2004;91:967-976.

[12] Davies JO, Hunt BJ. Myocardial infarction in young patients without coronary atherosclerosis: assume primary antiphospholipid syndrome until proved otherwise. *Int J Clin Pract*. 2007;61:379-384.

[13] Bili A, Moss AJ, Francis CW, Zareba W, Watelet LF, Sanz I Anticardiolipin antibodies and recurrent coronary events: a prospective study of 1150 patients. *Circulation.* 2000;102:1258-1263.

[14] Edwards CJ, Syddall H, Jameson K, Williams EL, Polosa R, Goswami R, Dennison EM, Arden NK, Cooper C; Hertfordshire Cohort Study Group. The presence of anticardiolipin antibodies in adults may be influenced by infections in infancy. *QJM.* 2008;101:41-47.

[15] Toyoshima M, Maegaki Y, Yotsumata K, Takei S, Kawano Y. Antiphospholipid syndrome associated with human herpesvirus-6 infection. *Pediatr Neurol.* 2007;37:449-451.

[16] Asherson RA, Cervera R. Antiphospholipid antibodies and infections. *Ann Rheum Dis*. 2003;62:388-393.

[17] Uthman IW, Gharavi AE. Viral infections and antiphospholipid antibodies. *Semin Arthritis Rheum.* 2002;31:256-263.

[18] Aydin K, Sert A, Ati Guzes E, Kiresi DA. Acute childhood hemiplegia associated with chickenpox and elevated anticardiolipin antibody. *J Child Neurol.* 2006; 21:890-893.

[19] Manco-Johnsn MJ, Nuss R. Lupus anticoagulant in children with thrombosis. *Am J Hematol.* 1995;48:240-243.

Index

A

B

C

D

F

G

H

I

J

K

L

M

N

O

P

Q

R

S

T

U

V